# EVERYDAY FASHIONS OF THE TWENTIES

## As Pictured in Sears and Other Catalogs

# EVERYDAY FASHIONS OF THE TWENTIES

## As Pictured in Sears and Other Catalogs

Edited and with Text by

**Stella Blum**

Curator, Costume Institute,
The Metropolitan Museum of Art

DOVER PUBLICATIONS, INC.
NEW YORK

Published in Canada by General Publishing Company, Ltd., 30 Lesmill Road, Don Mills, Toronto, Ontario.
Published in the United Kingdom by Constable and Company, Ltd., 10 Orange Street, London WC2H 7EG.

*Everyday Fashions of the Twenties as Pictured in Sears and Other Catalogs* is a new work, first published by Dover Publications, Inc., in 1981.

*International Standard Book Number: 0-486-24134-3*
*Library of Congress Catalog Card Number: 81-65205*

Manufactured in the United States of America
Dover Publications, Inc.
180 Varick Street
New York, N.Y. 10014

# INTRODUCTION

The first mail-order catalog was issued by Aaron Montgomery Ward in 1872; Sears, Roebuck and Co. produced their first in 1896. During the early part of the twentieth century innumerable firms joined the mail-marketing business and the volume of sales was prodigious. By the end of World War I, buying through the mails had grown into a firmly established American institution and the mail-order catalog had become the "Farmer's Bible" and the "Nation's Wishbook."

People living in isolated hamlets, on far-flung farms or in the less-affluent sections of the cities, awaited each new catalog with excited anticipation. Its arrival meant hours of entertainment, a fund of information, some dreams to be realized and others to be kept warm by the hope of being fulfilled in the future. Even those too poor to succumb to the temptations of the fashion pages could, through the purchase of some thread, a length of yard goods or a meager article of farm equipment, be assured of receiving the next catalog and news of the latest fashions. If there was no money to buy them ready-made, they could somehow be copied and sewn at home.

In 1925 Sears announced, "We have become the world's largest store" and stated that nine million families bought from them. Based on this claim, and since all mail-order houses included wearing apparel, the fashion sections of the mail-order catalogs must have been America's most popular and best-read fashion magazines.

In the 1920s the entire family could be dressed via the United States Postal Service system. The mail-order catalogs not only showed women's clothes but also consistently included fashions for children, teenagers and men. Although small children's fashions resembled in some measure those of the adults, there were now clothes specially designed for little boys and girls. Changes in men's fashions during this period were relatively slow and subtle. Nevertheless they were there and become quite obvious if one compares, for example, the fashions of 1919 with those of 1927.

Although today there is a great deal of buying through the mails on even the highest levels, it has become a popular notion that mail-order clothes of the past were purely utilitarian, having little flair of design or quality. While it is true that many pages were devoted to cheap, practical wearing apparel, and none to ballgowns or white ties and tails, the most impressive segment of these catalogs was the one devoted to fashions—clothes to be worn as Sunday best, for going out, sports, leisure times and for everyday wear. Even housedresses and workshirts had a modicum of style and were in tune with the times. Placed at the beginning of the catalog, carefully delineated drawings and photographs, many in color, gave the book excitement, life and eye appeal.

Mail-order merchandisers did not attempt to project fashion trends. What they promised was rapid delivery. As Sears, Roebuck boasted, "We are proud of our merchandise and proud of the service we give our customers. REAL 24-hour service. 99 out of every 100 orders we receive are shipped in less than 24 hours." These firms had to have a ready supply of whatever they offered for a specified time at the listed prices. Their investment was enormous and they could not afford to gamble with the untried or untested, especially in areas as unpredictable as next season's fashions. Yet, if the styles they featured did not have the élan or the ultra-chic avant-garde appearance of the latest fashions shown in New York or Paris, they did inform their readers of what was currently espoused and accepted. Fads and unsuccessful projections are minimal in these catalogs; anyone interested in knowing how the majority of Americans dressed during the period can feel secure in the knowledge that what was illustrated was pretty much what was generally worn.

Few periods demonstrate with such clarity the way fashions reflect their own times as do the 1960s and the 1920s; both periods have much in common and present many parallels. Each focused on social realignments and youth; each involved feminine liberation. In both cycles, wars and technological developments produced rapid changes that led to a quest for excitement, to restlessness and even to violence and destruction.

How was life in the 1920s reflected in the era's fashions? Improved production methods enabled a rapidly growing middle class, even those at its lower level, to participate in the world of fashion that previously had been the sole realm of a privileged few. Another important factor in the democratization of fashions came as a result of the interest among the members of the leisure group in more casual daytime wear. The war years had brought on harsh realities and evoked a desire to do one's bit that touched all levels of society. Even those who formerly had lived in glossy cocoons, where a minimum of physical exertion was a symbol of high station and wealth, sought to become involved in the war effort. After the war many of these people found their prior sedentary life boring and had little desire to return to it. The taste of activity as a release of energy appealed to them. To fit into the pattern of this new version of the good life, fashions became more informal and less complicated. Clothing manufacturers could now easily produce cheap versions that were within the price range of their fashion-hungry customers who had to work for a living.

All fashions reflected the new spirit as youthful, more carefree, ideals gradually replaced the earlier, more staid, models. But it was in fashions for women that the changes were most obvious. Feminine liberation found freedom in discarding the corset. For the first time in centuries women's legs were exposed and freed for mobility and action. To gain equality with men and to resemble them, women flattened their breasts and hips and cut their hair. The 1920s bob and boyish ideal were the period's own version of unisex. Aesthetically, the fashions mirrored the abstract elements of art movements of the period. Geometric in form, they relied on the motion of living women to breathe a shape and a sensuality into an otherwise sterile silhouette. All this was totally sympathetic with an era of pulsating dynamism bent on breaking down remaining restrictions based on the social, economic, political and moral concepts of the past century.

These were the forces that helped to create the fashions of the twenties. Yet, for all the violence, excesses, the licentiousness we have come to associate with this flamboyant period, as one looks through the pages of mail-order catalogs one finds that, although the changes are there, the progression is smooth and orderly. Long hair gave way to bobbed hair. Skirts gradually rose to the knees. Underwear diminished to accommodate the new mood and look. More and more space was devoted to cosmetics, and here and there pants for women were featured. Nowhere are there examples of the revealing, extravagantly low-cut gowns tantalizingly covered with fringes or sparkling beading. The few party dresses shown are very modest and demure, pictures of naive innocence (page 90). The "flapper" dresses, as they appear on page 92, are merely a timid, decorous reflection of the sophisticated sexuality of the so-called "Roaring Twenties," only a muted echo of the ragtime rhythms of the Jazz Age.

Men's coats and suits on the whole remained fairly conservative, only occasionally showing the collegiate "rah-rah" or the "razzmatazz" flashiness we have come to associate with the decade. The new concept found expression mainly in casual and sports clothes, accessories and in a wider range of designs available in work clothes.

Apparently revolution was the choice and privilege of a minority. The majority chose the safer path and course of evolution.

In the 1920s motion pictures exerted an ever-increasing impact on the American scene. Movie stars brought the viewers adventure, a shimmering aura of wealth, beauty and romance. Films gave a semblance of reality to fantasies and aroused the public to new hopes, tastes and appetites. Sensing this, Sears, Roebuck and Co. began to include fashions endorsed by such stars as Clara Bow (page 105), Gloria Swanson (page 56) and Joan Crawford (page 127). For men there were Western-style hats and boots (page 14); little boys could playact in cowboy and Indian costumes (page 118). Although the movies during this decade kept their audiences informed of the latest fashions, the female stars' most significant influence was on the face and figure, coiffure, posture and grooming. As a result beauty parlors and reducing regimens abounded, and the field of cosmetics became a major industry.

Women may have looked to Hollywood for goddesses to emulate, but the direction of fashion was set in Paris. As glamorous as the clothes appeared in the movies, they were in the main versions of what the French couture had proposed. This seems to have been no mystery to the staffs responsible for the fashions to be featured in the catalogs. References to movie stars were primarily to such details as hats and shoes. The bulk of the fashion merchandise, coats, suits and dresses claim to have their origins in New York or Paris. This is probably quite true because a well-trained eye can readily spot elements of the inventive creations of various French designers. The greatest single influence throughout the 1920s, however, was that of Coco Chanel. Her use of supple jerseys, simple ensembles consisting of jacket, blouse and skirt, costume accessories such as scarves and inexpensive jewelry, had a natural appeal for the active, practical American woman. The workmanship or quality certainly could not compare with that of the French couture. The degree of downgrading, however, is difficult to ascertain. The clientele of mail-order purchasing was hardly the sort to stockpile a wardrobe and leave it for posterity; they were more apt to wear out their clothes.

Sunday-best clothes would be updated through alterations or be downgraded for everyday wear. And when they were replaced, they would be passed on to younger or less-fortunate members of the family or community, if they were still useable. The Puritan ethic was still in force; to do otherwise would have been considered sinful. In any case, not enough examples have survived to make a valid comparison.

The common practice of placing time and life into tidy compartments by decades is a handy device used to pull together loosely the peak essences of an era. Actually, the fashions of the twenties can be split into two phases. As usual, changes occur somewhat earlier in the world of the haute couture (in this case 1919–1923 and 1924–1929). Those shown in mail-order catalogs break into the following two time spans: 1919–1924 and 1925–1931. Although neither period remained static, there is something homogenous about each segment and it is interesting to view them in that context.

# Part One: 1919-1924

In 1919, people in Europe and America, exhausted and depleted by World War I, longed to return to what they considered normalcy, to the way of life they had known before the war. Fashions reverted to those of 1913–1914, as though they had only been dropped for the duration. A new view of how women should dress had begun around 1909 and the course toward freedom, youth and equality was established even before 1914. By 1920, after a few steps backwards, the movement was accelerated by the experience and changes brought on by the war. During the next several years, the fashion ideal became younger and younger and proceeded to divest itself of many of the physical and mental trappings of the nineteenth century.

Growing urbanization, increased affluence, shorter working hours and paid vacations allowed for more leisure time and extra energy. As a result, interest in sports escalated, necessitating a whole range of special clothes designed for active and spectactor sports. Gradually this freer concept of dressing crept into daywear. Clothes became simpler and lighter in weight. Feminine curves, long a symbol of a woman's frailty, were negated by the fashion for the new streamlined vertical lines. These six years were essentially a transitional period in women's fashions. The new style was to emerge fully in 1925.

By 1919 pregnancy was no longer veiled in gowns for déshabillé or at-home robes. Maternity dresses designed in the styles of the period, along with maternity corsets, were illustrated graphically with explicit text explaining their function and virtues (page 7).

When one compares the fashions shown by Sears, Roebuck and Co. during this period with those in a French magazine such as *L'Art et la Mode* or with the American *Vogue* or *Harper's Bazaar*, it is interesting to note that there is only about a one-year lag in the overall aspect of the mail-order fashions. Yet, although the styles were not exactly the dernier cri or as handsomely presented as those in the high-fashion magazines, many fashions shown by Sears in 1919–24 reveal a surprising amount of chic and elegance. Not all of the clothes were inexpensive. Some coats and suits sold for almost $50, while some "better" dresses were priced over $30. Considering the purchasing power of a dollar in those days, it is apparent that those who could afford these prices were not confined to large cities and that mail-order catalogs catered not only to the rustic needs of farmers or the meager purses of the poorer classes. During these six years, the range of cost and taste was rather wide; the fashions presented must have been aimed at a broad spectrum of Americans.

## 1919

(pages 5-14)

The hobble skirt of the prewar period took on the "peg-top" look (pages 5 and 6) and the 1913 "barrel form" was shown along with pyramid shapes popular in 1915–16. The waistlines were either high or undefined. The bust retained the earlier low monobosom look. By our standards, the figure was quite full. The use of decorations, such as a proliferation of buttons, tassels and braid, was also a holdover from past fashions.

Although the current silhouette actually required little constriction, women, except for the most liberated, continued to wear corsets. There were even corsets for "children up to 12 years" (page 8). White cotton, trimmed with eyelet and lace, was popular for lingerie. Very pointed high shoes, laced or buttoned, with solid or spat tops and Louis or military heels were preferred. Stockings, which showed only when pumps were occasionally worn, were generally black or dark gray, although white was sometimes worn with white shoes. Hats, which had large crowns to accommodate long hair, were worn low, just above the eyebrows.

Male fashions reminiscent of the Edwardian styles are shown on models with large, square-jawed heads, and hair neatly plastered down. Their clothes had narrow shoulders and were slightly high-waisted, like the women's fashions. For sports there were Norfolk jackets and knickerbockers for golf or hiking and suits for riding.

The cosmetics available were limited to rouge, face powder and discreet lip rouge. One could buy a pencil to darken eyebrows, lashes and, for the men, beards and mustaches. For the nails there were cuticle removers, nail whites and polishing pastes.

## 1920
(pages 15-34)

Skirts became a little shorter, figures somewhat slimmer, bosoms smaller and the waistline was more naturally placed. Suits appeared sleeker and more tailored. Middy and overblouses, now an important item, figured prominently in modified forms into the 1930s. Lingerie—petticoats, chemises, bloomers—were shown in a profusion of colored silks in purple, flesh, blue, green, plum and black. Bandeaux or brassieres began to displace the camisole.

Automobile dusters were included in the menswear section. Although jackets for youths and boys were similar to those for men, suits for boys 9 to 17 were shown with knickerbockers.

## 1921
(pages 35-48)

There was a further simplicity this year. Dresses on page 38 were designed to fall in an unbroken line from shoulder to hem. Worn loose, slightly belted at the normal waist, this was to be the silhouette of most of the decade. Although dresses remained below calf length, coats became shorter. Heavy trimming began to disappear. Some hair was obviously cut but was kept soft-looking with side curls (page 38). High shoes and spats were still worn but there was in increase in the popularity of pumps and oxfords. Stockings remained dark. The Japanese-style kimono as well as sleeping suits (pajamas for women) made their appearance. Men's outerwear included chesterfields, town ulsters and reversible rubber interlined raincoats. Shirts with detachable collars were popular. The separate collars could be either stiff or soft, and some, called "rubber collars," were made of celluloid.

## 1922
(pages 49-66)

Skirts reached mid-calf length. Coats continued to hold to the earlier style with full or dolman sleeves and were trimmed with some braid, tassels, embroidery and buttons. Suits, however, generally had a more male look. They were worn either beltless or with belts placed a little below the waist. Dresses showed the effects of the styles by the French designer, Paul Poiret—especially his use of peasant-type embroidery (page 50). Touches of Jeanne Lanvin can also be detected in the dresses worn by the two center figures on page 50. The echoes of Chanel's designs are too numerous to mention since much of the knitwear and classically simple clothes of the 1920s must be attributed to her influence.

Moving toward the new slimness, foundations began to accent hip and bust flattening. As hemlines rose, footwear became decorative: T-strap slippers and fashions for gaiters, galoshes and "arctics." Stockings, though still on the dark side, developed clocks and fancy heels. Rayon stockings made the silken look for legs available at a low price (78¢ as opposed to $2.69 for a pair of silk stockings with clocks.)

Sweaters for men were featured in a wide range of colors, patterns and details, such as shawl collars and turtlenecks. Sports clothes received added attention. For bathing, men were offered one piece knit suits with attached skirts while women could choose from several dressmaker-type costumes that were worn over an undergarment. There were also suits for football, hockey, skiing, golf and shooting. Underwear for men took on an athletic tone in the form of boxer shorts.

## 1923
(pages 67-76)

The waistline now has slipped down to the top of the hips. But, as though there was still some doubt or uneasiness about the future, this year's fashions harked back not so much to those of 1913 but all the way to those of 1909. A matronly silhouette—with wide sleeves, tassel and braid trimming, lower hemlines nearly ankle length—seems to have come back. In dresses, Lanvin's *robe de style*, with its low-waisted bodice and long full skirt, was shown in many adopted versions (page 69, right figure). Accessories now included mesh purses and silver-plated compacts.

## 1924
(pages 77-84)

Fashions this year were a blend of the old and the new (page 78). The waistline descended to the hips. There was a hint of the surface decoration and geometric insertions that would serve to break up the stark simplicity of the coming rectangular silhouette (page 77). Beltless jackets were shorter and worn with slim untrimmed skirts. Page 83 shows sports pants outfits; page 82 advertises "Bob" hats for women with bobbed hair.

# Women's Attractive Fur Coats and Capes

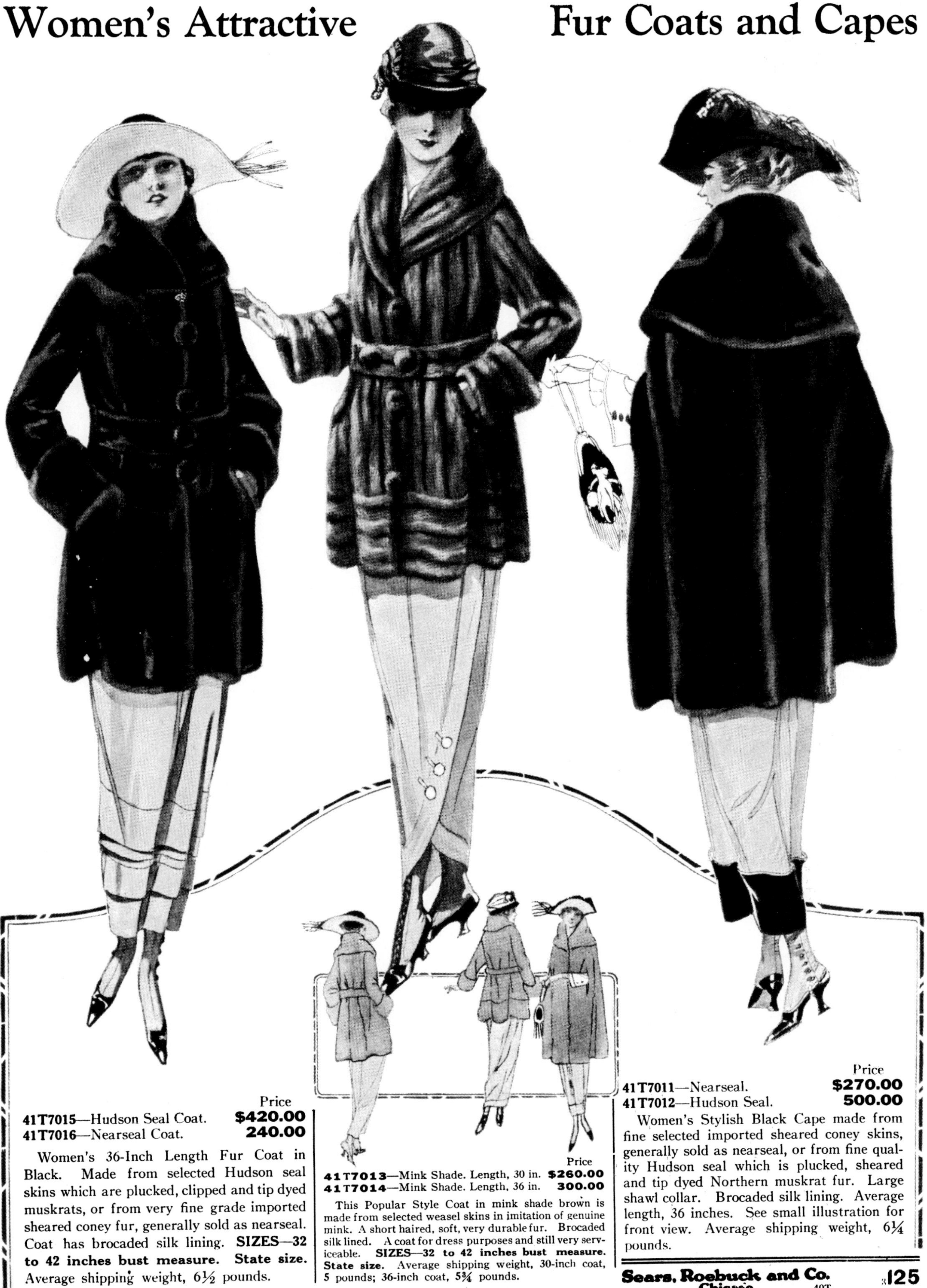

41T7015—Hudson Seal Coat. Price $420.00
41T7016—Nearseal Coat. 240.00

Women's 36-Inch Length Fur Coat in Black. Made from selected Hudson seal skins which are plucked, clipped and tip dyed muskrats, or from very fine grade imported sheared coney fur, generally sold as nearseal. Coat has brocaded silk lining. **SIZES—32 to 42 inches bust measure. State size.** Average shipping weight, 6½ pounds.

41T7013—Mink Shade. Length, 30 in. Price $260.00
41T7014—Mink Shade. Length, 36 in. 300.00

This Popular Style Coat in mink shade brown is made from selected weasel skins in imitation of genuine mink. A short haired, soft, very durable fur. Brocaded silk lined. A coat for dress purposes and still very serviceable. **SIZES—32 to 42 inches bust measure. State size.** Average shipping weight, 30-inch coat, 5 pounds; 36-inch coat, 5¾ pounds.

41T7011—Nearseal. Price $270.00
41T7012—Hudson Seal. 500.00

Women's Stylish Black Cape made from fine selected imported sheared coney skins, generally sold as nearseal, or from fine quality Hudson seal which is plucked, sheared and tip dyed Northern muskrat fur. Large shawl collar. Brocaded silk lining. Average length, 36 inches. See small illustration for front view. Average shipping weight, 6¼ pounds.

# Women's Imported Coney Fur Sets

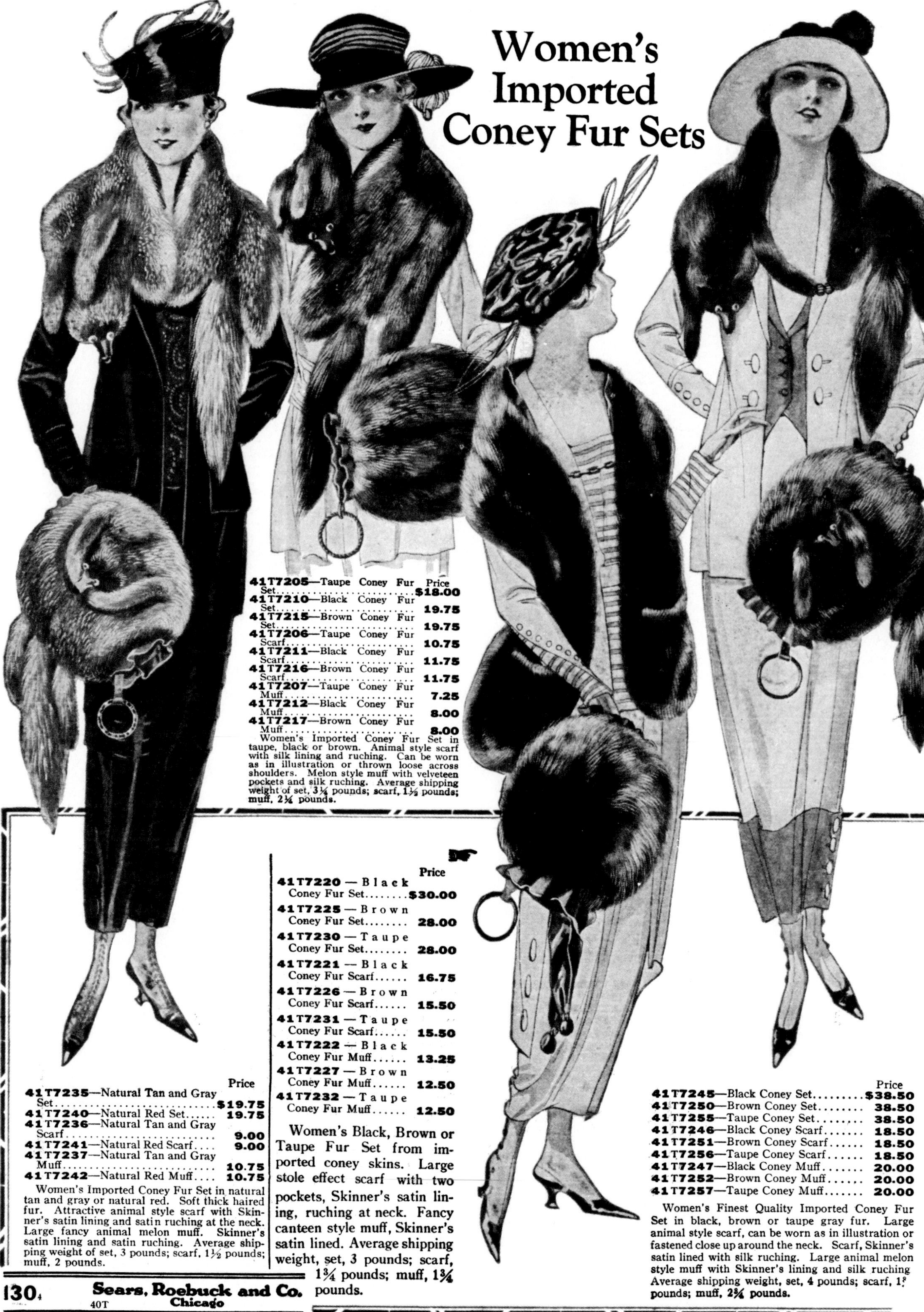

| | Price |
|---|---|
| 41T7205—Taupe Coney Fur Set | $18.00 |
| 41T7210—Black Coney Fur Set | 19.75 |
| 41T7215—Brown Coney Fur Set | 19.75 |
| 41T7206—Taupe Coney Fur Scarf | 10.75 |
| 41T7211—Black Coney Fur Scarf | 11.75 |
| 41T7216—Brown Coney Fur Scarf | 11.75 |
| 41T7207—Taupe Coney Fur Muff | 7.25 |
| 41T7212—Black Coney Fur Muff | 8.00 |
| 41T7217—Brown Coney Fur Muff | 8.00 |

Women's Imported Coney Fur Set in taupe, black or brown. Animal style scarf with silk lining and ruching. Can be worn as in illustration or thrown loose across shoulders. Melon style muff with velveteen pockets and silk ruching. Average shipping weight of set, 3¼ pounds; scarf, 1½ pounds; muff, 2¼ pounds.

| | Price |
|---|---|
| 41T7235—Natural Tan and Gray Set | $19.75 |
| 41T7240—Natural Red Set | 19.75 |
| 41T7236—Natural Tan and Gray Scarf | 9.00 |
| 41T7241—Natural Red Scarf | 9.00 |
| 41T7237—Natural Tan and Gray Muff | 10.75 |
| 41T7242—Natural Red Muff | 10.75 |

Women's Imported Coney Fur Set in natural tan and gray or natural red. Soft thick haired fur. Attractive animal style scarf with Skinner's satin lining and satin ruching at the neck. Large fancy animal melon muff. Skinner's satin lining and satin ruching. Average shipping weight of set, 3 pounds; scarf, 1½ pounds; muff, 2 pounds.

| | Price |
|---|---|
| 41T7220—Black Coney Fur Set | $30.00 |
| 41T7225—Brown Coney Fur Set | 28.00 |
| 41T7230—Taupe Coney Fur Set | 28.00 |
| 41T7221—Black Coney Fur Scarf | 16.75 |
| 41T7226—Brown Coney Fur Scarf | 15.50 |
| 41T7231—Taupe Coney Fur Scarf | 15.50 |
| 41T7222—Black Coney Fur Muff | 13.25 |
| 41T7227—Brown Coney Fur Muff | 12.50 |
| 41T7232—Taupe Coney Fur Muff | 12.50 |

Women's Black, Brown or Taupe Fur Set from imported coney skins. Large stole effect scarf with two pockets, Skinner's satin lining, ruching at neck. Fancy canteen style muff, Skinner's satin lined. Average shipping weight, set, 3 pounds; scarf, 1¾ pounds; muff, 1¾ pounds.

| | Price |
|---|---|
| 41T7245—Black Coney Set | $38.50 |
| 41T7250—Brown Coney Set | 38.50 |
| 41T7255—Taupe Coney Set | 38.50 |
| 41T7246—Black Coney Scarf | 18.50 |
| 41T7251—Brown Coney Scarf | 18.50 |
| 41T7256—Taupe Coney Scarf | 18.50 |
| 41T7247—Black Coney Muff | 20.00 |
| 41T7252—Brown Coney Muff | 20.00 |
| 41T7257—Taupe Coney Muff | 20.00 |

Women's Finest Quality Imported Coney Fur Set in black, brown or taupe gray fur. Large animal style scarf, can be worn as in illustration or fastened close up around the neck. Scarf, Skinner's satin lined with silk ruching. Large animal melon style muff with Skinner's lining and silk ruching Average shipping weight, set, 4 pounds; scarf, 1⅞ pounds; muff, 2¾ pounds.

# Comfortable *and* Stylish Maternity Dresses

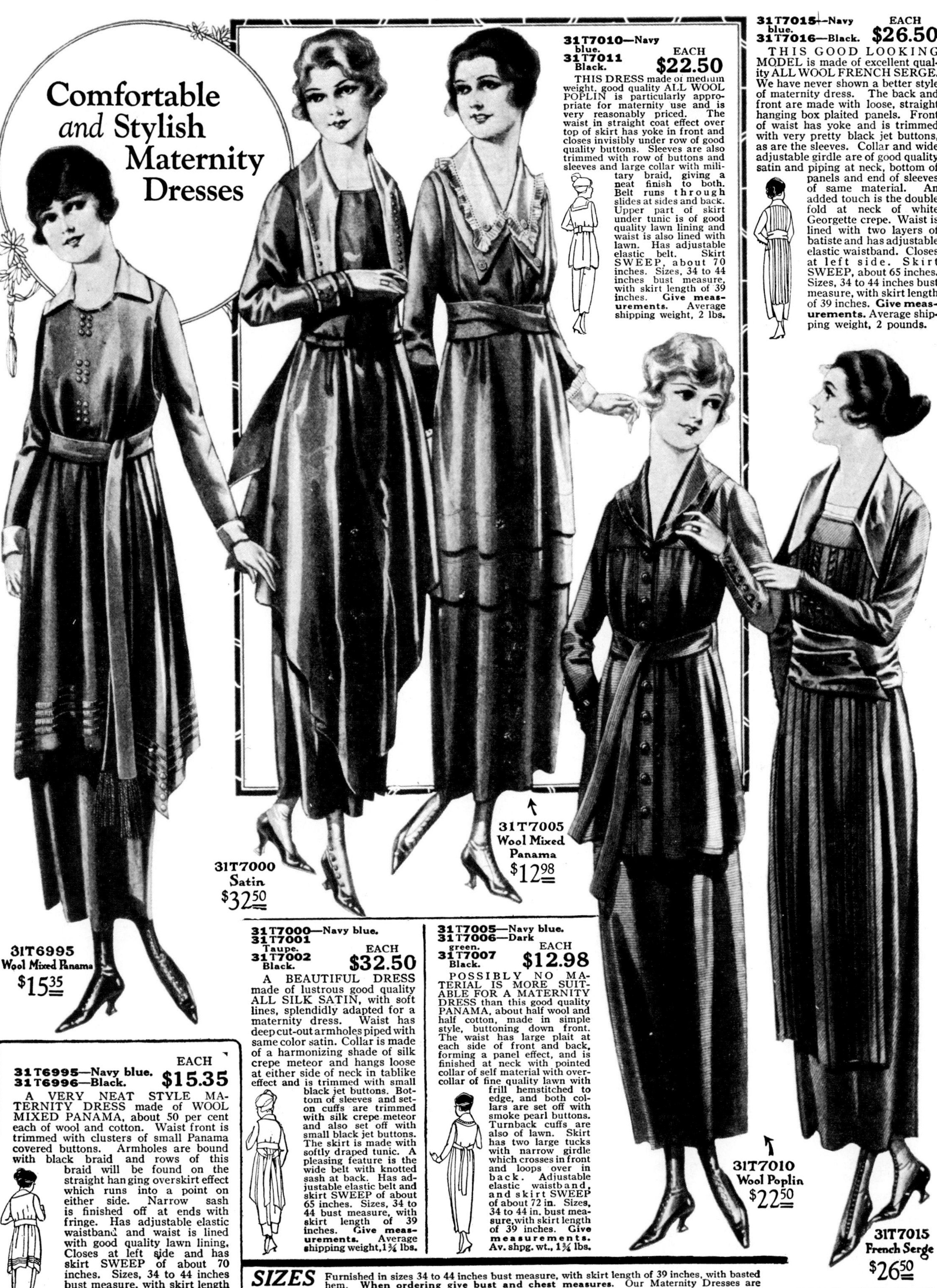


**31T7010—Navy blue.**
**31T7011 Black.** EACH **$22.50**

THIS DRESS made of medium weight, good quality ALL WOOL POPLIN is particularly appropriate for maternity use and is very reasonably priced. The waist in straight coat effect over top of skirt has yoke in front and closes invisibly under row of good quality buttons. Sleeves are also trimmed with row of buttons and sleeves and large collar with military braid, giving a neat finish to both. Belt runs through slides at sides and back. Upper part of skirt under tunic is of good quality lawn lining and waist is also lined with lawn. Has adjustable elastic belt. Skirt SWEEP, about 70 inches. Sizes, 34 to 44 inches bust measure, with skirt length of 39 inches. **Give measurements.** Average shipping weight, 2 lbs.

**31T7015—Navy blue.**
**31T7016—Black.** EACH **$26.50**

THIS GOOD LOOKING MODEL is made of excellent quality ALL WOOL FRENCH SERGE. We have never shown a better style of maternity dress. The back and front are made with loose, straight hanging box plaited panels. Front of waist has yoke and is trimmed with very pretty black jet buttons, as are the sleeves. Collar and wide adjustable girdle are of good quality satin and piping at neck, bottom of panels and end of sleeves of same material. An added touch is the double fold at neck of white Georgette crepe. Waist is lined with two layers of batiste and has adjustable elastic waistband. Closes at left side. Skirt SWEEP, about 65 inches. Sizes, 34 to 44 inches bust measure, with skirt length of 39 inches. **Give measurements.** Average shipping weight, 2 pounds.

**31T6995—Navy blue.**
**31T6996—Black.** EACH **$15.35**

A VERY NEAT STYLE MATERNITY DRESS made of WOOL MIXED PANAMA, about 50 per cent each of wool and cotton. Waist front is trimmed with clusters of small Panama covered buttons. Armholes are bound with black braid and rows of this braid will be found on the straight hanging overskirt effect which runs into a point on either side. Narrow sash is finished off at ends with fringe. Has adjustable elastic waistband and waist is lined with good quality lawn lining. Closes at left side and has skirt SWEEP of about 70 inches. Sizes, 34 to 44 inches bust measure, with skirt length of 39 inches. **Give measurements.** Average shipping wt., 2 pounds.

**31T7000—Navy blue.**
**31T7001 Taupe.**
**31T7002 Black.** EACH **$32.50**

A BEAUTIFUL DRESS made of lustrous good quality ALL SILK SATIN, with soft lines, splendidly adapted for a maternity dress. Waist has deep cut-out armholes piped with same color satin. Collar is made of a harmonizing shade of silk crepe meteor and hangs loose at either side of neck in tablike effect and is trimmed with small black jet buttons. Bottom of sleeves and set-on cuffs are trimmed with silk crepe meteor and also set off with small black jet buttons. The skirt is made with softly draped tunic. A pleasing feature is the wide belt with knotted sash at back. Has adjustable elastic belt and skirt SWEEP of about 65 inches. Sizes, 34 to 44 bust measure, with skirt length of 39 inches. **Give measurements.** Average shipping weight, 1¾ lbs.

**31T7005—Navy blue.**
**31T7006—Dark green.**
**31T7007 Black.** EACH **$12.98**

POSSIBLY NO MATERIAL IS MORE SUITABLE FOR A MATERNITY DRESS than this good quality PANAMA, about half wool and half cotton, made in simple style, buttoning down front. The waist has large plait at each side of front and back, forming a panel effect, and is finished at neck with pointed collar of self material with overcollar of fine quality lawn with frill hemstitched to edge, and both collars are set off with smoke pearl buttons. Turnback cuffs are also of lawn. Skirt has two large tucks with narrow girdle which crosses in front and loops over in back. Adjustable elastic waistband, and skirt SWEEP of about 72 in. Sizes, 34 to 44 in. bust measure, with skirt length of 39 inches. **Give measurements.** Av. shpg. wt., 1¾ lbs.

***SIZES*** Furnished in sizes 34 to 44 inches bust measure, with skirt length of 39 inches, with basted hem. **When ordering give bust and chest measures.** Our Maternity Dresses are cut along lines that will give the most comfort during the pregnant period. The adjustable waistband expands with the figure and does not allow the skirt to pull up from the bottom in an unsightly manner or draw across the abdomen. THESE DRESSES CAN BE WORN AFTER CONFINEMENT WITH SLIGHT, IF ANY, ALTERATIONS.

# Special Value Corsets, Waists and Hip Confiners

Read page 279 about size. There's a reason.

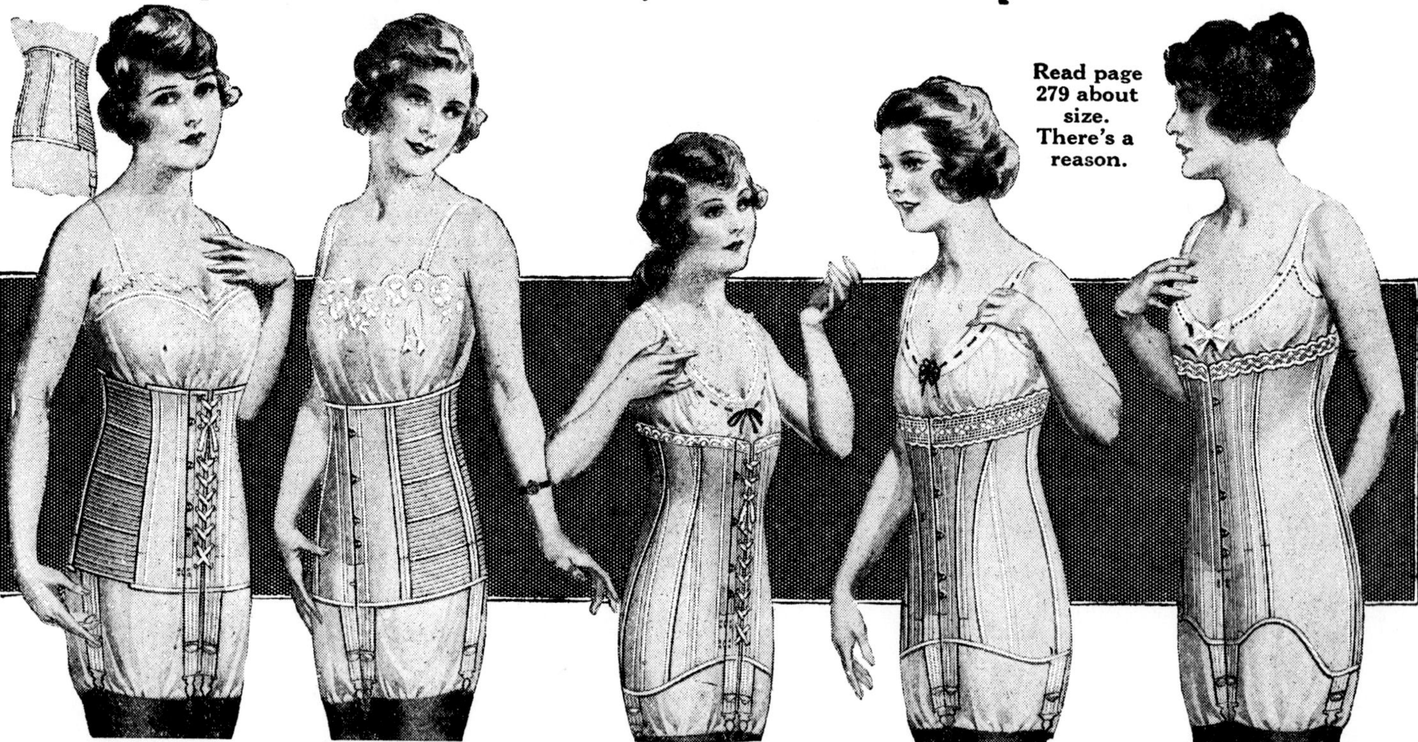

**Front Lacing Topless Corset or Hip Confiner.**

**18T110 $1.79**

*Clasp, 8 in. Corset sizes, 19 to 28.*

Very popular model, made of strong elastic and coutil. Lightly boned, but will give good support and allow plenty of freedom to wearer. Four long hose supporters. **State corset size.**

**Back Lacing Topless Corset or Hip Confiner.**

**18T111 $1.65**

*Clasp, 7½ in. Corset sizes, 19 to 26.*

Made of good quality elastic webbing and strong coutil. Light weight, flexible boning placed to give support and still allow plenty of freedom. Four good hose supporters. **State corset size.**

**Front Lacing. For Misses and Slender Women.**

**18T140 $1.59**

*Medium bust, 3½ in. above waistline. Clasp, 9½ in. Sizes, 19 to 28.*

Made of good quality coutil. Pliable boning carefully placed to give support. Neat trimming. Four hose supporters. **State corset size.** See our instructions on page 279.

**Back Lacing. For Misses and Slender Women.**

**18T121 $1.48**

*Medium bust, 3½ in. above waistline. Clasp, 10 in. Sizes, 19 to 26.*

A splendid corset for growing girls. Well made of good quality batiste. Lightly boned, but will give good support. Neat braid trimming. Four good hose supporters. **State corset size.**

**Back Lacing. For Slender to Average Figures.**

**18T120 $1.59**

*Medium bust, 4 in. above waistline. Clasp, 10½ in. Sizes, 19 to 26.*

Long skirted corset, made of medium quality coutil. Lightly boned; no pressure over hips. Neat embroidery trimming. Four good quality hose supporters. **State corset size** after reading instructions on page 279.

Average shipping weight of corsets on this page, about 1½ pounds.

QUALITY GUARANTEED

CHS — COMFORT HEALTH STYLE

TRADE MARK

Our Own Trade Mark—Registered in U. S. Patent Office.

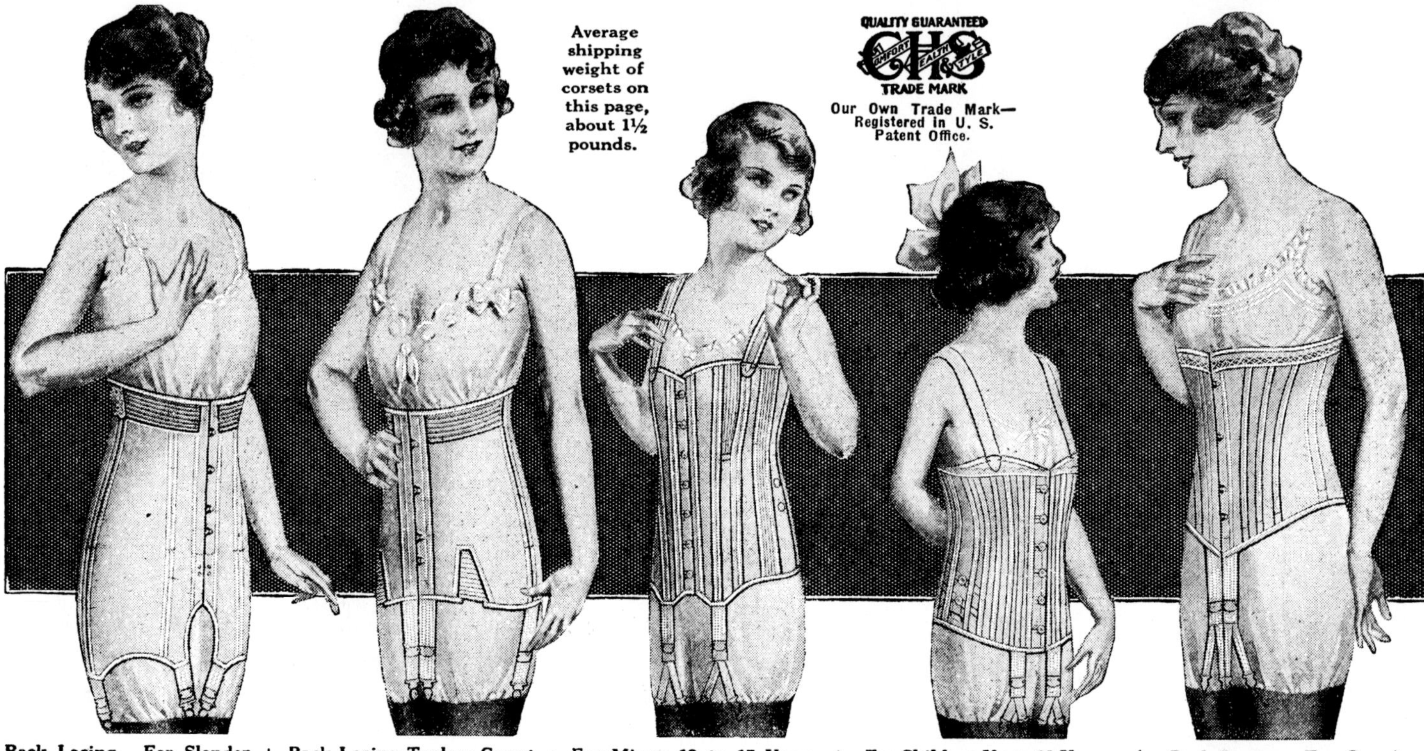

**Back Lacing. For Slender and Average Figures.**

**18T117 $1.79**

*Very low bust, 2 in. above waistline. Clasp, 8 in. Sizes, 19 to 28.*

Made of good quality coutil. Wide elastic sections in bust. Long skirt. Lightly boned; no pressure over hips. Neat embroidery trimming. Four good hose supporters. Read page 279, then **state corset size.**

**Back Lacing Topless Corset for Slender Women.**

**18T116 $1.19**

*Clasp, 9 in. Corset sizes, 19 to 28.*

Made of good quality coutil with wide elastic sections at waistline. Two small elastic inserts in skirt. Lightly boned. Four hose supporters. Popular for athletic and general wear. Read page 279 about giving corset size. **State size.**

**For Misses 12 to 17 Years.**

**18T275 $1.29**

*Comes in sizes 18 to 28.*

Made of strong corset jean, well reinforced and closely corded. Soft plaited bust. Good bone buttons, strongly attached. One pair of two-button hose supporters. Do not order by age. Measure your girl's waist and subtract 1 inch for spread of lacing. Thus, if girl's waist measure is 24 inches, order size 23. **State size.**

**For Children Up to 12 Years.**

**18T265 $1.29**

*Comes in sizes 18 to 28.*

Made of durable corset material, strongly corded and reinforced. Neat braid trimming. Button front with good bone buttons. One pair of two-button hose supporters. Do not order by age. Measure your child's waist and subtract 1 inch for spread of lacing. Thus, if a child's waist measure is 24 inches, order size 23. **State size.**

**Back Lacing. For Growing Girls and Slender Women.**

**18T139 98c**

*Clasp, 9½ in. Corset sizes, 18 to 26.*

Made of good quality batiste. Very short skirt. High in bust. Recommended as a first corset for growing girls. Pliable boning. Neat braid trimming. One pair of two-button hose supporters.

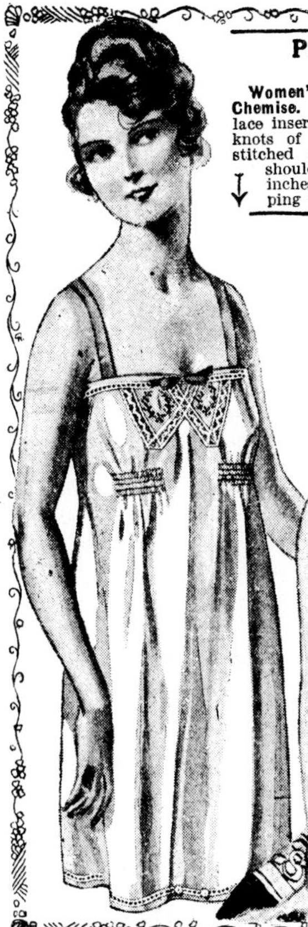

# BEST IN THEIR CLASS *Phillis* BRAND UNDERMUSLINS

REG. U.S. PAT. OFF.

"Phillis" Brand Undermuslins are specially made for us from the latest and most attractive designs. Only very fine quality nainsooks and cambrics are used, while the laces and embroideries are of exceptional quality. The workmanship throughout is the best that we can secure. The sizes are accurate and full.

Each garment is carefully inspected, folded, wrapped in tissue paper and packed in a separate box, thus reaching the customer in the best condition.

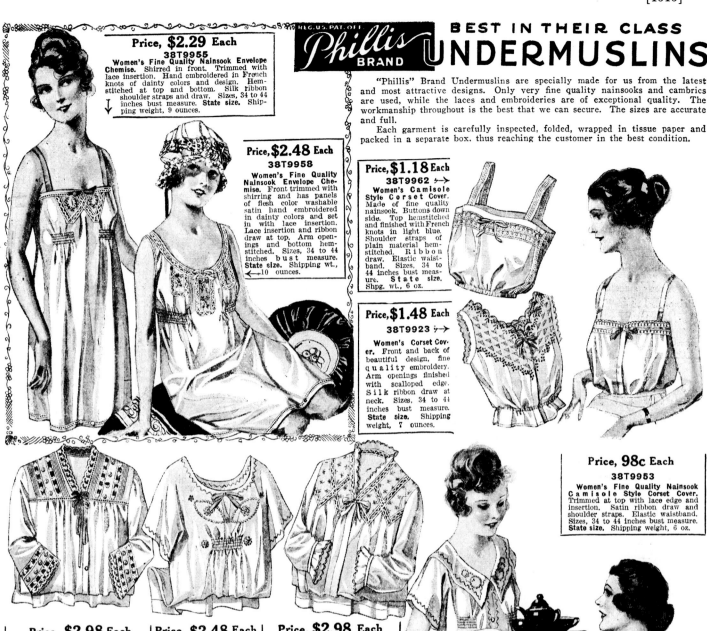

**Price, $2.29 Each**
**38T9955**
**Women's Fine Quality Nainsook Envelope Chemise.** Shirred in front. Trimmed with lace insertion. Hand embroidered in French knots of dainty colors and design. Hemstitched at top and bottom. Silk ribbon shoulder straps and draw. Sizes, 34 to 44 inches bust measure. **State size.** Shipping weight, 9 ounces.

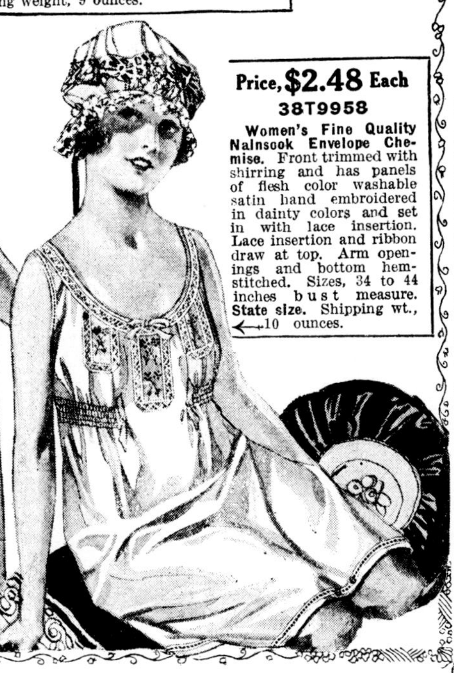

**Price, $2.48 Each**
**38T9958**
**Women's Fine Quality Nainsook Envelope Chemise.** Front trimmed with shirring and has panels of flesh color washable satin hand embroidered in dainty colors and set in with lace insertion. Lace insertion and ribbon draw at top. Arm openings and bottom hemstitched. Sizes, 34 to 44 inches bust measure. **State size.** Shipping wt., 10 ounces.

**Price, $1.18 Each**
**38T9962**
**Women's Camisole Style Corset Cover.** Made of fine quality nainsook. Buttons down side. Top hemstitched and finished with French knots in light blue. Shoulder straps of plain material hemstitched. Ribbon draw. Elastic waistband. Sizes, 34 to 44 inches bust measure. **State size.** Shpg. wt., 6 oz.

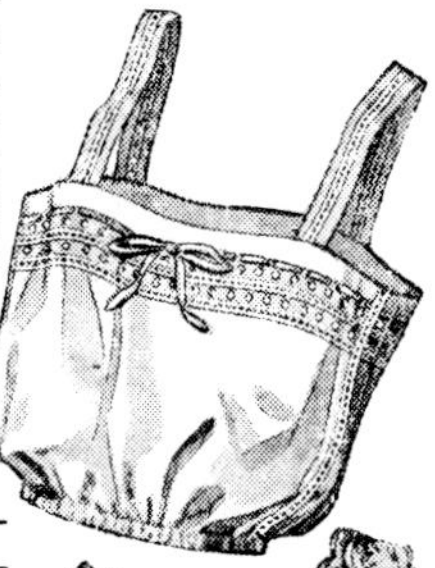

**Price, $1.48 Each**
**38T9923**
**Women's Corset Cover.** Front and back of beautiful design, fine quality embroidery. Arm openings finished with scalloped edge. Silk ribbon draw at neck. Sizes, 34 to 44 inches bust measure. **State size.** Shipping weight, 7 ounces.

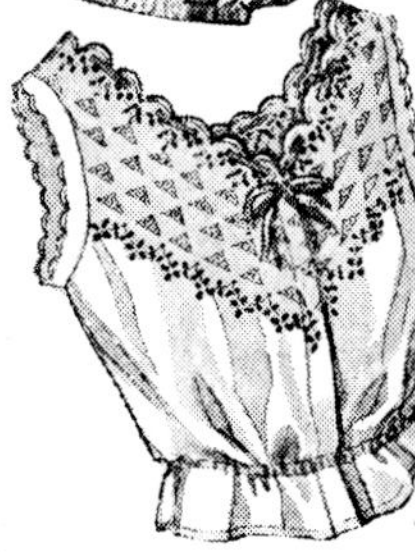

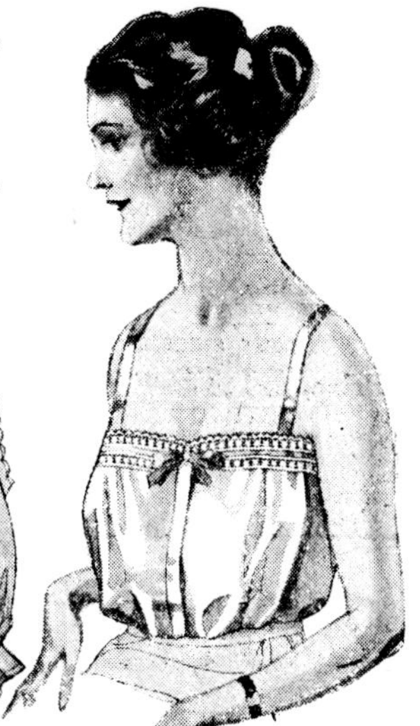

**Price, 98c Each**
**38T9953**
**Women's Fine Quality Nainsook Camisole Style Corset Cover.** Trimmed at top with lace edge and insertion. Satin ribbon draw and shoulder straps. Elastic waistband. Sizes, 34 to 44 inches bust measure. **State size.** Shipping weight, 6 oz.

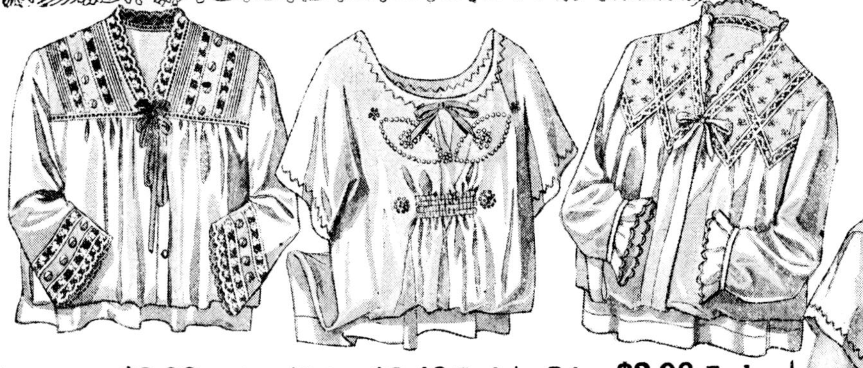

**Price, $2.98 Each**
**38T9960**
**Women's Fine Quality Nainsook Nightgown.** Front yoke made of organdy panels, embroidered in dainty colors, set in with lace insertion and tucks. Narrow beading joins the yoke to body of garment. Neck finished with beading and lace. Bell shaped sleeves, trimmed to match yoke. Has fancy rosette. Sizes, 34 to 44 inches bust measure. **State size.** Shipping weight, 15 oz.

**Price, $2.48 Each**
**38T9959**
**Women's Fine Quality Nainsook Slipover Nightgown.** Front shirred and hand embroidered in French knots of dainty colors. Neck and short sleeves featherstitched. Ribbon draw. Sizes, 34 to 44 inches bust measure. **State size.** Shpg. weight, 15 ounces.

**Price, $2.98 Each**
**38T9957**
**Women's Fine Quality Nainsook Nightgown.** Front yoke made up of beautiful pattern allover embroidery panels, set in with embroidery insertion. Neck and long sleeves finished with well made scalloped embroidered edge. Has silk ribbon bow. Sizes, 34 to 44 inches bust measure. **State size.** Shipping weight, 15 ounces.

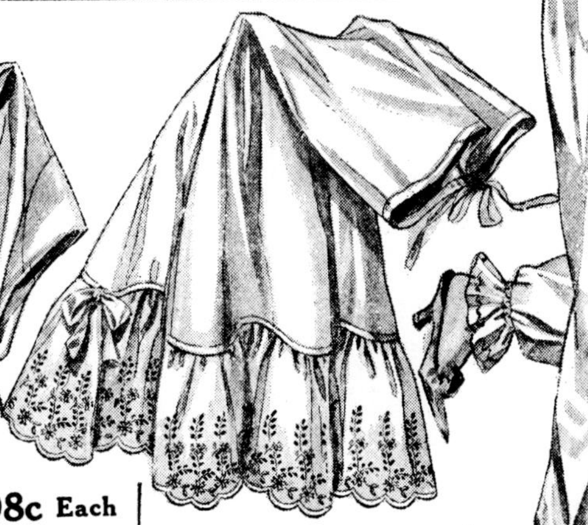

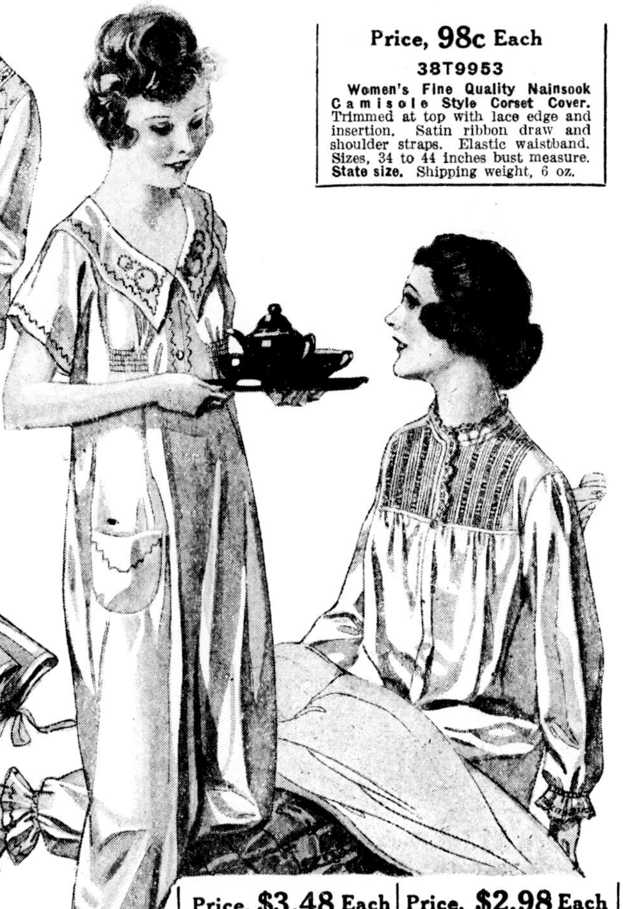

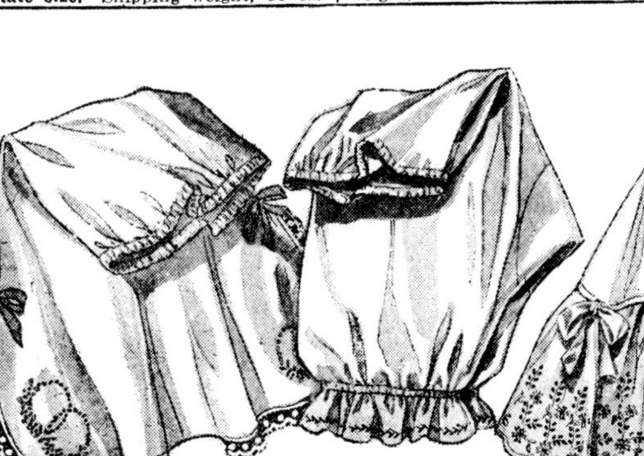

**Price, $1.78 Each**
**38T9956**
**Women's Step-In Umbrella Style Drawers.** Made of fine quality nainsook. Bottoms edged with good quality Valenciennes lace. Trimmed with hand embroidery in floral design, and ribbon bows. Elastic at waistband. Sizes, medium and large. **State size.** Shipping weight, 10 ounces.

**Price, 98c Each**
**38T9961**—Flesh color. **Women's Fine Quality Nainsook Bloomers.** Bottoms trimmed with light colors in a fancy stitch. Reinforced at crotch. Elastic at waist and knees. Sizes, small, medium and large. **State size.** Shipping weight, 10 ounces.

**Price, $2.39 Each**
**38T9951**
**Women's Fine Quality Cambric Underskirt.** Flounce of neat pattern high grade embroidery, trimmed with silk ribbon bow. String top. Has underlay. Lengths, 34 to 42 inches. **State length.** Shipping weight, 15 ounces.

**Price, $3.48 Each**
**38T9952**
**Women's Fine Quality Nainsook "Billie Burke."** Has fancy collar, hand embroidered with French knots in colors. Featherstitching on collar, front opening, short sleeves, pocket and bottoms. Shirred in front. Open crotch. Elastic at ankles. Sizes, 34 to 44 inches bust measure. **State size.** Shipping weight, 14 oz.

**Price, $2.98 Each**
**38T9954**
**Women's Fine Quality Cambric High Neck Nightgown.** Yoke tucked and trimmed with dainty pattern embroidery insertion. Neck finished with embroidery edge to match. Long sleeves trimmed with insertion and embroidery edge. Sizes, 34 to 44 inches bust measure. **State size.** Shipping wt., 1⅛ lbs.

# Women's Dress Shoes

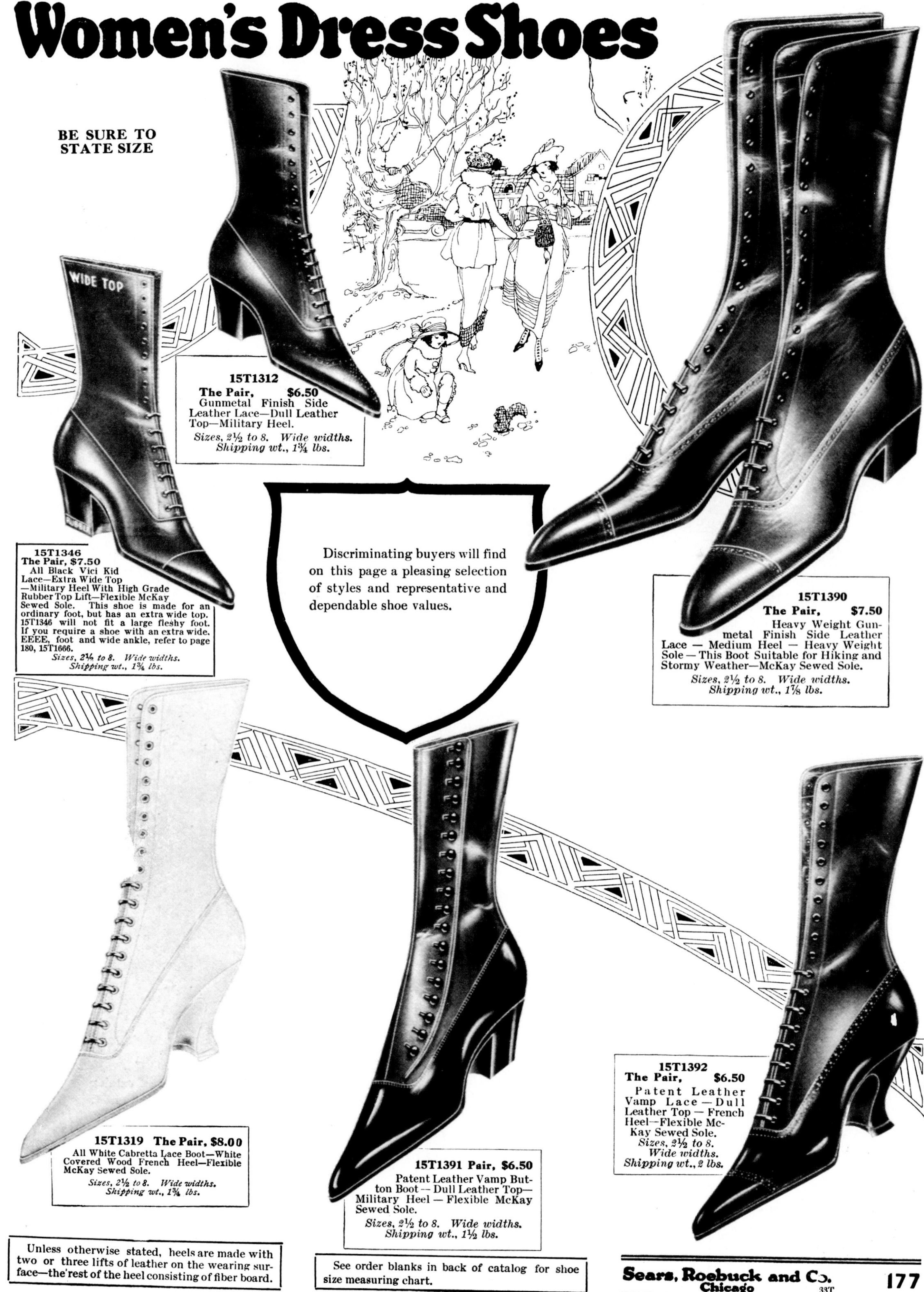


**BE SURE TO STATE SIZE**

**15T1312**
**The Pair, $6.50**
Gunmetal Finish Side Leather Lace—Dull Leather Top—Military Heel.
*Sizes, 2½ to 8. Wide widths.*
*Shipping wt., 1¾ lbs.*

**15T1346**
**The Pair, $7.50**
All Black Vici Kid Lace—Extra Wide Top—Military Heel With High Grade Rubber Top Lift—Flexible McKay Sewed Sole. This shoe is made for an ordinary foot, but has an extra wide top. 15T1346 will not fit a large fleshy foot. If you require a shoe with an extra wide, EEEE, foot and wide ankle, refer to page 180, 15T1666.
*Sizes, 2½ to 8. Wide widths.*
*Shipping wt., 1¾ lbs.*

Discriminating buyers will find on this page a pleasing selection of styles and representative and dependable shoe values.

**15T1390**
**The Pair, $7.50**
Heavy Weight Gunmetal Finish Side Leather Lace — Medium Heel — Heavy Weight Sole — This Boot Suitable for Hiking and Stormy Weather—McKay Sewed Sole.
*Sizes, 2½ to 8. Wide widths.*
*Shipping wt., 1⅞ lbs.*

**15T1319 The Pair, $8.00**
All White Cabretta Lace Boot—White Covered Wood French Heel—Flexible McKay Sewed Sole.
*Sizes, 2½ to 8. Wide widths.*
*Shipping wt., 1¾ lbs.*

**15T1391 Pair, $6.50**
Patent Leather Vamp Button Boot — Dull Leather Top—Military Heel — Flexible McKay Sewed Sole.
*Sizes, 2½ to 8. Wide widths.*
*Shipping wt., 1½ lbs.*

**15T1392**
**The Pair, $6.50**
Patent Leather Vamp Lace — Dull Leather Top — French Heel—Flexible McKay Sewed Sole.
*Sizes, 2½ to 8.*
*Wide widths.*
*Shipping wt., 2 lbs.*

Unless otherwise stated, heels are made with two or three lifts of leather on the wearing surface—the rest of the heel consisting of fiber board.

See order blanks in back of catalog for shoe size measuring chart.

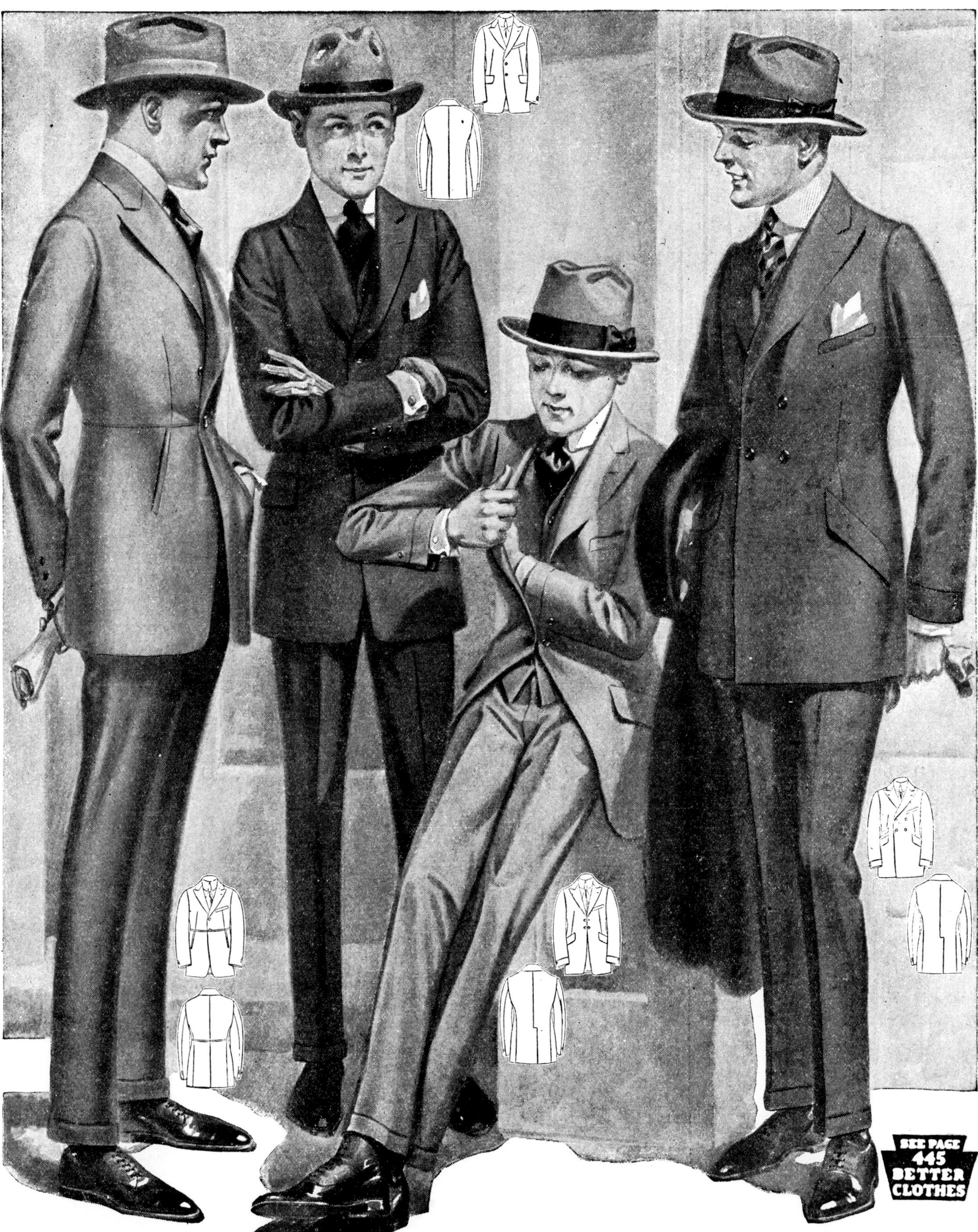


**Model 5**

This is a very stylish waist seam coat—slanting slash pockets, a flaring skirt, and high peaked lapels. Open vent in back. The coat closes with two buttons; the vest with five. The pants are fairly close fitting, made with cuff bottoms and belt loops. For color reproductions of fabrics made in this style see opposite page.

**Model 7**

One of our best models—suitable for any well dressed man or young man. It is medium close fitting, with peaked lapels, three buttons and lower pockets with flap. Closed back. The vest is made without collar and closes with five buttons. The pants have cuff bottoms, tunnel belt loops and are made in young man's style. See the opposite page for color reproductions of fabrics made in this style.

**Model 8**

A two-button coat, made with a lower link button and usually worn as shown in the illustration above. Peaked lapels, cuff on sleeves, and slanting pockets with flap. Open vent sleeve and open vent in back. The pants are made with cuff bottoms and tunnel belt loops. Five-button vest. A very stylish suit any man can wear. Made in a variety of good fabrics reproduced in color on the opposite page.

**Model 9**

This is a very smart two-button double breasted coat—slanting lower pockets, high peaked lapels, separate cuffs, with open vent. Long skirt effect. Open vent in back. Young men's style pants with cuff bottoms and tunnel belt loops. Five-button vest, made without collar. See opposite page for color reproductions of fabrics in which this suit is made.

# Chester·field

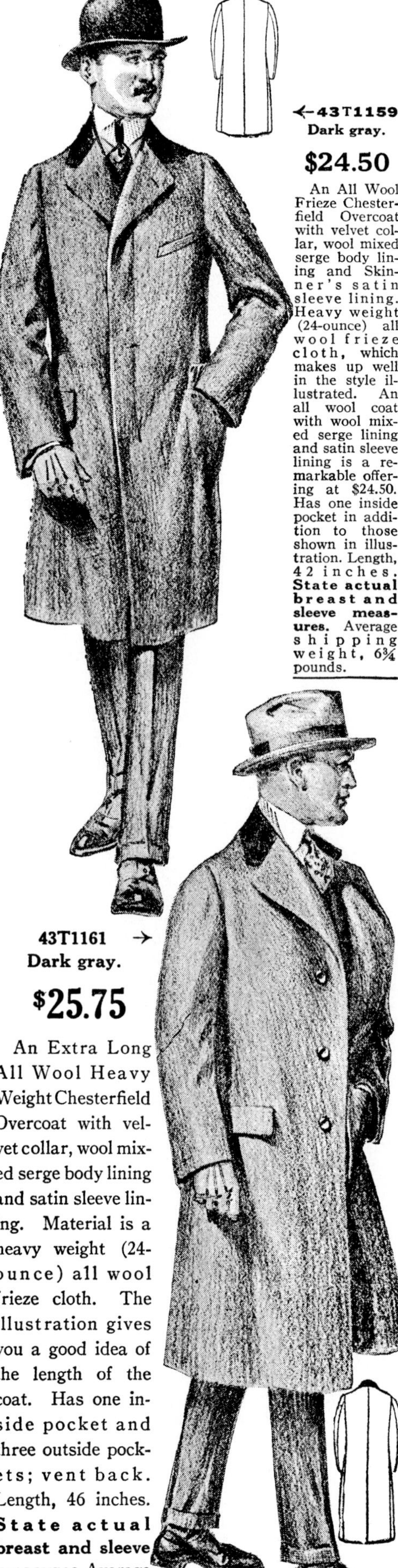

←43T1159
**Dark gray.**

**$24.50**

An All Wool Frieze Chesterfield Overcoat with velvet collar, wool mixed serge body lining and Skinner's satin sleeve lining. Heavy weight (24-ounce) all wool frieze cloth, which makes up well in the style illustrated. An all wool coat with wool mixed serge lining and satin sleeve lining is a remarkable offering at $24.50. Has one inside pocket in addition to those shown in illustration. Length, 42 inches. **State actual breast and sleeve measures.** Average shipping weight, 6¾ pounds.

**43T1161** →
**Dark gray.**

**$25.75**

An Extra Long All Wool Heavy Weight Chesterfield Overcoat with velvet collar, wool mixed serge body lining and satin sleeve lining. Material is a heavy weight (24-ounce) all wool frieze cloth. The illustration gives you a good idea of the length of the coat. Has one inside pocket and three outside pockets; vent back. Length, 46 inches. **State actual breast and sleeve measures.** Average shipping weight, 7 pounds.

**43T1157**—Oxford gray.
**43T1158**—Black.

**$21.50**

An Inexpensive Chesterfield Melton Overcoat. Material is about 85 per cent wool and 15 per cent cotton melton heavy weight (25-oz.) overcoating. Neat velvet collar. The body and sleeves are lined throughout with a fine finished twill. The material will be found durable and good looking. Note the three outside pockets; also has one inside pocket. A splendid coat for the price asked. Length, 43 inches. **State actual breast and sleeve measures.** Average shipping weight, 6½ pounds.

**43T1163**—Black.
**43T1164**—Dark brown.

**$26.75**

Heavy Weight All Wool Fine Melton Chesterfield Overcoat with velvet collar. Material is a tight woven fine finished heavy weight (26-ounce) all wool melton. Body of coat is lined throughout with wool mixed serge and satin sleeve lining. A very dressy coat. Has one inside pocket in addition to those shown in illustration; vent back. Length, 42 inches. **State actual breast and sleeve measures.** Average shipping weight, 6¾ pounds.

***SIZES*** 34 to 48 inches breast measure. **State actual breast and sleeve measures,** for coats are made several inches larger to allow for clothing worn underneath. **If you are a stout size give waist measure also.** For simple measuring instructions see order blanks in back of catalog. If you want to see cloth samples of these coats before ordering, write us a letter giving the catalog numbers of the coats in which you are especially interested.

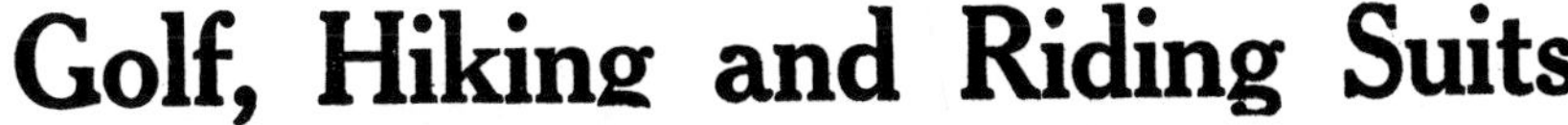

# Golf, Hiking and Riding Suits

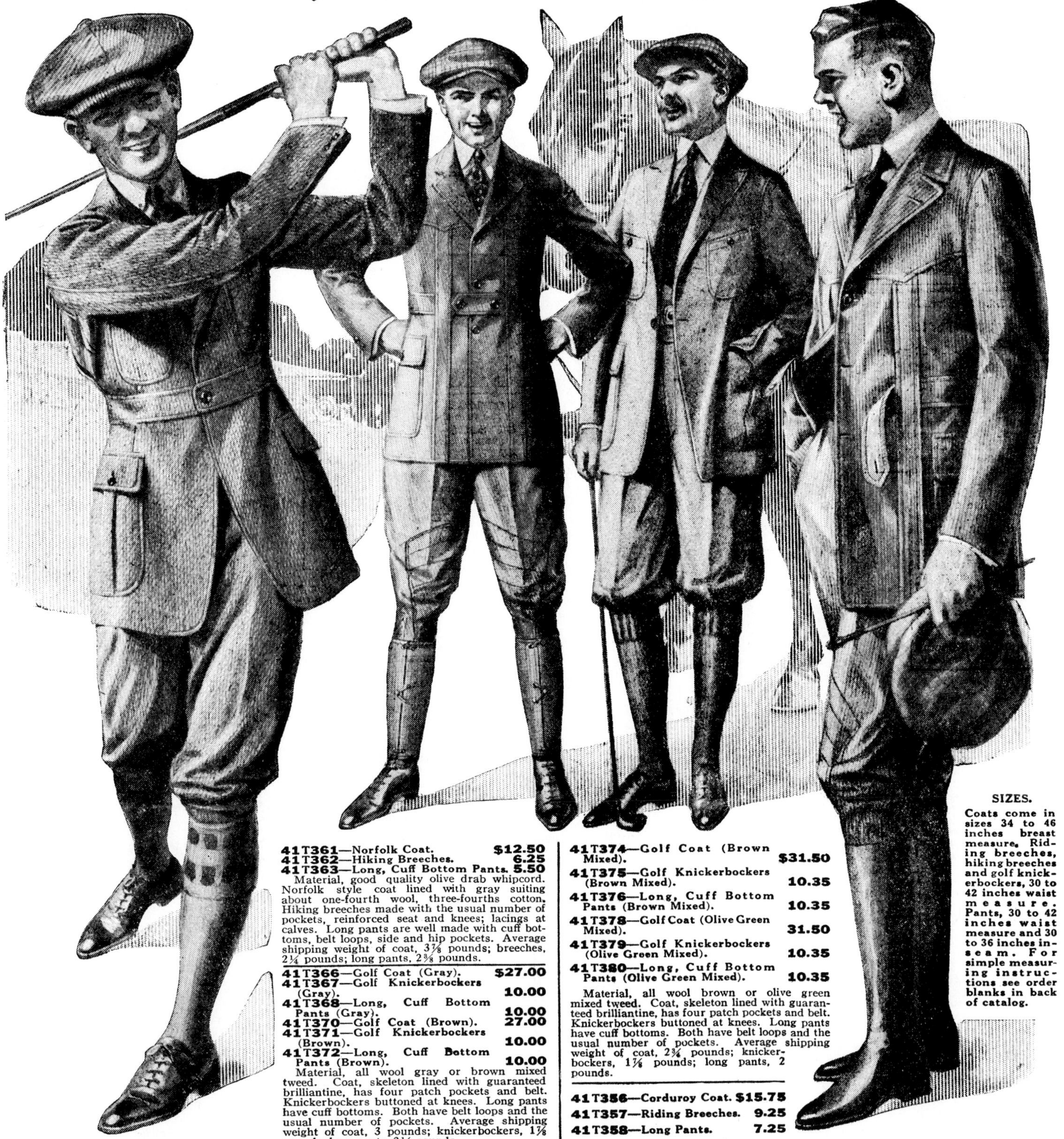

**41T361**—Norfolk Coat. **$12.50**
**41T362**—Hiking Breeches. **6.25**
**41T363**—Long, Cuff Bottom Pants. **5.50**

Material, good quality olive drab whipcord. Norfolk style coat lined with gray suiting about one-fourth wool, three-fourths cotton. Hiking breeches made with the usual number of pockets, reinforced seat and knees; lacings at calves. Long pants are well made with cuff bottoms, belt loops, side and hip pockets. Average shipping weight of coat, 3⅞ pounds; breeches, 2¼ pounds; long pants, 2⅜ pounds.

**41T366**—Golf Coat (Gray). **$27.00**
**41T367**—Golf Knickerbockers (Gray). **10.00**
**41T368**—Long, Cuff Bottom Pants (Gray). **10.00**
**41T370**—Golf Coat (Brown). **27.00**
**41T371**—Golf Knickerbockers (Brown). **10.00**
**41T372**—Long, Cuff Bottom Pants (Brown). **10.00**

Material, all wool gray or brown mixed tweed. Coat, skeleton lined with guaranteed brilliantine, has four patch pockets and belt. Knickerbockers buttoned at knees. Long pants have cuff bottoms. Both have belt loops and the usual number of pockets. Average shipping weight of coat, 3 pounds; knickerbockers, 1⅞ pounds; long pants, 2⅛ pounds.

**Golf Stockings in All Wool Heather Mixtures.**

**41T381**—Brown predominating. **$3.60**
**41T384**—Green predominating. **3.60**
**41T395**—Oxford Gray predominating. **3.60**

Sizes, 9½ to 11. Average shipping weight, 12 ounces.

**41T374**—Golf Coat (Brown Mixed). **$31.50**
**41T375**—Golf Knickerbockers (Brown Mixed). **10.35**
**41T376**—Long, Cuff Bottom Pants (Brown Mixed). **10.35**
**41T378**—Golf Coat (Olive Green Mixed). **31.50**
**41T379**—Golf Knickerbockers (Olive Green Mixed). **10.35**
**41T380**—Long, Cuff Bottom Pants (Olive Green Mixed). **10.35**

Material, all wool brown or olive green mixed tweed. Coat, skeleton lined with guaranteed brilliantine, has four patch pockets and belt. Knickerbockers buttoned at knees. Long pants have cuff bottoms. Both have belt loops and the usual number of pockets. Average shipping weight of coat, 2¾ pounds; knickerbockers, 1⅞ pounds; long pants, 2 pounds.

**41T356**—Corduroy Coat. **$15.75**
**41T357**—Riding Breeches. **9.25**
**41T358**—Long Pants. **7.25**

Material, good quality heavy weight olive drab narrow wale thickset corduroy. Norfolk style coat lined with moleskin cloth. Riding breeches have reinforced seat and lacings at calves. Cut large and roomy. Long pants have cuff bottoms, usual number of pockets and welt seams. Average shipping weight of coat, 4⅛ pounds; riding breeches, 2⅝ pounds; long pants, 2⅝ pounds.

**SIZES.**

**Coats come in sizes 34 to 46 inches breast measure. Riding breeches, hiking breeches and golf knickerbockers, 30 to 42 inches waist measure. Pants, 30 to 42 inches waist measure and 30 to 36 inches inseam. For simple measuring instructions see order blanks in back of catalog.**

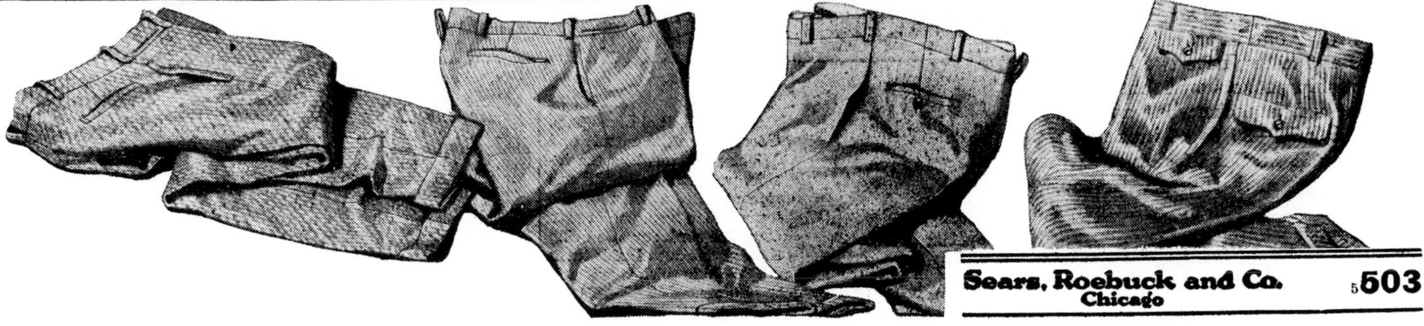

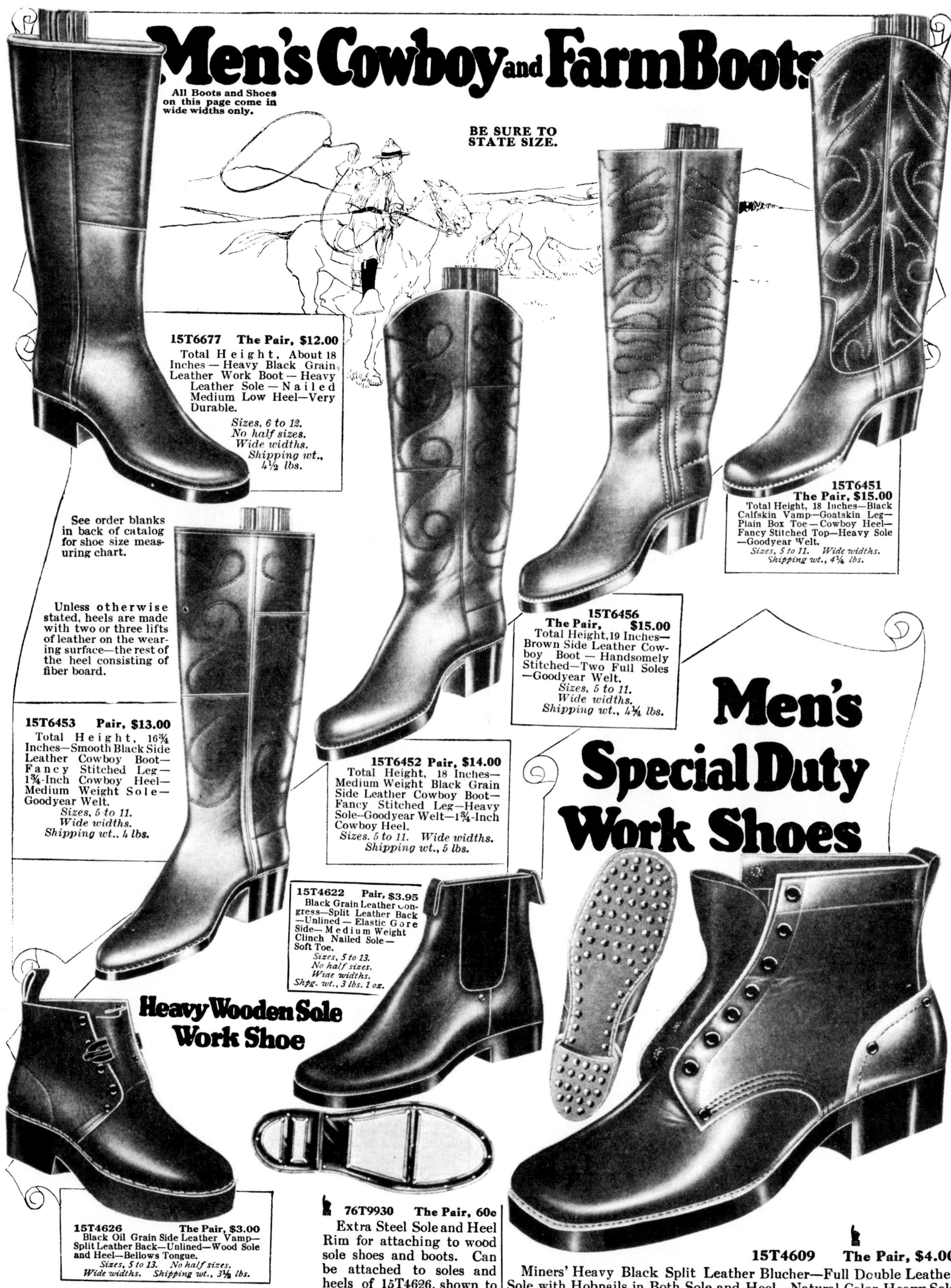
Men's Cowboy and Farm Boots
All Boots and Shoes on this page come in wide widths only.
BE SURE TO STATE SIZE.
15T6677 The Pair, $12.00
Total Height, About 18 Inches — Heavy Black Grain Leather Work Boot — Heavy Leather Sole — Nailed Medium Low Heel—Very Durable.
Sizes, 6 to 12. No half sizes. Wide widths. Shipping wt., 4½ lbs.
15T6451 The Pair, $15.00
Total Height, 18 Inches—Black Calfskin Vamp—Goatskin Leg—Plain Box Toe—Cowboy Heel—Fancy Stitched Top—Heavy Sole—Goodyear Welt.
Sizes, 5 to 11. Wide widths. Shipping wt., 4¼ lbs.
See order blanks in back of catalog for shoe size measuring chart.
Unless otherwise stated, heels are made with two or three lifts of leather on the wearing surface—the rest of the heel consisting of fiber board.
15T6456 The Pair, $15.00
Total Height, 19 Inches—Brown Side Leather Cowboy Boot — Handsomely Stitched—Two Full Soles—Goodyear Welt.
Sizes, 5 to 11. Wide widths. Shipping wt., 4¼ lbs.
15T6453 Pair, $13.00
Total Height, 16¾ Inches—Smooth Black Side Leather Cowboy Boot—Fancy Stitched Leg—1¾-Inch Cowboy Heel—Medium Weight Sole—Goodyear Welt.
Sizes, 5 to 11. Wide widths. Shipping wt., 4 lbs.
15T6452 Pair, $14.00
Total Height, 18 Inches—Medium Weight Black Grain Side Leather Cowboy Boot—Fancy Stitched Leg—Heavy Sole—Goodyear Welt—1¾-Inch Cowboy Heel.
Sizes, 5 to 11. Wide widths. Shipping wt., 5 lbs.
Men's Special Duty Work Shoes
15T4622 Pair, $3.95
Black Grain Leather Congress—Split Leather Back—Unlined — Elastic Gore Side— Medium Weight Clinch Nailed Sole—Soft Toe.
Sizes, 5 to 13. No half sizes. Wide widths. Shpg. wt., 3 lbs. 1 oz.
Heavy Wooden Sole Work Shoe
15T4626 The Pair, $3.00
Black Oil Grain Side Leather Vamp—Split Leather Back—Unlined—Wood Sole and Heel—Bellows Tongue.
Sizes, 5 to 13. No half sizes. Wide widths. Shipping wt., 3½ lbs.
76T9930 The Pair, 60c

Extra Steel Sole and Heel Rim for attaching to wood sole shoes and boots. Can be attached to soles and heels of 15T4626, shown to the left.

*Sizes, 5 to 13. No half sizes.*
*Shipping wt., 14 oz.*

**15T4609 The Pair, $4.00**

Miners' Heavy Black Split Leather Blucher—Full Double Leather Sole with Hobnails in Both Sole and Heel—Natural Color Heavy Sole Leather Outside Counter—Waxed Thread Sewed and Riveted.

*Sizes, 5 to 12. No half sizes. Wide widths.*
*Shipping wt., 4 lbs.*

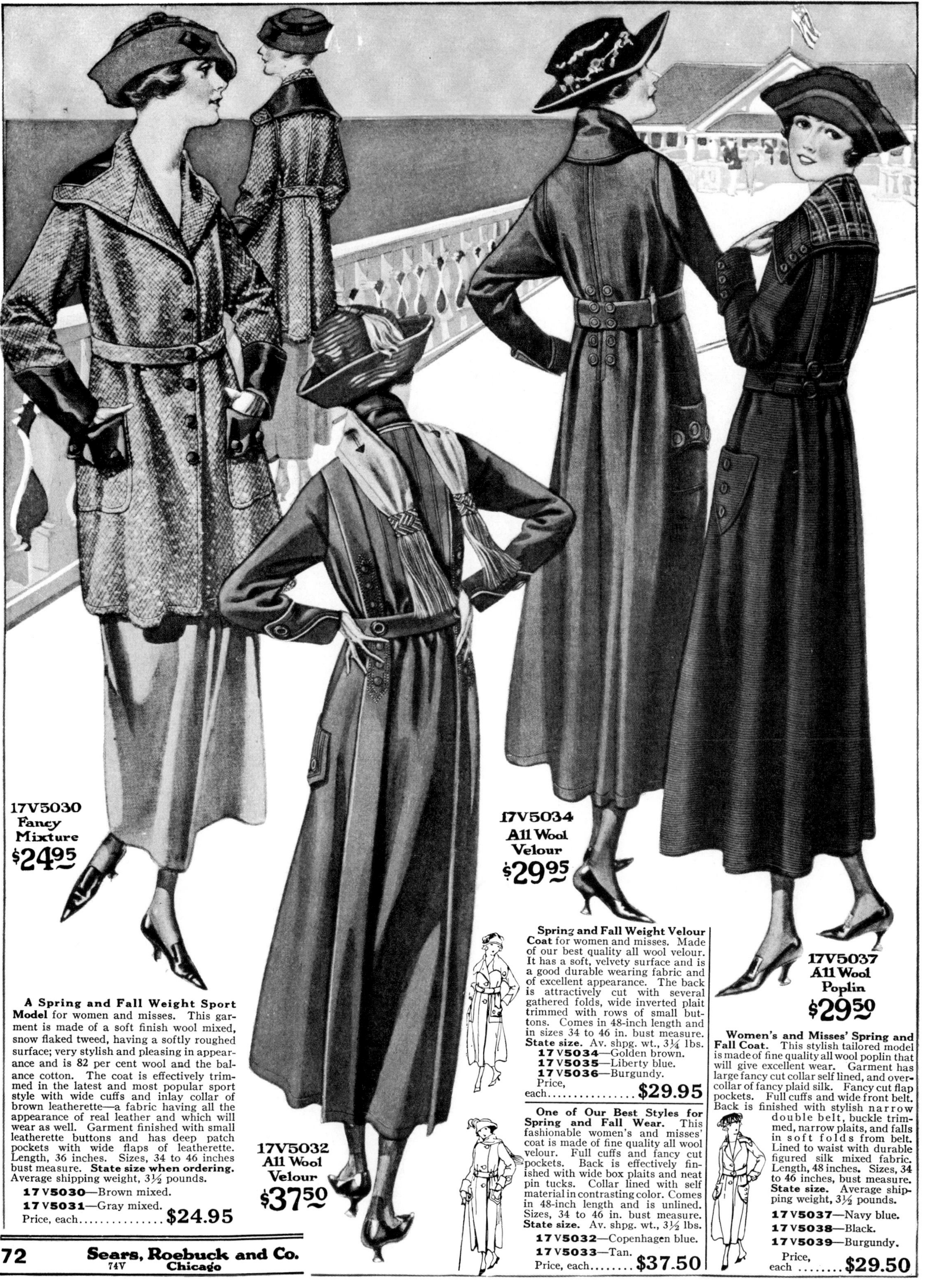


**A Spring and Fall Weight Sport Model** for women and misses. This garment is made of a soft finish wool mixed, snow flaked tweed, having a softly roughed surface; very stylish and pleasing in appearance and is 82 per cent wool and the balance cotton. The coat is effectively trimmed in the latest and most popular sport style with wide cuffs and inlay collar of brown leatherette—a fabric having all the appearance of real leather and which will wear as well. Garment finished with small leatherette buttons and has deep patch pockets with wide flaps of leatherette. Length, 36 inches. Sizes, 34 to 46 inches bust measure. **State size when ordering.** Average shipping weight, 3½ pounds.

**17 V5030**—Brown mixed.
**17 V5031**—Gray mixed.
Price, each............... **$24.95**

**Spring and Fall Weight Velour Coat** for women and misses. Made of our best quality all wool velour. It has a soft, velvety surface and is a good durable wearing fabric and of excellent appearance. The back is attractively cut with several gathered folds, wide inverted plait trimmed with rows of small buttons. Comes in 48-inch length and in sizes 34 to 46 in. bust measure. **State size.** Av. shpg. wt., 3¼ lbs.

**17 V5034**—Golden brown.
**17 V5035**—Liberty blue.
**17 V5036**—Burgundy.
Price, each................ **$29.95**

**One of Our Best Styles for Spring and Fall Wear.** This fashionable women's and misses' coat is made of fine quality all wool velour. Full cuffs and fancy cut pockets. Back is effectively finished with wide box plaits and neat pin tucks. Collar lined with self material in contrasting color. Comes in 48-inch length and is unlined. Sizes, 34 to 46 in. bust measure. **State size.** Av. shpg. wt., 3½ lbs.

**17 V5032**—Copenhagen blue.
**17 V5033**—Tan.
Price, each........ **$37.50**

**Women's and Misses' Spring and Fall Coat.** This stylish tailored model is made of fine quality all wool poplin that will give excellent wear. Garment has large fancy cut collar self lined, and overcollar of fancy plaid silk. Fancy cut flap pockets. Full cuffs and wide front belt. Back is finished with stylish narrow double belt, buckle trimmed, narrow plaits, and falls in soft folds from belt. Lined to waist with durable figured silk mixed fabric. Length, 48 inches. Sizes, 34 to 46 inches, bust measure. **State size.** Average shipping weight, 3½ pounds.

**17 V5037**—Navy blue.
**17 V5038**—Black.
**17 V5039**—Burgundy.
Price, each ........ **$29.50**

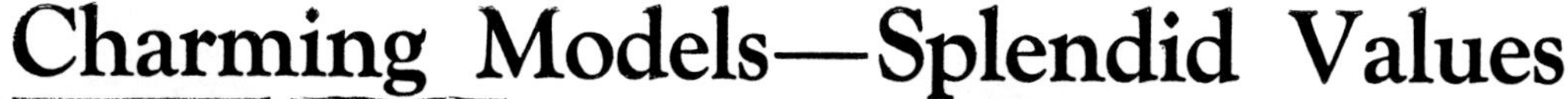

# Charming Models—Splendid Values

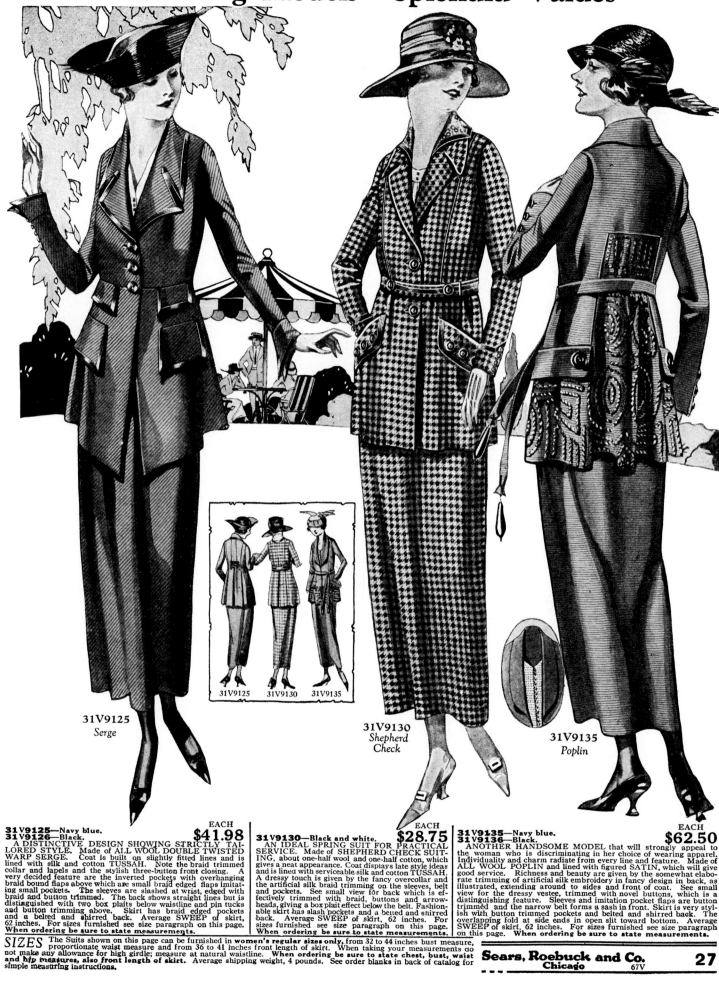

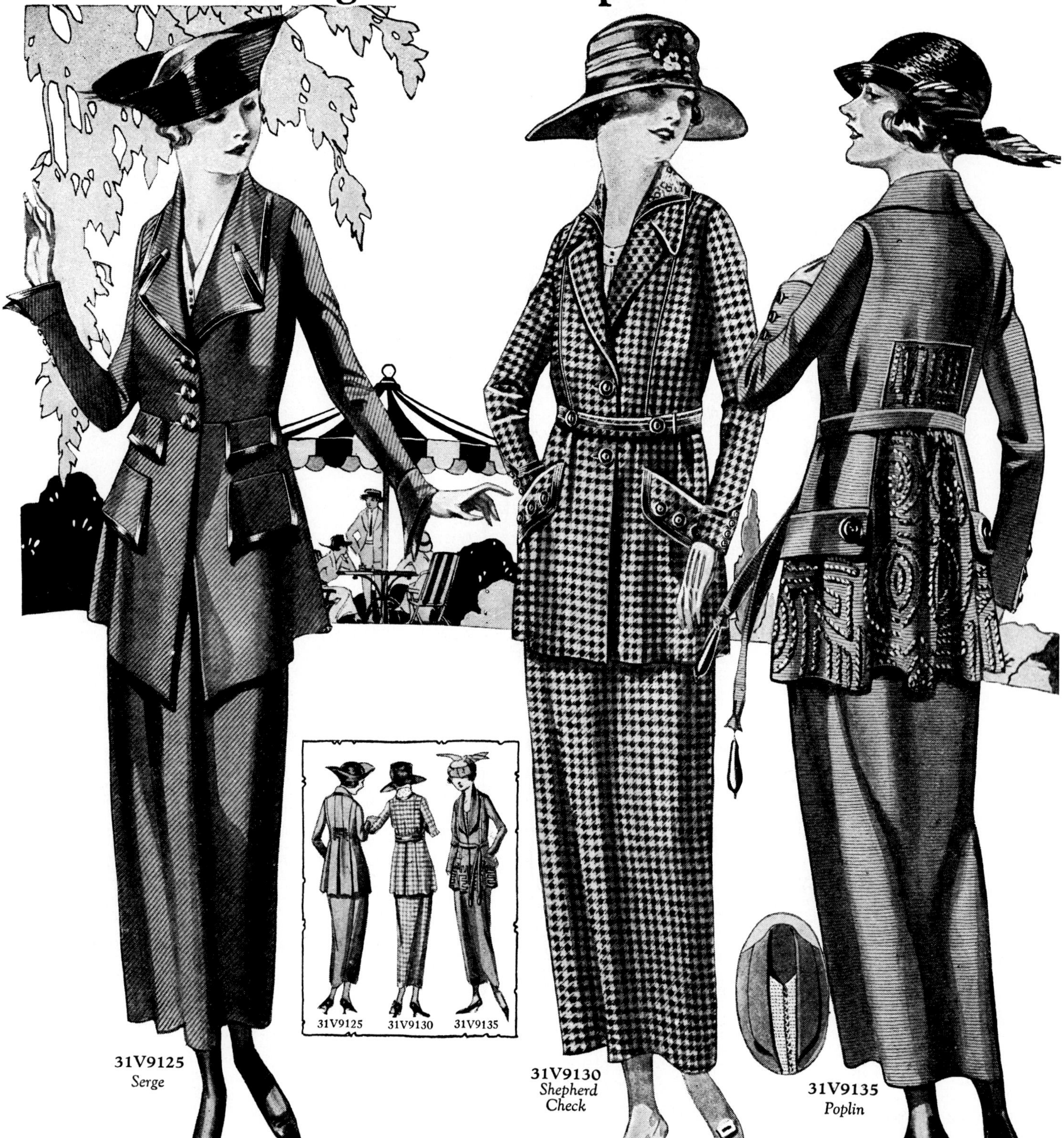

31V9125 31V9130 31V9135

31V9125
*Serge*

31V9130
*Shepherd Check*

31V9135
*Poplin*

**31V9125—Navy blue.**
**31V9126—Black.**

EACH **$41.98**

A DISTINCTIVE DESIGN SHOWING STRICTLY TAILORED STYLE. Made of ALL WOOL DOUBLE TWISTED WARP SERGE. Coat is built on slightly fitted lines and is lined with silk and cotton TUSSAH. Note the braid trimmed collar and lapels and the stylish three-button front closing. A very decided feature are the inverted pockets with overhanging braid bound flaps above which are small braid edged flaps imitating small pockets. The sleeves are slashed at wrist, edged with braid and button trimmed. The back shows straight lines but is distinguished with two box plaits below waistline and pin tucks and button trimming above. Skirt has braid edged pockets and a belted and shirred back. Average SWEEP of skirt, 62 inches. For sizes furnished see size paragraph on this page. **When ordering be sure to state measurements.**

**31V9130—Black and white.**

EACH **$28.75**

AN IDEAL SPRING SUIT FOR PRACTICAL SERVICE. Made of SHEPHERD CHECK SUITING, about one-half wool and one-half cotton, which gives a neat appearance. Coat displays late style ideas and is lined with serviceable silk and cotton TUSSAH. A dressy touch is given by the fancy overcollar and the artificial silk braid trimming on the sleeves, belt and pockets. See small view for back which is effectively trimmed with braid, buttons and arrowheads, giving a box plait effect below the belt. Fashionable skirt has slash pockets and a belted and shirred back. Average SWEEP of skirt, 62 inches. For sizes furnished see size paragraph on this page. **When ordering be sure to state measurements.**

**31V9135—Navy blue.**
**31V9136—Black.**

EACH **$62.50**

ANOTHER HANDSOME MODEL that will strongly appeal to the woman who is discriminating in her choice of wearing apparel. Individuality and charm radiate from every line and feature. Made of ALL WOOL POPLIN and lined with figured SATIN, which will give good service. Richness and beauty are given by the somewhat elaborate trimming of artificial silk embroidery in fancy design in back, as illustrated, extending around to sides and front of coat. See small view for the dressy vestee, trimmed with novel buttons, which is a distinguishing feature. Sleeves and imitation pocket flaps are button trimmed and the narrow belt forms a sash in front. Skirt is very stylish with button trimmed pockets and belted and shirred back. The overlapping fold at side ends in open slit toward bottom. Average SWEEP of skirt, 62 inches. For sizes furnished see size paragraph on this page. **When ordering be sure to state measurements.**

*SIZES* The Suits shown on this page can be furnished in **women's regular sizes only,** from 32 to 44 inches bust measure, proportionate waist measure and from 36 to 41 inches front length of skirt. When taking your measurements do not make any allowance for high girdle; measure at natural waistline. **When ordering be sure to state chest, bust, waist and hip measures, also front length of skirt.** Average shipping weight, 4 pounds. See order blanks in back of catalog for simple measuring instructions.

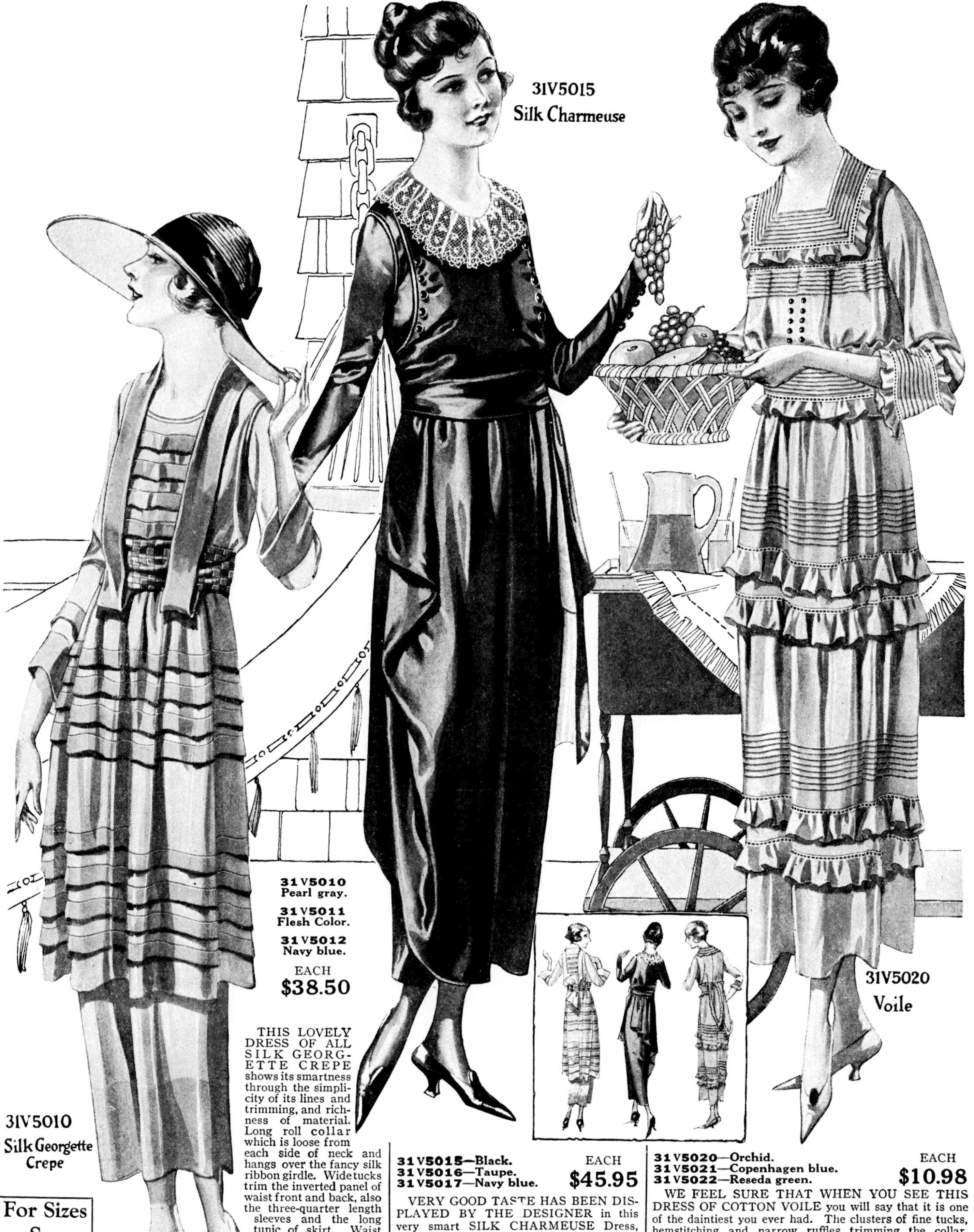


**31 V5010**
**Pearl gray.**
**31 V5011**
**Flesh Color.**
**31 V5012**
**Navy blue.**

EACH
**$38.50**

THIS LOVELY DRESS OF ALL SILK GEORGETTE CREPE shows its smartness through the simplicity of its lines and trimming, and richness of material. Long roll collar which is loose from each side of neck and hangs over the fancy silk ribbon girdle. Wide tucks trim the inverted panel of waist front and back, also the three-quarter length sleeves and the long tunic of skirt. Waist lining and foundation skirt are of Jap silk. Fastens at left side and has skirt SWEEP of about 52 in. Women's sizes, 32 to 44 inches bust measure. **Give measurements.** Average shipping weight, 1¾ pounds.

For Sizes See Page 2

**31 V5015—Black.**
**31 V5016—Taupe.**
**31 V5017—Navy blue.**

EACH
**$45.95**

VERY GOOD TASTE HAS BEEN DISPLAYED BY THE DESIGNER in this very smart SILK CHARMEUSE Dress, made with the one sided drapery on the skirt forming graduated tunic in back. The self material button trimmed front section of waist is made in basque effect, which continues from sides to back, forming the girdle which can be looped over at side, showing the dainty contrasting color Georgette crepe lining. Close fitting sleeves are also trimmed with self covered buttons, and neck is finished with lace frill. Jap silk waist lining. Fastens at left side and has skirt SWEEP of about 50 inches. Women's sizes, 32 to 44 inches bust measure. **Give measurements..** Av. shpg. wt., 1¾ lbs.

**31 V5020—Orchid.**
**31 V5021—Copenhagen blue.**
**31 V5022—Reseda green.**

EACH
**$10.98**

WE FEEL SURE THAT WHEN YOU SEE THIS DRESS OF COTTON VOILE you will say that it is one of the daintiest you ever had. The clusters of fine tucks, hemstitching and narrow ruffles trimming the collar, sleeves, wide girdle and skirt are particular features. The square collar is new and stylish. Front of waist is set off with pretty pearl buttons, harmonizing in shade with the color of the dress. Girdle forms sash at back, and dress fastens at back. Has skirt SWEEP of about 60 inches. Women's sizes, 32 to 44 inches bust measure. **Give measurements.** Average shipping weight, 1¾ pounds.

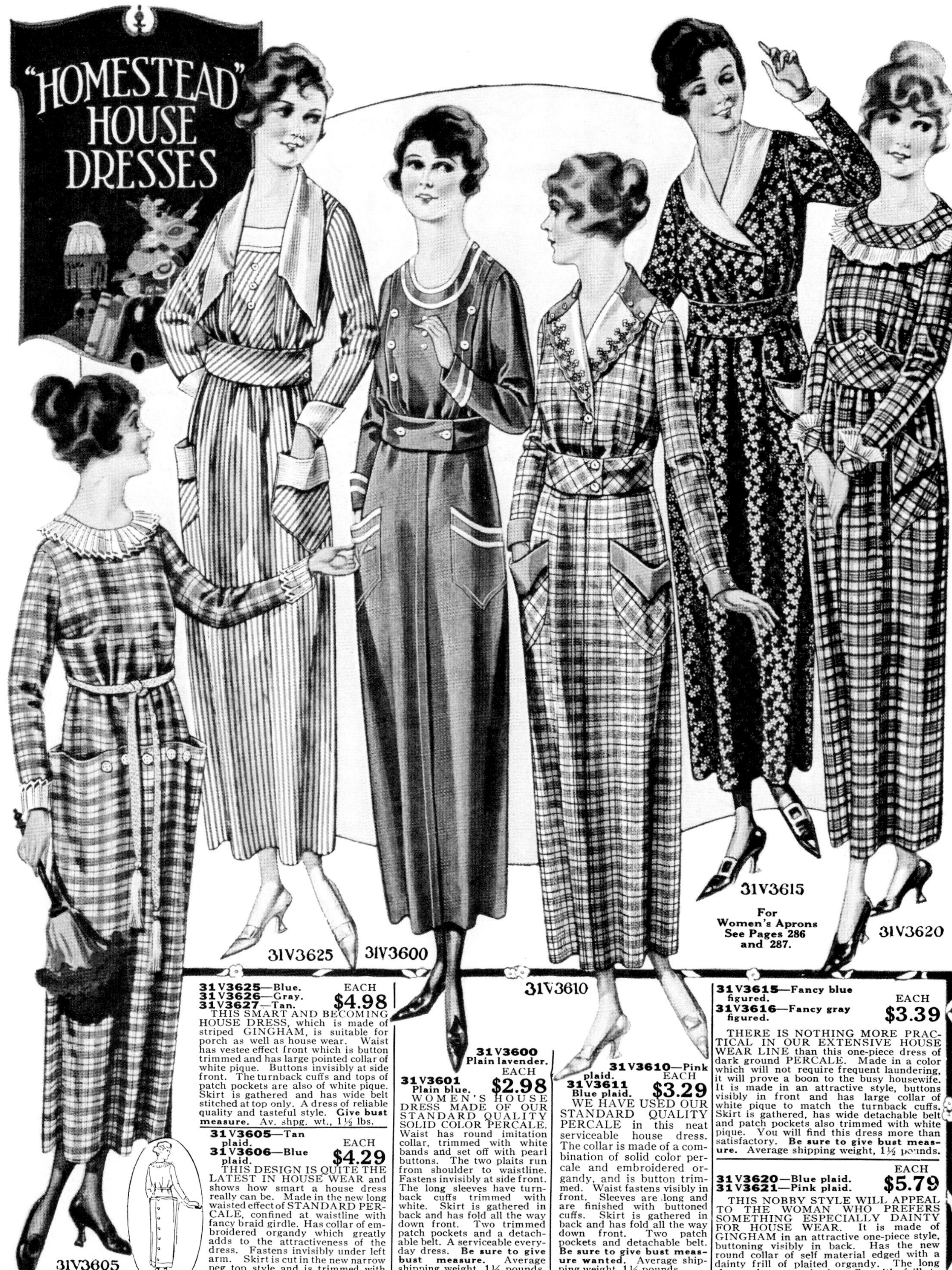


For Women's Aprons See Pages 286 and 287.

**31V3625**—Blue. **31V3626**—Gray. **31V3627**—Tan. EACH **$4.98**

THIS SMART AND BECOMING HOUSE DRESS, which is made of striped GINGHAM, is suitable for porch as well as house wear. Waist has vestee effect front which is button trimmed and has large pointed collar of white pique. Buttons invisibly at side front. The turnback cuffs and tops of patch pockets are also of white pique. Skirt is gathered and has wide belt stitched at top only. A dress of reliable quality and tasteful style. **Give bust measure.** Av. shpg. wt., 1½ lbs.

**31V3605**—Tan plaid. **31V3606**—Blue plaid. EACH **$4.29**

THIS DESIGN IS QUITE THE LATEST IN HOUSE WEAR and shows how smart a house dress really can be. Made in the new long waisted effect of STANDARD PERCALE, confined at waistline with fancy braid girdle. Has collar of embroidered organdy which greatly adds to the attractiveness of the dress. Fastens invisibly under left arm. Skirt is cut in the new narrow peg top style and is trimmed with pearl buttons. **Be sure to give bust measure wanted.** Average shipping weight, 1½ lbs.

**31V3600** Plain lavender. **31V3601** Plain blue. EACH **$2.98**

WOMEN'S HOUSE DRESS MADE OF OUR STANDARD QUALITY SOLID COLOR PERCALE. Waist has round imitation collar, trimmed with white bands and set off with pearl buttons. The two plaits run from shoulder to waistline. Fastens invisibly at side front. The long sleeves have turnback cuffs trimmed with white. Skirt is gathered in back and has fold all the way down front. Two trimmed patch pockets and a detachable belt. A serviceable everyday dress. **Be sure to give bust measure.** Average shipping weight, 1½ pounds.

**31V3610**—Pink plaid. **31V3611** Blue plaid. EACH **$3.29**

WE HAVE USED OUR STANDARD QUALITY PERCALE in this neat serviceable house dress. The collar is made of a combination of solid color percale and embroidered organdy, and is button trimmed. Waist fastens visibly in front. Sleeves are long and are finished with buttoned cuffs. Skirt is gathered in back and has fold all the way down front. Two patch pockets and detachable belt. **Be sure to give bust measure wanted.** Average shipping weight, 1¼ pounds.

**31V3615**—Fancy blue figured. **31V3616**—Fancy gray figured. EACH **$3.39**

THERE IS NOTHING MORE PRACTICAL IN OUR EXTENSIVE HOUSE WEAR LINE than this one-piece dress of dark ground PERCALE. Made in a color which will not require frequent laundering, it will prove a boon to the busy housewife. It is made in an attractive style, buttons visibly in front and has large collar of white pique to match the turnback cuffs. Skirt is gathered, has wide detachable belt and patch pockets also trimmed with white pique. You will find this dress more than satisfactory. **Be sure to give bust measure.** Average shipping weight, 1½ pounds.

**31V3620**—Blue plaid. **31V3621**—Pink plaid. EACH **$5.79**

THIS NOBBY STYLE WILL APPEAL TO THE WOMAN WHO PREFERS SOMETHING ESPECIALLY DAINTY FOR HOUSE WEAR. It is made of GINGHAM in an attractive one-piece style, buttoning visibly in back. Has the new round collar of self material edged with a dainty frill of plaited organdy. The long sleeves have turnback cuffs with frill to match collar. The pointed belt is button trimmed. Skirt is gathered all the way around and has two patch pockets. **Be sure to give bust measure wanted.** Average shipping weight, 1½ pounds.

***SIZES*** House dresses on this page are furnished in sizes 34 to 46 inches bust measure, with full length skirt. Sweeps run from 72 to 82 inches according to size, with the exception of 31V3605 which has the narrow sweep necessary in a garment of this style.

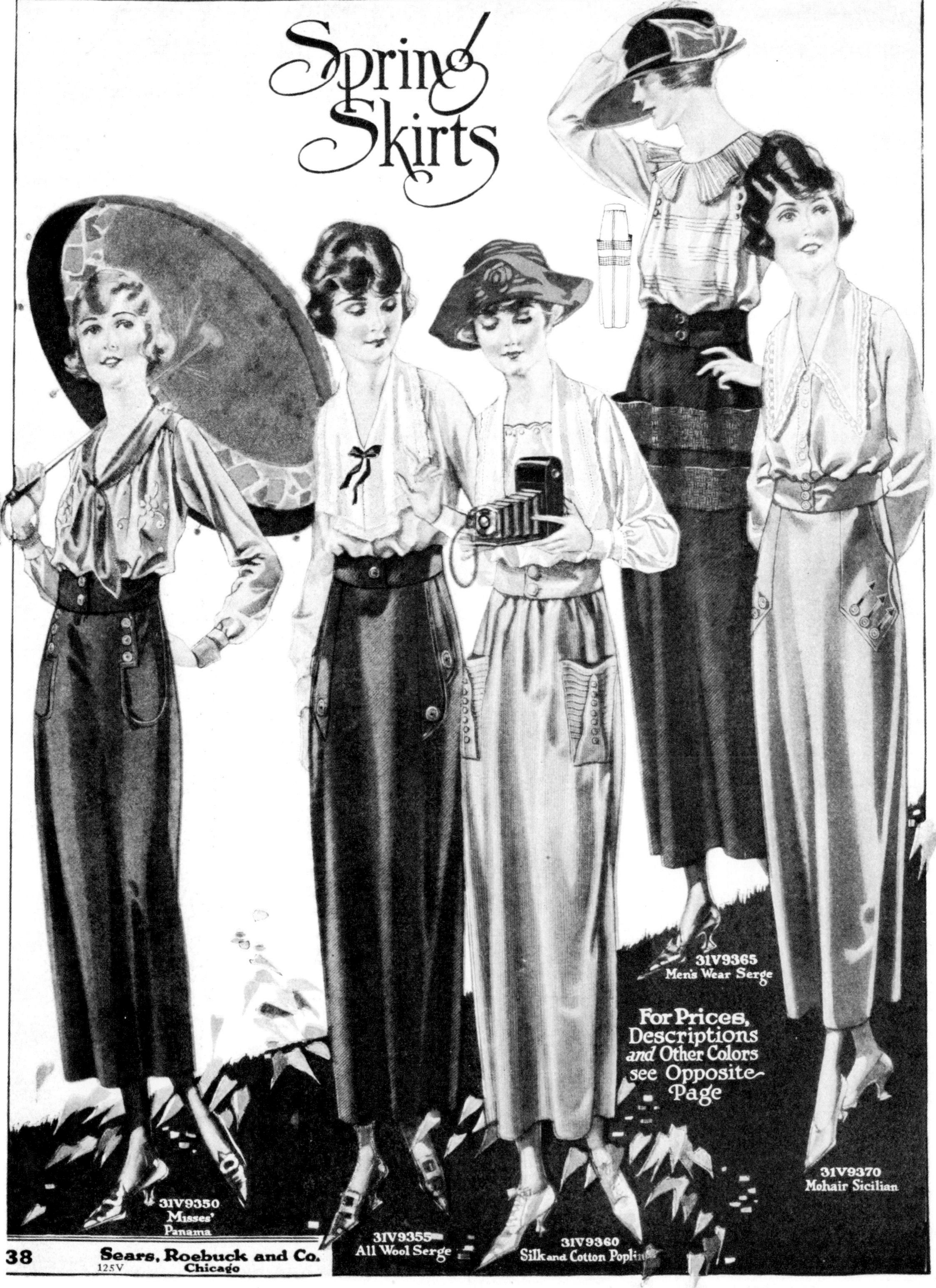
Spring Skirts
31V9350
Misses' Panama
31V9355
All Wool Serge
31V9360
Silk and Cotton Poplin
31V9365
Men's Wear Serge
31V9370
Mohair Sicilian
For Prices, Descriptions and Other Colors see Opposite Page
38
Sears, Roebuck and Co.
125V
Chicago

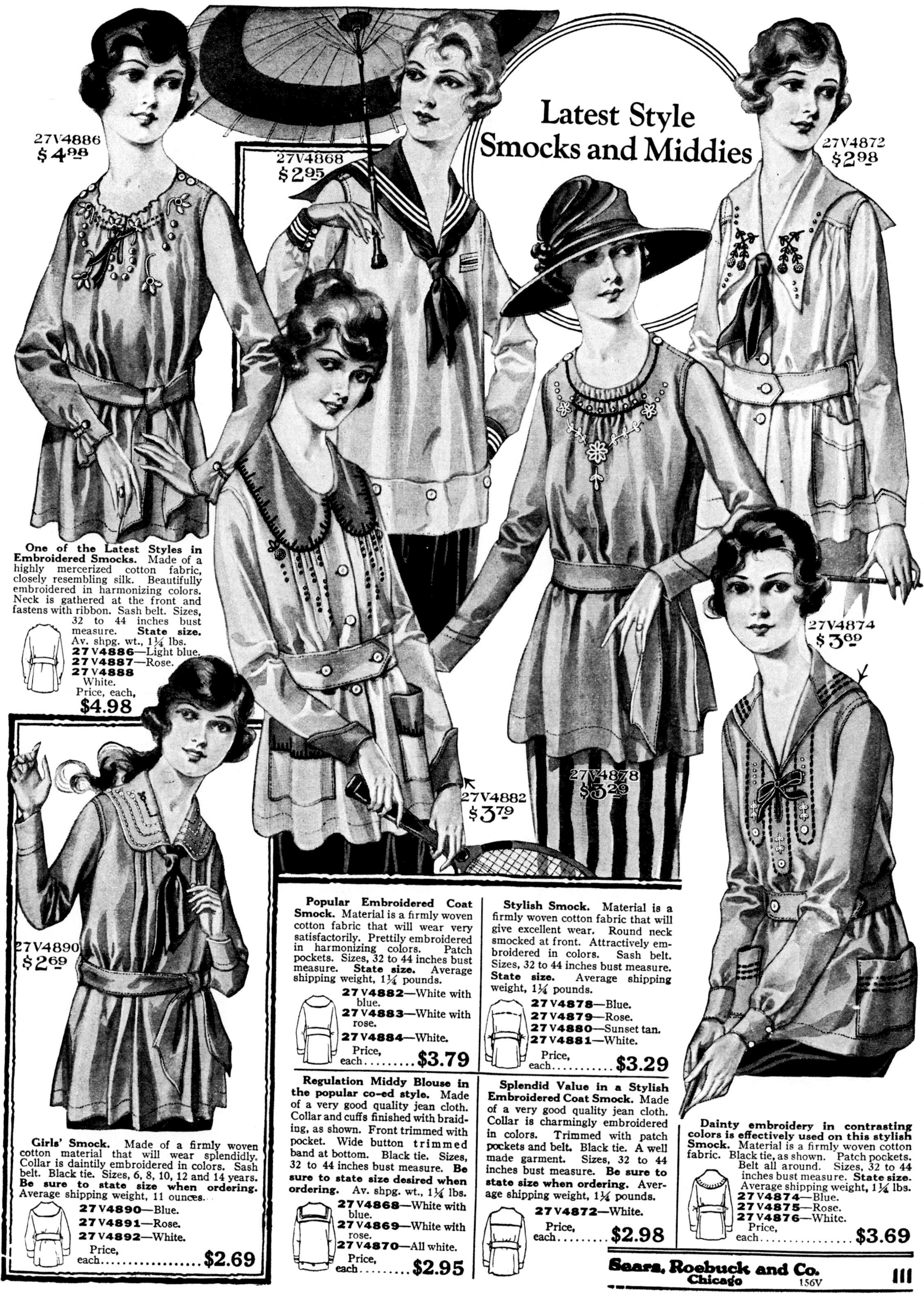
Latest Style
Smocks and Middies
27V4886
$4.98
27V4868
$2.95
27V4872
$2.98
27V4874
$3.69
27V4878
$3.29
27V4882
$3.79
27V4890
$2.69
One of the Latest Styles in Embroidered Smocks. Made of a highly mercerized cotton fabric, closely resembling silk. Beautifully embroidered in harmonizing colors. Neck is gathered at the front and fastens with ribbon. Sash belt. Sizes, 32 to 44 inches bust measure. State size. Av. shpg. wt., 1¼ lbs.
27V4886—Light blue.
27V4887—Rose.
27V4888
White.
Price, each, $4.98
Girls' Smock. Made of a firmly woven cotton material that will wear splendidly. Collar is daintily embroidered in colors. Sash belt. Black tie. Sizes, 6, 8, 10, 12 and 14 years. Be sure to state size when ordering. Average shipping weight, 11 ounces.
27V4890—Blue.
27V4891—Rose.
27V4892—White.
Price, each.................. $2.69
Popular Embroidered Coat Smock. Material is a firmly woven cotton fabric that will wear very satisfactorily. Prettily embroidered in harmonizing colors. Patch pockets. Sizes, 32 to 44 inches bust measure. State size. Average shipping weight, 1¼ pounds.
27V4882—White with blue.
27V4883—White with rose.
27V4884—White.
Price, each......... $3.79
Stylish Smock. Material is a firmly woven cotton fabric that will give excellent wear. Round neck smocked at front. Attractively embroidered in colors. Sash belt. Sizes, 32 to 44 inches bust measure. State size. Average shipping weight, 1¼ pounds.
27V4878—Blue.
27V4879—Rose.
27V4880—Sunset tan.
27V4881—White.
Price, each........... $3.29
Regulation Middy Blouse in the popular co-ed style. Made of a very good quality jean cloth. Collar and cuffs finished with braiding, as shown. Front trimmed with pocket. Wide button trimmed band at bottom. Black tie. Sizes, 32 to 44 inches bust measure. Be sure to state size desired when ordering. Av. shpg. wt., 1¼ lbs.
27V4868—White with blue.
27V4869—White with rose.
27V4870—All white.
Price, each......... $2.95
Splendid Value in a Stylish Embroidered Coat Smock. Made of a very good quality jean cloth. Collar is charmingly embroidered in colors. Trimmed with patch pockets and belt. Black tie. A well made garment. Sizes, 32 to 44 inches bust measure. Be sure to state size when ordering. Average shipping weight, 1¼ pounds.
27V4872—White.
Price, each......... $2.98
Dainty embroidery in contrasting colors is effectively used on this stylish Smock. Material is a firmly woven cotton fabric. Black tie, as shown. Patch pockets. Belt all around. Sizes, 32 to 44 inches bust measure. State size. Average shipping weight, 1¼ lbs.
27V4874—Blue.
27V4875—Rose.
27V4876—White.
Price, each................ $3.69
Sears, Roebuck and Co.
Chicago
156V
111

# STYLISH AND SERVICEABLE COLORED DRESSES

To fit sizes 2 to 6 years. For sizes 7 to 14 years see pages 54 to 59.

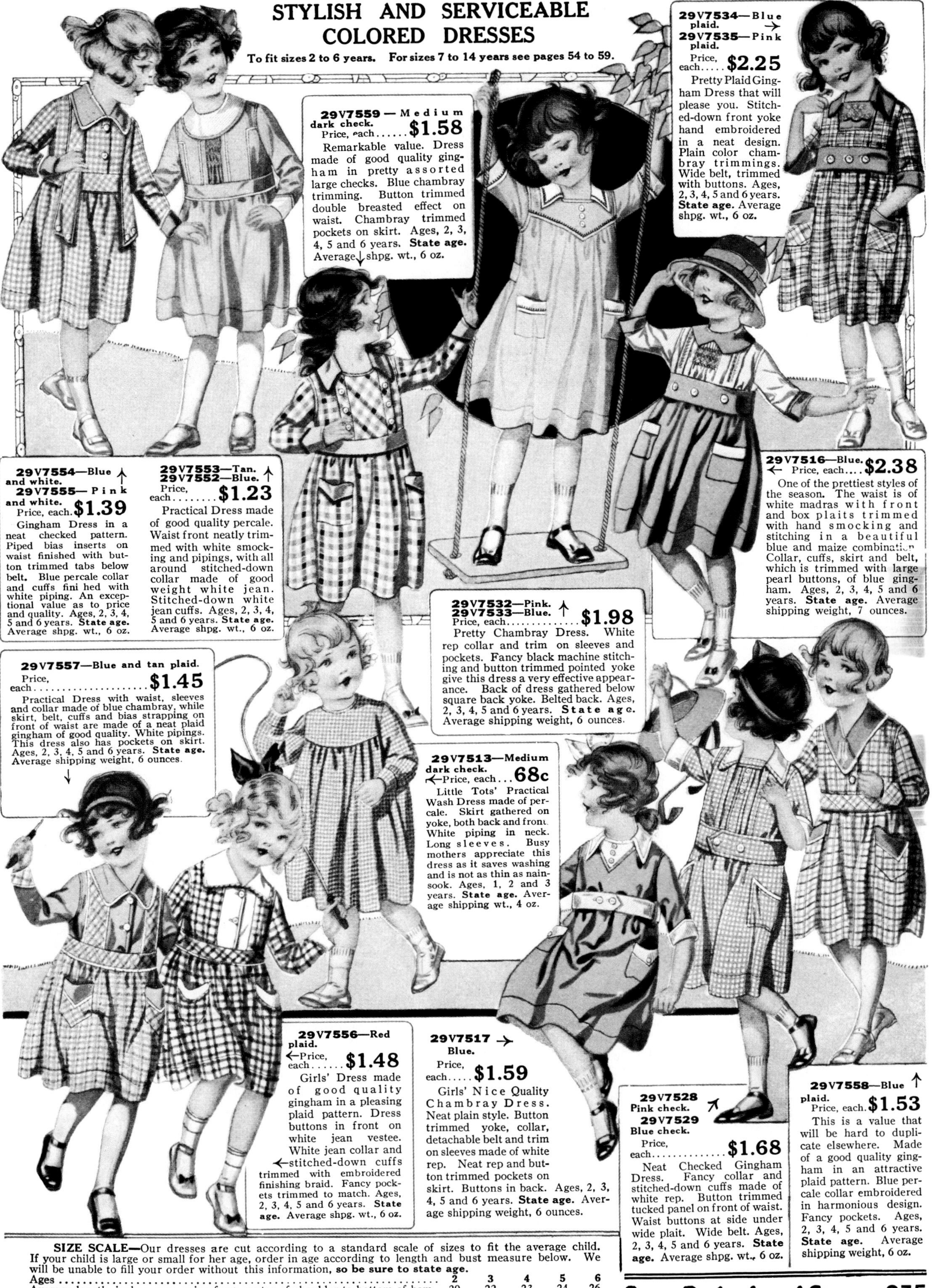

**29V7559—Medium dark check.** Price, each......**$1.58**
Remarkable value. Dress made of good quality gingham in pretty assorted large checks. Blue chambray trimming. Button trimmed double breasted effect on waist. Chambray trimmed pockets on skirt. Ages, 2, 3, 4, 5 and 6 years. **State age.** Average shpg. wt., 6 oz.

**29V7534—Blue plaid.**
**29V7535—Pink plaid.**
Price, each.....**$2.25**
Pretty Plaid Gingham Dress that will please you. Stitched-down front yoke hand embroidered in a neat design. Plain color chambray trimmings. Wide belt, trimmed with buttons. Ages, 2, 3, 4, 5 and 6 years. **State age.** Average shpg. wt., 6 oz.

**29V7554—Blue and white.**
**29V7555—Pink and white.**
Price, each.**$1.39**
Gingham Dress in a neat checked pattern. Piped bias inserts on waist finished with button trimmed tabs below belt. Blue percale collar and cuffs fini hed with white piping. An exceptional value as to price and quality. Ages, 2, 3, 4, 5 and 6 years. **State age.** Average shpg. wt., 6 oz.

**29V7553—Tan.**
**29V7552—Blue.**
Price, each........**$1.23**
Practical Dress made of good quality percale. Waist front neatly trimmed with white smocking and pipings, with all around stitched-down collar made of good weight white jean. Stitched-down white jean cuffs. Ages, 2, 3, 4, 5 and 6 years. **State age.** Average shpg. wt., 6 oz.

**29V7516—Blue.** Price, each....**$2.38**
One of the prettiest styles of the season. The waist is of white madras with front and box plaits trimmed with hand smocking and stitching in a beautiful blue and maize combination. Collar, cuffs, skirt and belt, which is trimmed with large pearl buttons, of blue gingham. Ages, 2, 3, 4, 5 and 6 years. **State age.** Average shipping weight, 7 ounces.

**29V7532—Pink.**
**29V7533—Blue.**
Price, each..............**$1.98**
Pretty Chambray Dress. White rep collar and trim on sleeves and pockets. Fancy black machine stitching and button trimmed pointed yoke give this dress a very effective appearance. Back of dress gathered below square back yoke. Belted back. Ages, 2, 3, 4, 5 and 6 years. **State age.** Average shipping weight, 6 ounces.

**29V7557—Blue and tan plaid.**
Price, each.....................**$1.45**
Practical Dress with waist, sleeves and collar made of blue chambray, while skirt, belt, cuffs and bias strapping on front of waist are made of a neat plaid gingham of good quality. White pipings. This dress also has pockets on skirt. Ages, 2, 3, 4, 5 and 6 years. **State age.** Average shipping weight, 6 ounces.

**29V7513—Medium dark check.**
Price, each...**68c**
Little Tots' Practical Wash Dress made of percale. Skirt gathered on yoke, both back and front. White piping in neck. Long sleeves. Busy mothers appreciate this dress as it saves washing and is not as thin as nainsook. Ages, 1, 2 and 3 years. **State age.** Average shipping wt., 4 oz.

**29V7556—Red plaid.**
Price, each......**$1.48**
Girls' Dress made of good quality gingham in a pleasing plaid pattern. Dress buttons in front on white jean vestee. White jean collar and stitched-down cuffs trimmed with embroidered finishing braid. Fancy pockets trimmed to match. Ages, 2, 3, 4, 5 and 6 years. **State age.** Average shpg. wt., 6 oz.

**29V7517 Blue.**
Price, each.....**$1.59**
Girls' Nice Quality Chambray Dress. Neat plain style. Button trimmed yoke, collar, detachable belt and trim on sleeves made of white rep. Neat rep and button trimmed pockets on skirt. Buttons in back. Ages, 2, 3, 4, 5 and 6 years. **State age.** Average shipping weight, 6 ounces.

**29V7528 Pink check.**
**29V7529 Blue check.**
Price, each.............**$1.68**
Neat Checked Gingham Dress. Fancy collar and stitched-down cuffs made of white rep. Button trimmed tucked panel on front of waist. Waist buttons at side under wide plait. Wide belt. Ages, 2, 3, 4, 5 and 6 years. **State age.** Average shpg. wt., 6 oz.

**29V7558—Blue plaid.**
Price, each.**$1.53**
This is a value that will be hard to duplicate elsewhere. Made of a good quality gingham in an attractive plaid pattern. Blue percale collar embroidered in harmonious design. Fancy pockets. Ages, 2, 3, 4, 5 and 6 years. **State age.** Average shipping weight, 6 oz.

**SIZE SCALE**—Our dresses are cut according to a standard scale of sizes to fit the average child. If your child is large or small for her age, order in age according to length and bust measure below. We will be unable to fill your order without this information, **so be sure to state age.**

| Ages | 2 | 3 | 4 | 5 | 6 |
|---|---|---|---|---|---|
| Average length, inches, measuring from center of shoulder to bottom of hem | 20 | 22 | 23 | 24 | 26 |
| Average bust measure, inches | 26 | 26½ | 27 | 27½ | 28 |

# FINE QUALITY

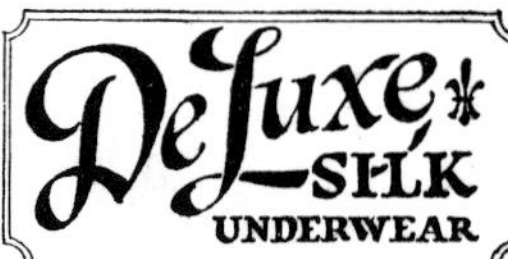


We ask that our customers give special attention to the high grade silk crepe de chine, messalines, satins and laces used on all our silk underwear. These, combined with excellent workmanship, make our silk line one which will offer service and satisfaction. We are showing conservative but latest styles, which will charm the wearer of silk underwear.

**Price, Each $3.48**
**38E9740**—Flesh.
**Women's Fine Quality Silk Crepe de Chine Envelope Chemise.** Front and back trimmed with insertions of good quality lace and silk satin. Top and bottom neatly edged with lace. Attractively finished in front with two rows of shirring. Has silk ribbon draw and rosettes. Sizes, 34 to 44 inches bust measure. **State size.** Shipping weight, ← 12 ounces.

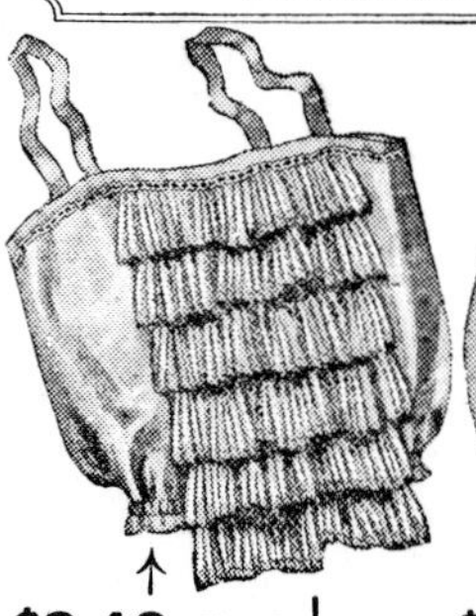

**Price, $2.48 Each**
**38E9776**—White.
**Women's Vestee.** Body made of good quality crepe de chine. Front made with plaited ruffles of high grade net and finished at top with row of hemstitching. Ribbon shoulder straps and draw. Elastic at waist. A very popular garment which may be worn in place of a waist with a suit or sweater. Sizes, 34 to 44 inches bust measure. **State size.** Shipping weight, 10 oz.

**Price, $1.38 Each**
**38E4598**—Flesh.
**Women's Silk Satin Bandeau.** Trimmed in front with neat pattern good quality lace and edged at top with lace to match. Ribbon shoulder straps and draw string. Elastic in back. Closes in back with hooks and eyes. Sizes, 32 to 48 inches bust measure. **State size.** Shipping wt., 10 oz.

**Price, $1.49 Each**
**38E4599**—Flesh.
**Women's Bandeau.** Made of good quality washable satin. Front and sides neatly shirred. Top and front trimmed with lace edging. Has rosette and ribbon shoulder straps. Rustproof boning. Elastic in back. Closes in back with hooks and eyes. A very attractive bandeau. Sizes, 32 to 48 inches bust measure. **State size.** Shipping weight, 10 ounces.

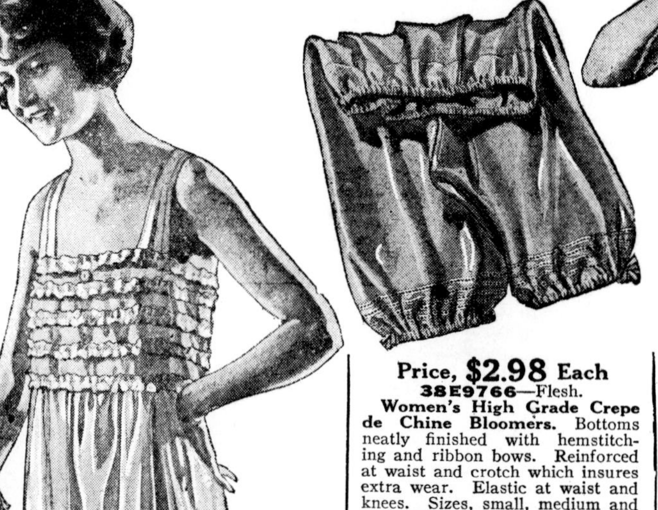

**Price, $2.98 Each**
**38E9766**—Flesh.
**Women's High Grade Crepe de Chine Bloomers.** Bottoms neatly finished with hemstitching and ribbon bows. Reinforced at waist and crotch which insures extra wear. Elastic at waist and knees. Sizes, small, medium and large. **State size.** Shipping weight, 14 ounces.

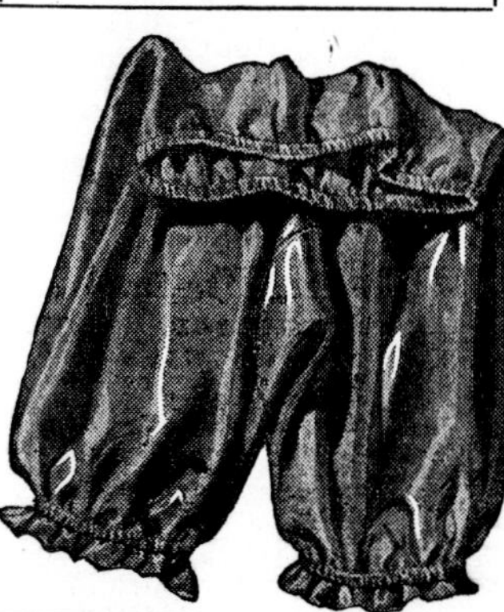

**Price, $3.58 Each** ↑
**38E9713**—Flesh.
**Women's High Grade Washable Satin Bloomers.** Neatly finished at bottoms with elastic and hemstitched ruffles. Have elastic at waist and knees. Reinforced at crotch. Sizes, small, medium and large. **State size.** Shipping weight, 1⅛ pounds.

↖ **Price, $3.98 Each**
**38E9743**—Flesh.
**Women's Fine Quality Silk Crepe de Chine Combination.** Front and back attractively finished with shirred white satin ribbon. Closes at side. Double shoulder straps of same material. Ribbon draw. Front set off with rosettes. Bottoms have elastic at knees and ruffles edged with satin ribbon and trimmed with rosettes. Crotch closes with snap fasteners. Sizes, 34 to 44 inches bust measure. **State size.** Shipping weight, 14 ounces.

**Price, $3.98 Each**
**38E9708**—Brown and shamrock changeable.
**38E9709**—Purple.
**38E9710**—Navy blue.
**38E9711**—Flesh.
**Women's High Grade Silk Messaline Bloomers.** Reinforced at crotch. Elastic at waist and at knees. Finished at bottoms with small ruffles. Length, 27 inches. Shipping weight, 1 pound.

**Price, $4.98 Each**
**38E9755**—Flesh.
**38E9756**—Black.
**38E9757**—Navy blue.
**38E9758**—Copenhagen blue.
**38E9759**—Blue and green changeable.
**38E9760**—Plum.
**Women's High Grade Three-Quarter Length Messaline Silk Bloomers.** Neatly finished at bottom with two rows of elastic. Elastic waistband. Reinforced crotch. Length, 33 inches. Shipping weight, 1 pound.

# SPRING STYLES

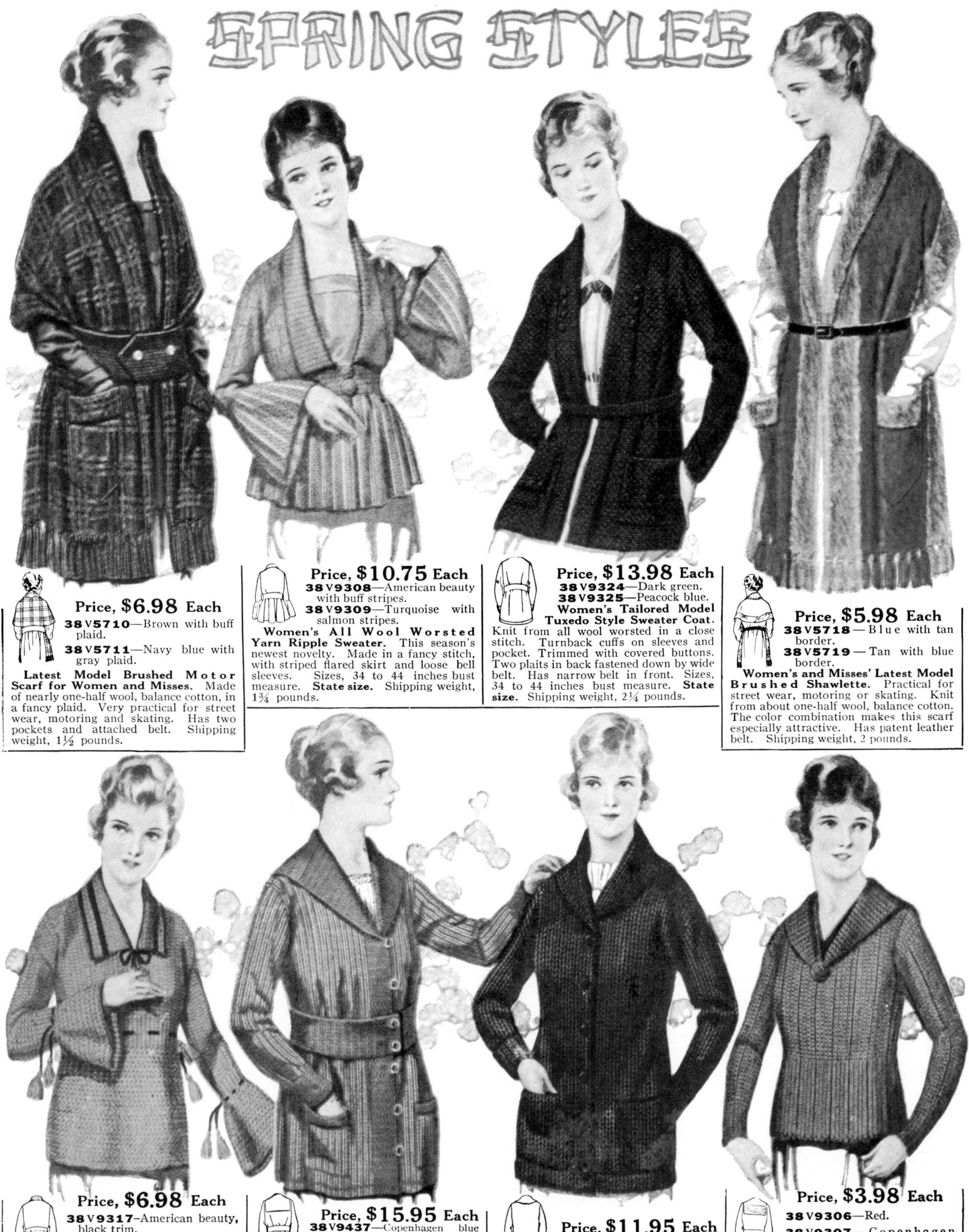

Price, $6.98 Each
**38V5710**—Brown with buff plaid.
**38V5711**—Navy blue with gray plaid.
**Latest Model Brushed Motor Scarf for Women and Misses.** Made of nearly one-half wool, balance cotton, in a fancy plaid. Very practical for street wear, motoring and skating. Has two pockets and attached belt. Shipping weight, 1½ pounds.

Price, $10.75 Each
**38V9308**—American beauty with buff stripes.
**38V9309**—Turquoise with salmon stripes.
**Women's All Wool Worsted Yarn Ripple Sweater.** This season's newest novelty. Made in a fancy stitch, with striped flared skirt and loose bell sleeves. Sizes, 34 to 44 inches bust measure. **State size.** Shipping weight, 1¾ pounds.

Price, $13.98 Each
**38V9324**—Dark green.
**38V9325**—Peacock blue.
**Women's Tailored Model Tuxedo Style Sweater Coat.** Knit from all wool worsted in a close stitch. Turnback cuffs on sleeves and pocket. Trimmed with covered buttons. Two plaits in back fastened down by wide belt. Has narrow belt in front. Sizes, 34 to 44 inches bust measure. **State size.** Shipping weight, 2¼ pounds.

Price, $5.98 Each
**38V5718**—Blue with tan border.
**38V5719**—Tan with blue border.
**Women's and Misses' Latest Model Brushed Shawlette.** Practical for street wear, motoring or skating. Knit from about one-half wool, balance cotton. The color combination makes this scarf especially attractive. Has patent leather belt. Shipping weight, 2 pounds.

Price, $6.98 Each
**38V9317**—American beauty, black trim.
**38V9318**—Peacock blue, tan trim.
**Women's Slipover Sweater.** Knit from about one-half wool, balance cotton. Collar attractively striped and finished with tie and tassel. Loose bell sleeves and waist have ties and tassels. Sizes, 34 to 44 inches bust measure. **State size.** Shipping weight, 1½ pounds.

Price, $15.95 Each
**38V9437**—Copenhagen blue and gold.
**38V9458**—Rose and Copenhagen blue.
**38V9459**—American beauty and buff.
**Women's Artificial Silk Sweater Coat.** Knit in two-toned color effect from artificial silk and reinforced with mercerized cotton. Has large sailor collar, two pockets, turnback cuffs and full belt. A very beautiful sweater. Sizes, 34 to 44 in. bust measure. **State size.** Shipping weight, 1¾ pounds.

Price, $11.95 Each
**38V9344**—Maroon.
**38V9346**—Dark green.
**38V9434**—Navy blue.
**Women's Heavy Weight Shaker Knit Sweater Coat.** Knit from all worsted wool outside and wool inside. Has wide double shawl collar and two pockets. Exceptionally well made and will give great warmth. This sweater is splendid for outdoor sports wear. Sizes, 34 to 44 inches bust measure. **State size.** Shipping weight, 3 pounds.

Price, $3.98 Each
**38V9306**—Red.
**38V9307**—Copenhagen blue.
**Women's Slip-On Sweater.** Knit from about one-third worsted wool, balance cotton, in a neat ribbed stitch. Sailor collar trimmed with stripes in contrasting colors. Has pompon. Sizes, 34 to 44 inches bust measure. **State size.** Shipping weight, 1½ pounds.

# WOMEN'S OXFORDS

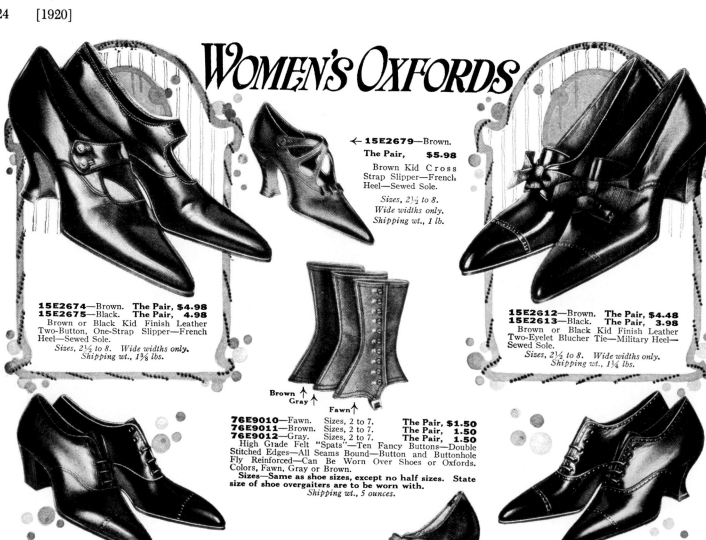

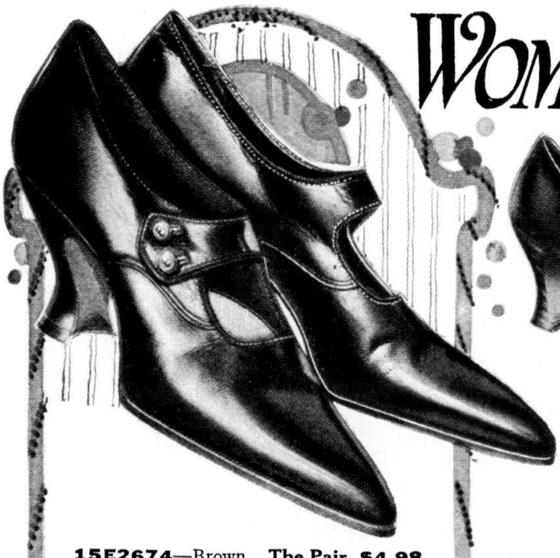

**15E2674**—Brown. **The Pair, $4.98**
**15E2675**—Black. **The Pair, 4.98**
Brown or Black Kid Finish Leather Two-Button, One-Strap Slipper—French Heel—Sewed Sole.
*Sizes, 2½ to 8. Wide widths only.*
*Shipping wt., 1⅜ lbs.*

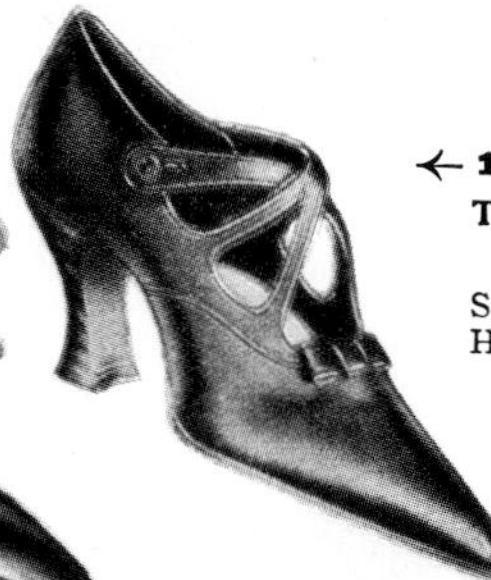

← **15E2679**—Brown.
**The Pair, $5.98**
Brown Kid Cross Strap Slipper—French Heel—Sewed Sole.
*Sizes, 2½ to 8.*
*Wide widths only.*
*Shipping wt., 1 lb.*

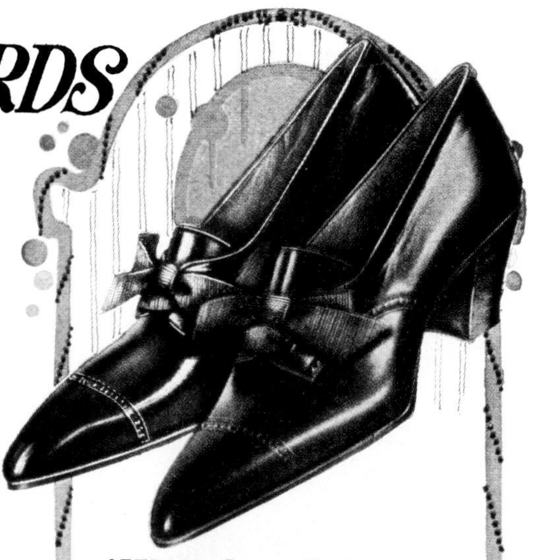

**15E2612**—Brown. **The Pair, $4.48**
**15E2613**—Black. **The Pair, 3.98**
Brown or Black Kid Finish Leather Two-Eyelet Blucher Tie—Military Heel—Sewed Sole.
*Sizes, 2½ to 8. Wide widths only.*
*Shipping wt., 1¼ lbs.*

**Brown** ↑ **Gray** ↑ **Fawn** ↑

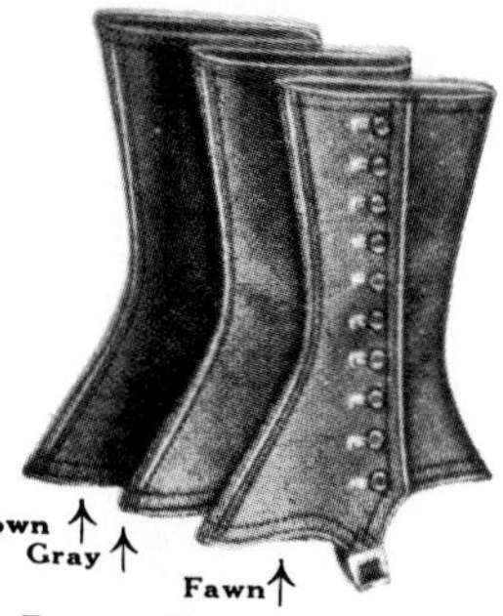

**76E9010**—Fawn. Sizes, 2 to 7. **The Pair, $1.50**
**76E9011**—Brown. Sizes, 2 to 7. **The Pair, 1.50**
**76E9012**—Gray. Sizes, 2 to 7. **The Pair, 1.50**
High Grade Felt "Spats"—Ten Fancy Buttons—Double Stitched Edges—All Seams Bound—Button and Buttonhole Fly Reinforced—Can Be Worn Over Shoes or Oxfords. Colors, Fawn, Gray or Brown.
**Sizes—Same as shoe sizes, except no half sizes. State size of shoe overgaiters are to be worn with.**
*Shipping wt., 5 ounces.*

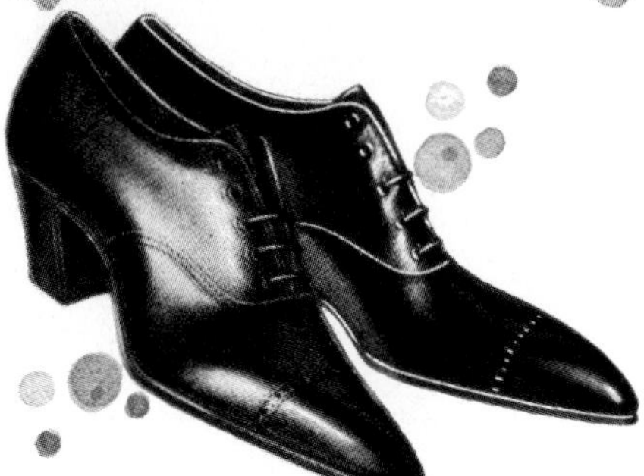

**15E2625**—Brown. **The Pair, $4.98**
**15E2626**—Black. **The Pair, 4.48**
Brown or Black Kid Finish Leather Lace Oxford—Military Heel—Sewed Sole.
*Sizes, 2½ to 8. Wide widths only.*
*Shipping wt., 1½ lbs.*

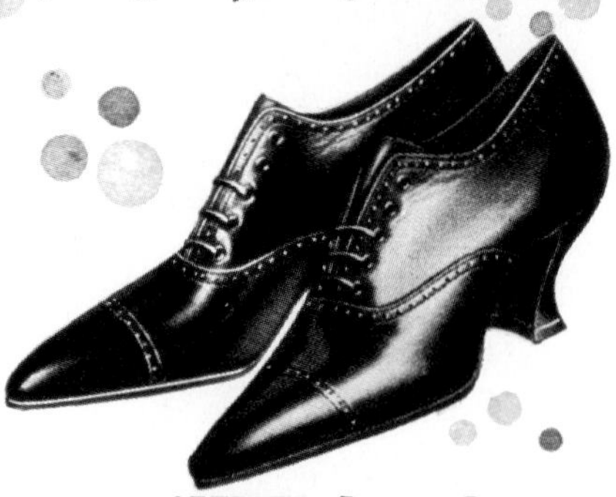

**15E2671**—Brown. **Pair, $4.48**
**15E2672**—Black. **Pair, 3.98**
Brown or Black Kid Finish Leather Lace Oxford — French Heel — Sewed Sole.
*Sizes, 2½ to 8. Wide widths only.*
*Shipping wt., 1¼ lbs.*

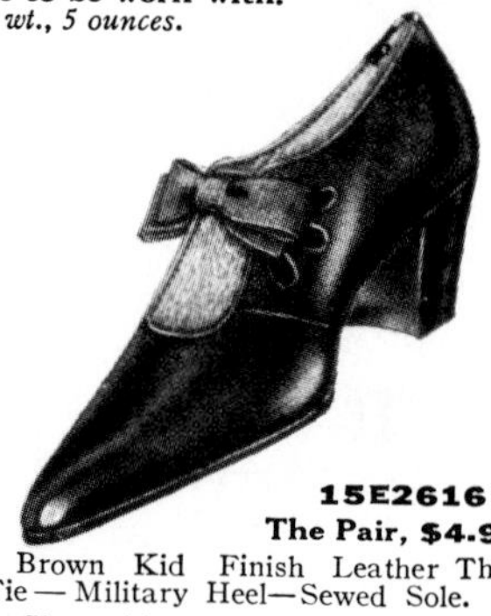

**15E2616**
**The Pair, $4.98**
Brown Kid Finish Leather Theo Tie — Military Heel—Sewed Sole.
*Sizes, 2½ to 8. Wide widths only.*
*Shipping wt., 1¼ lbs.*

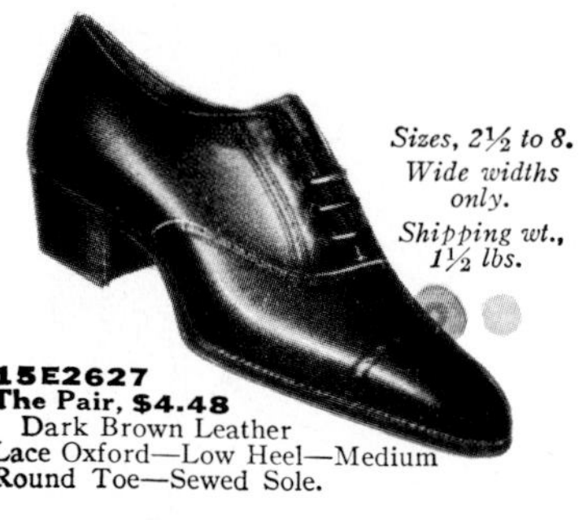

*Sizes, 2½ to 8.*
*Wide widths only.*
*Shipping wt., 1½ lbs.*

**15E2627**
**The Pair, $4.48**
Dark Brown Leather Lace Oxford—Low Heel—Medium Round Toe—Sewed Sole.

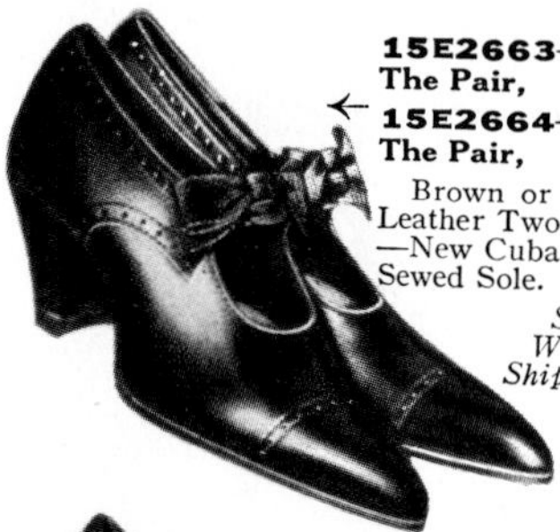

← **15E2663**—Brown.
**The Pair, $4.98**
**15E2664**—Black.
**The Pair, 4.48**
Brown or Black Kid Finish Leather Two-Eyelet Instep Tie —New Cuban Military Heel—Sewed Sole.
*Sizes, 2½ to 8.*
*Wide widths only.*
*Shipping wt., 1¼ lbs.*

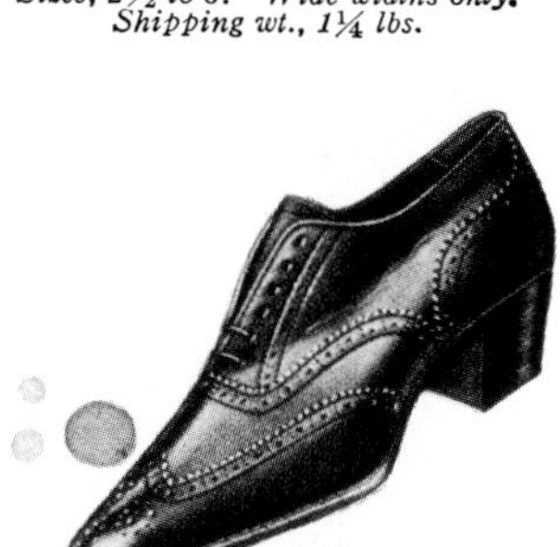

**15E2604** **The Pair, $4.95**
Dark Brown Leather Brogue Oxford —Fancy Perforations—Military Heel —Sewed Sole.
*Sizes, 2½ to 8. Wide widths only.*
*Shipping wt., 1¼ lbs.*

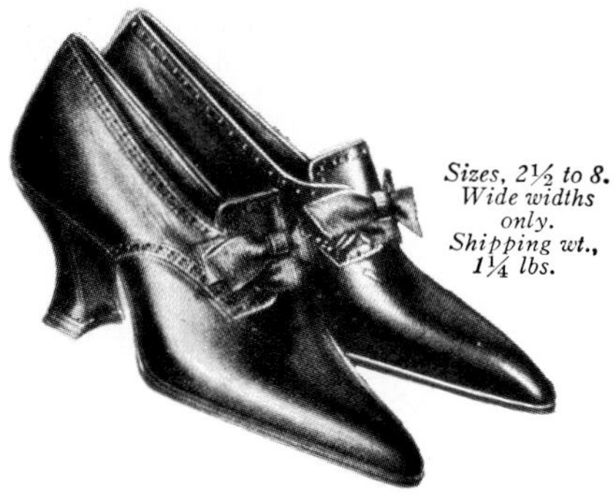

*Sizes, 2½ to 8.*
*Wide widths only.*
*Shipping wt., 1¼ lbs.*

**15E2623**—Brown. **The Pair, $4.48**
**15E2624**—Black. **The Pair, 3.98**
Brown or Black Kid Finish Leather Two-Eyelet Blucher Tie—French Heel—Sewed Sole.

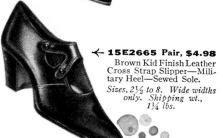

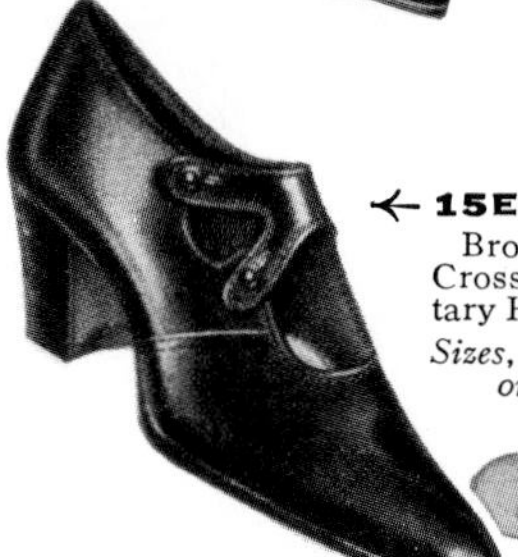

← **15E2665 Pair, $4.98**
Brown Kid Finish Leather Cross Strap Slipper—Military Heel—Sewed Sole.
*Sizes, 2½ to 8. Wide widths only. Shipping wt., 1¼ lbs.*

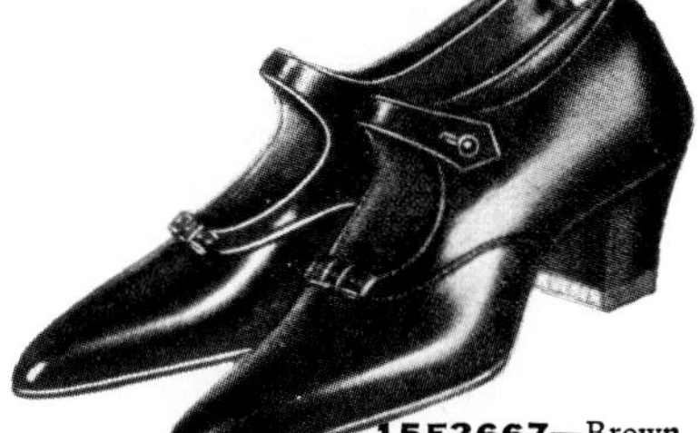

**15E2667**—Brown.
**The Pair, $4.98**
**15E2668**—Black.
**The Pair, $4.48**
Brown or Black Kid Finish Leather One-Strap Dress Slipper—Military Heel With Rubber Top Lift—Sewed Sole.
*Sizes, 2½ to 8. Wide widths only.*
*Shipping wt., 1 lb.*

# Young Men's Fine Suits

***SIZES*** **All suits shown on this page are furnished in sizes 34 to 42 inches chest measure, 29 to 40 inches waist measure and 29 to 35 inches inseam measure.** We placed a special order blank opposite this page for your convenience. If it has been used you'll find other order blanks in back of this catalog.

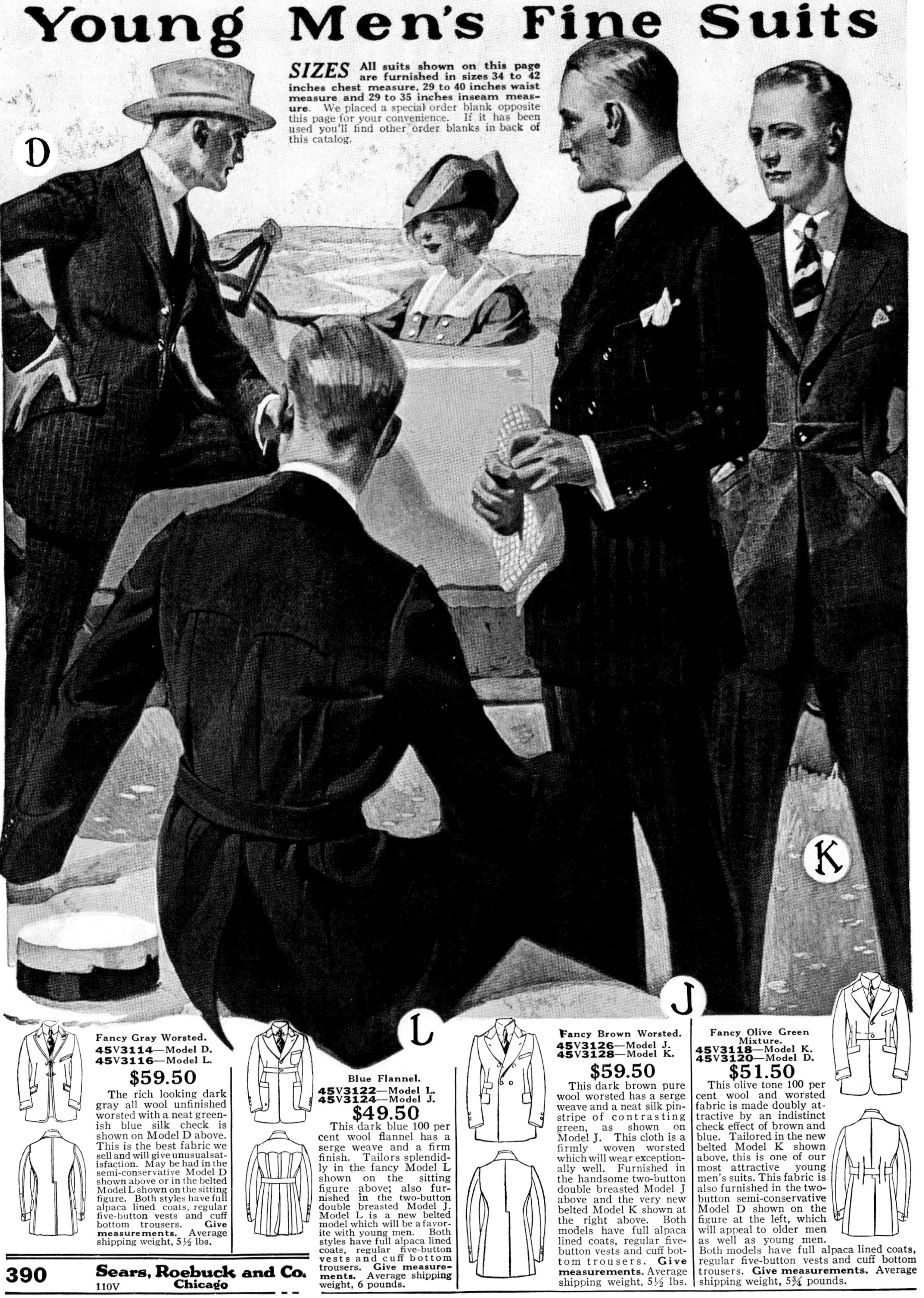


**Fancy Gray Worsted.**
**45V3114**—Model D.
**45V3116**—Model L.

## $59.50

The rich looking dark gray all wool unfinished worsted with a neat greenish blue silk check is shown on Model D above. This is the best fabric we sell and will give unusual satisfaction. May be had in the semi-conservative Model D shown above or in the belted Model L shown on the sitting figure. Both styles have full alpaca lined coats, regular five-button vests and cuff bottom trousers. **Give measurements.** Average shipping weight, 5½ lbs.

**Blue Flannel.**
**45V3122**—Model L.
**45V3124**—Model J.

## $49.50

This dark blue 100 per cent wool flannel has a serge weave and a firm finish. Tailors splendidly in the fancy Model L shown on the sitting figure above; also furnished in the two-button double breasted Model J. Model L is a new belted model which will be a favorite with young men. Both styles have full alpaca lined coats, regular five-button vests and cuff bottom trousers. **Give measurements.** Average shipping weight, 6 pounds.

**Fancy Brown Worsted.**
**45V3126**—Model J.
**45V3128**—Model K.

## $59.50

This dark brown pure wool worsted has a serge weave and a neat silk pinstripe of contrasting green, as shown on Model J. This cloth is a firmly woven worsted which will wear exceptionally well. Furnished in the handsome two-button double breasted Model J above and the very new belted Model K shown at the right above. Both models have full alpaca lined coats, regular five-button vests and cuff bottom trousers. **Give measurements.** Average shipping weight, 5½ lbs.

**Fancy Olive Green Mixture.**
**45V3118**—Model K.
**45V3120**—Model D.

## $51.50

This olive tone 100 per cent wool and worsted fabric is made doubly attractive by an indistinct check effect of brown and blue. Tailored in the new belted Model K shown above, this is one of our most attractive young men's suits. This fabric is also furnished in the two-button semi-conservative Model D shown on the figure at the left, which will appeal to older men as well as young men. Both models have full alpaca lined coats, regular five-button vests and cuff bottom trousers. **Give measurements.** Average shipping weight, 5¾ pounds.

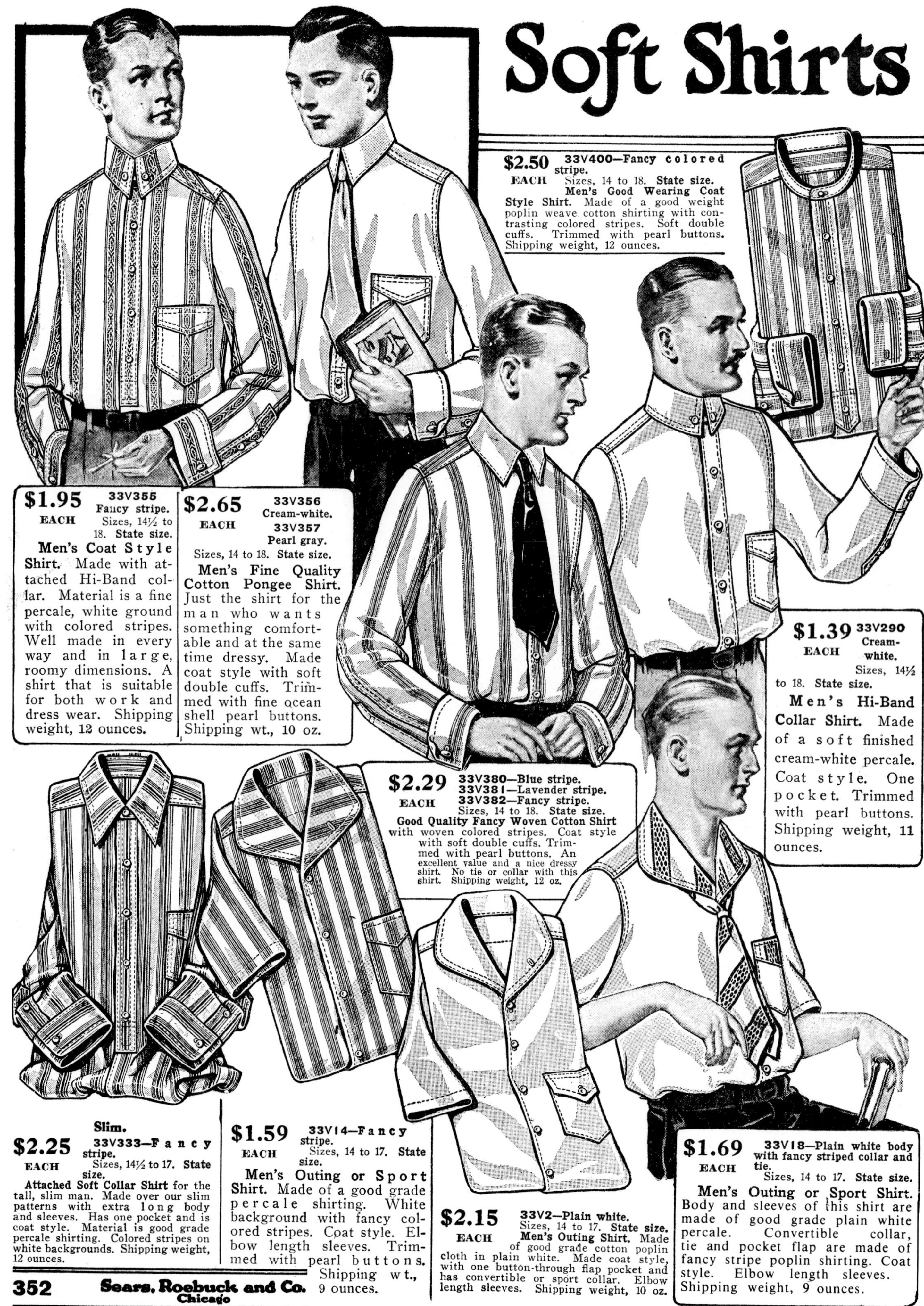
Soft Shirts
$2.50 EACH 33V400—Fancy colored stripe.
Sizes, 14 to 18. State size.
Men's Good Wearing Coat Style Shirt. Made of a good weight poplin weave cotton shirting with contrasting colored stripes. Soft double cuffs. Trimmed with pearl buttons. Shipping weight, 12 ounces.
$1.95 EACH 33V355 Fancy stripe.
Sizes, 14½ to 18. State size.
Men's Coat Style Shirt. Made with attached Hi-Band collar. Material is a fine percale, white ground with colored stripes. Well made in every way and in large, roomy dimensions. A shirt that is suitable for both work and dress wear. Shipping weight, 12 ounces.
$2.65 EACH 33V356 Cream-white. 33V357 Pearl gray.
Sizes, 14 to 18. State size.
Men's Fine Quality Cotton Pongee Shirt. Just the shirt for the man who wants something comfortable and at the same time dressy. Made coat style with soft double cuffs. Trimmed with fine ocean shell pearl buttons. Shipping wt., 10 oz.
$1.39 EACH 33V290 Cream-white.
Sizes, 14½ to 18. State size.
Men's Hi-Band Collar Shirt. Made of a soft finished cream-white percale. Coat style. One pocket. Trimmed with pearl buttons. Shipping weight, 11 ounces.
$2.29 EACH 33V380—Blue stripe. 33V381—Lavender stripe. 33V382—Fancy stripe.
Sizes, 14 to 18. State size.
Good Quality Fancy Woven Cotton Shirt with woven colored stripes. Coat style with soft double cuffs. Trimmed with pearl buttons. An excellent value and a nice dressy shirt. No tie or collar with this shirt. Shipping weight, 12 oz.
$2.25 EACH Slim. 33V333—Fancy stripe.
Sizes, 14½ to 17. State size.
Attached Soft Collar Shirt for the tall, slim man. Made over our slim patterns with extra long body and sleeves. Has one pocket and is coat style. Material is good grade percale shirting. Colored stripes on white backgrounds. Shipping weight, 12 ounces.
$1.59 EACH 33V14—Fancy stripe.
Sizes, 14 to 17. State size.
Men's Outing or Sport Shirt. Made of a good grade percale shirting. White background with fancy colored stripes. Coat style. Elbow length sleeves. Trimmed with pearl buttons. Shipping wt., 9 ounces.
$2.15 EACH 33V2—Plain white.
Sizes, 14 to 17. State size.
Men's Outing Shirt. Made of good grade cotton poplin cloth in plain white. Made coat style, with one button-through flap pocket and has convertible or sport collar. Elbow length sleeves. Shipping weight, 10 oz.
$1.69 EACH 33V18—Plain white body with fancy striped collar and tie.
Sizes, 14 to 17. State size.
Men's Outing or Sport Shirt. Body and sleeves of this shirt are made of good grade plain white percale. Convertible collar, tie and pocket flap are made of fancy stripe poplin shirting. Coat style. Elbow length sleeves. Shipping weight, 9 ounces.
352 Sears, Roebuck and Co. Chicago

**$2.75 A SUIT**
**33V950**
**Cream color.**
**Men's Pajamas.** Made of good quality medium weight pajama cloth. Trimmed with four frog fasteners and pearl buttons. Sizes, 15, 16, 17, 18 and 19. **State size.** Shipping weight, 1 pound.

# Men's Sleeping Garments

**$2.50 EACH**
**33V918—White.**
**Extra Quality Fine Yarn Cambric Nightshirt.** Made collarless style and trimmed with first quality pearl buttons. Length, 56 inches. Large and roomy. Sizes, 14, 15, 16, 17, 18, 19 and 20. **State size.** Shipping weight, 14 ounces.

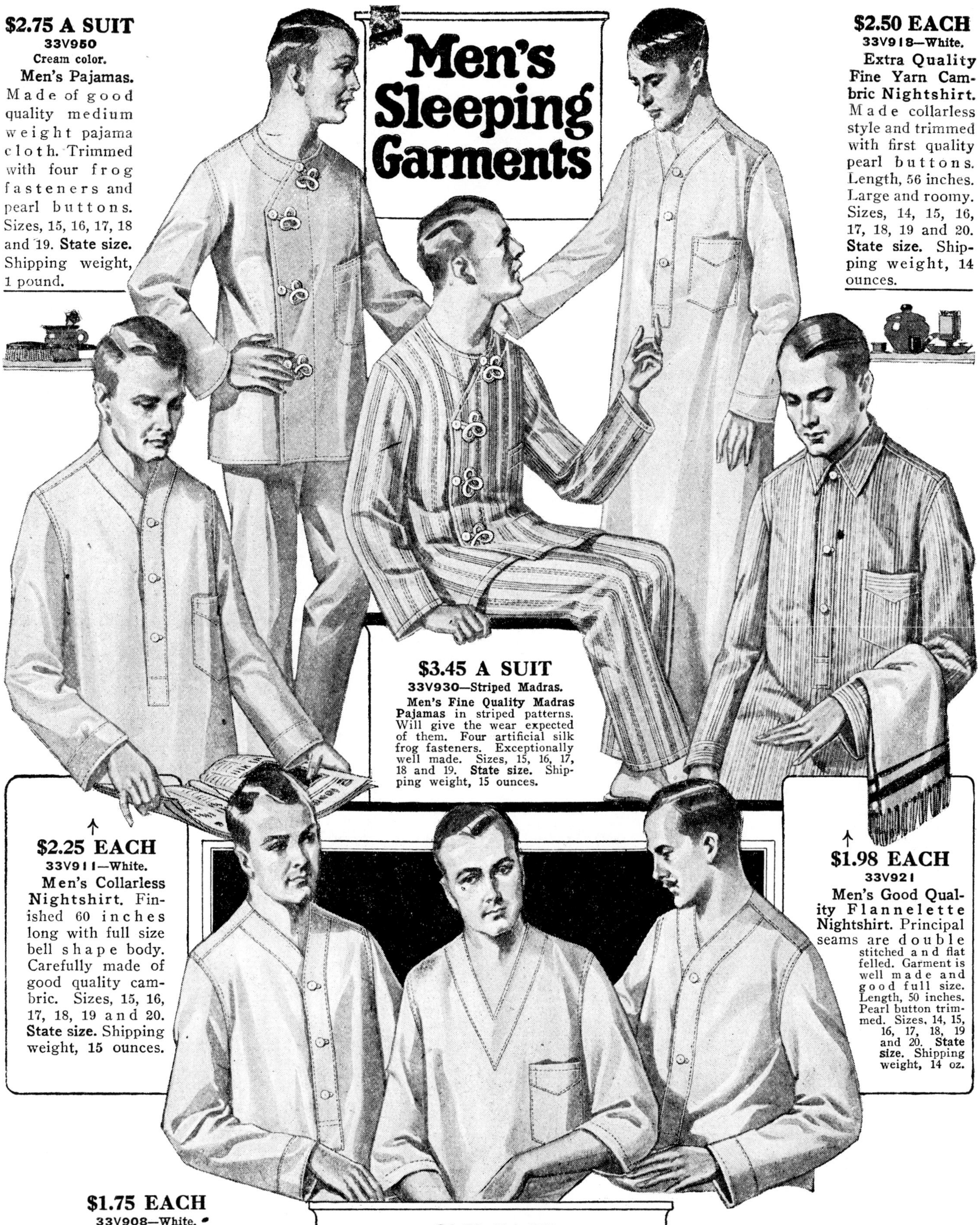

**$3.45 A SUIT**
**33V930—Striped Madras.**
**Men's Fine Quality Madras Pajamas** in striped patterns. Will give the wear expected of them. Four artificial silk frog fasteners. Exceptionally well made. Sizes, 15, 16, 17, 18 and 19. **State size.** Shipping weight, 15 ounces.

↑
**$2.25 EACH**
**33V911—White.**
**Men's Collarless Nightshirt.** Finished 60 inches long with full size bell shape body. Carefully made of good quality cambric. Sizes, 15, 16, 17, 18, 19 and 20. **State size.** Shipping weight, 15 ounces.

↑
**$1.98 EACH**
**33V921**
**Men's Good Quality Flannelette Nightshirt.** Principal seams are double stitched and flat felled. Garment is well made and good full size. Length, 50 inches. Pearl button trimmed. Sizes, 14, 15, 16, 17, 18, 19 and 20. **State size.** Shipping weight, 14 oz.

**$1.75 EACH**
**33V908—White.**
**Men's Good Quality White Muslin Nightgown.** Made collarless style. Full length and width body. Sizes, 14, 15, 16, 17, 18, 19 and 20. **State size.** Shipping weight, 12 ounces.

**$1.79 EACH**
**33V945—White.**
**Buttonless Nightshirt,** made V neck without buttons. This is a great advantage because there are no buttons to bother with. Elbow length sleeves. Made of extra quality white muslin. Sizes, 15, 16, 17, 18, 19 and 20. **State size.** Shipping weight, 12 ounces.

**$1.39 EACH**
**33V910—White.**
**Men's White Muslin Nightshirt.** Made collarless style. Well made and finished, 50 inches long. Principal seams are double stitched. Sizes, 14, 15, 16, 17, 18, 19 and 20. **State size.** Shipping weight, 11 oz.

See special measuring instructions between pages 374 and 375, 390 and 391.

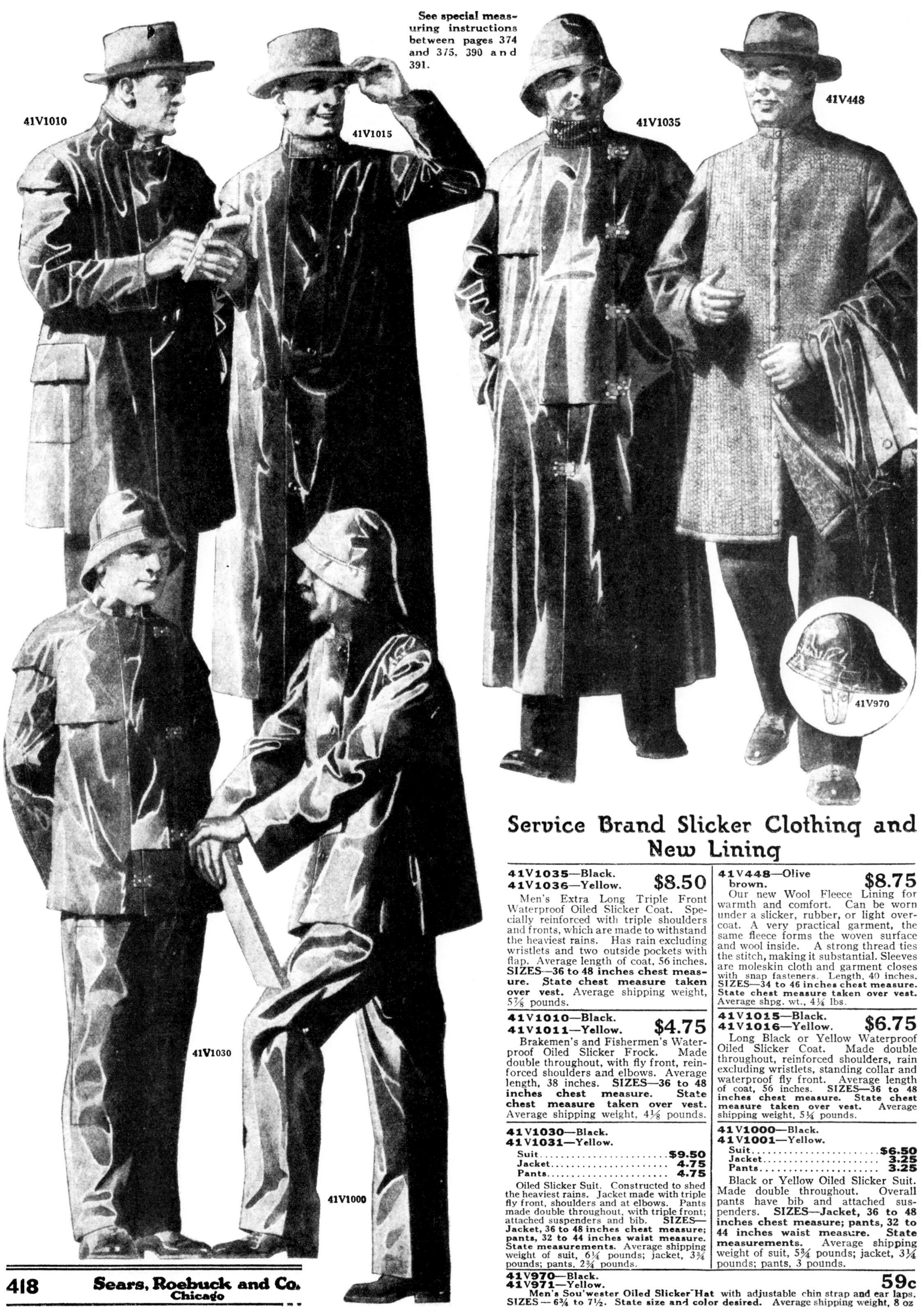


# Service Brand Slicker Clothing and New Lining

**41V1035—Black.**
**41V1036—Yellow.** **$8.50**
Men's Extra Long Triple Front Waterproof Oiled Slicker Coat. Specially reinforced with triple shoulders and fronts, which are made to withstand the heaviest rains. Has rain excluding wristlets and two outside pockets with flap. Average length of coat, 56 inches. **SIZES—36 to 48 inches chest measure. State chest measure taken over vest.** Average shipping weight, 5⅞ pounds.

**41V448—Olive brown.** **$8.75**
Our new Wool Fleece Lining for warmth and comfort. Can be worn under a slicker, rubber, or light overcoat. A very practical garment, the same fleece forms the woven surface and wool inside. A strong thread ties the stitch, making it substantial. Sleeves are moleskin cloth and garment closes with snap fasteners. Length, 40 inches. **SIZES—34 to 46 inches chest measure. State chest measure taken over vest.** Average shpg. wt., 4¼ lbs.

**41V1010—Black.**
**41V1011—Yellow.** **$4.75**
Brakemen's and Fishermen's Waterproof Oiled Slicker Frock. Made double throughout, with fly front, reinforced shoulders and elbows. Average length, 38 inches. **SIZES—36 to 48 inches chest measure. State chest measure taken over vest.** Average shipping weight, 4⅛ pounds.

**41V1015—Black.**
**41V1016—Yellow.** **$6.75**
Long Black or Yellow Waterproof Oiled Slicker Coat. Made double throughout, reinforced shoulders, rain excluding wristlets, standing collar and waterproof fly front. Average length of coat, 56 inches. **SIZES—36 to 48 inches chest measure. State chest measure taken over vest.** Average shipping weight, 5¼ pounds.

**41V1030—Black.**
**41V1031—Yellow.**

| | |
|---|---|
| Suit | **$9.50** |
| Jacket | **4.75** |
| Pants | **4.75** |

Oiled Slicker Suit. Constructed to shed the heaviest rains. Jacket made with triple fly front, shoulders and at elbows. Pants made double throughout, with triple front; attached suspenders and bib. **SIZES—Jacket, 36 to 48 inches chest measure; pants, 32 to 44 inches waist measure. State measurements.** Average shipping weight of suit, 6¼ pounds; jacket, 3¾ pounds; pants, 2¾ pounds.

**41V1000—Black.**
**41V1001—Yellow.**

| | |
|---|---|
| Suit | **$6.50** |
| Jacket | **3.25** |
| Pants | **3.25** |

Black or Yellow Oiled Slicker Suit. Made double throughout. Overall pants have bib and attached suspenders. **SIZES—Jacket, 36 to 48 inches chest measure; pants, 32 to 44 inches waist measure. State measurements.** Average shipping weight of suit, 5¾ pounds; jacket, 3¼ pounds; pants, 3 pounds.

**41V970—Black.**
**41V971—Yellow.** **59c**
**Men's Sou'wester Oiled Slicker Hat with adjustable chin strap and ear laps. SIZES — 6¾ to 7½. State size and color desired.** Average shipping weight, 8 oz

# NECKWEAR

## Our Tie Fabrics.

Our ties are made of standard fabrics such as are used by all reputable tie manufacturers. Unless otherwise stated they are made of silk and cotton or occasionally of artificial silk and cotton. The silk is always woven on the face of the material, combining that desired silky effect with durability.

Average shipping weight of ties on this page, 2 ounces.

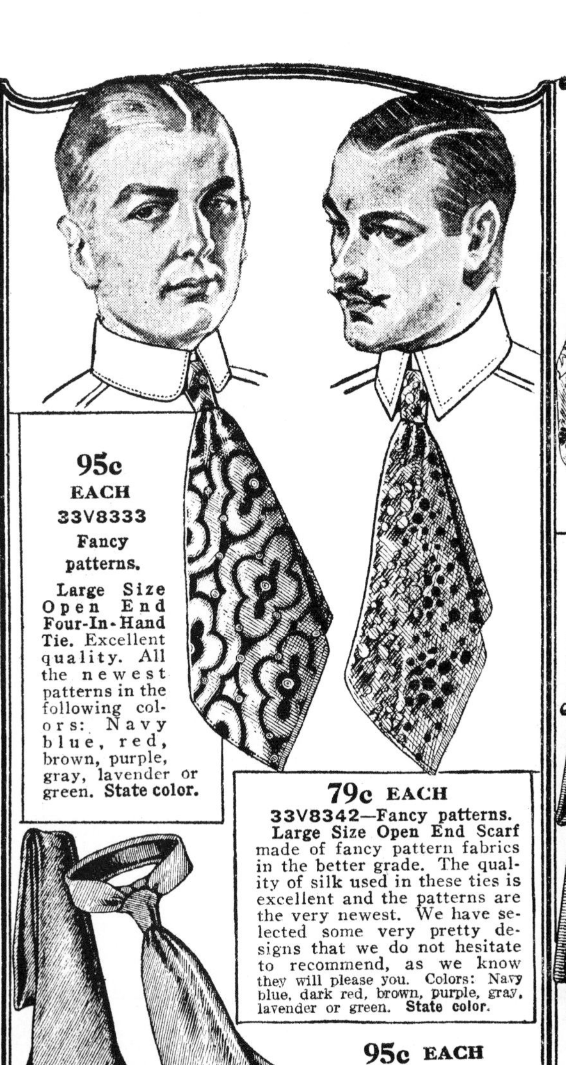

**95c EACH** 33V8333 Fancy patterns. Large Size Open End Four-In-Hand Tie. Excellent quality. All the newest patterns in the following colors: Navy blue, red, brown, purple, gray, lavender or green. State color.

**79c EACH** 33V8342—Fancy patterns. Large Size Open End Scarf made of fancy pattern fabrics in the better grade. The quality of silk used in these ties is excellent and the patterns are the very newest. We have selected some very pretty designs that we do not hesitate to recommend, as we know they will please you. Colors: Navy blue, dark red, brown, purple, gray, lavender or green. State color.

**95c EACH** 33V8403—Plain colors. Large Size Open End Four-In-Hand Tie. Material is of very fine quality. In plain colors only. Navy blue, red, brown, purple, gray, lavender, green, white or black. State color.

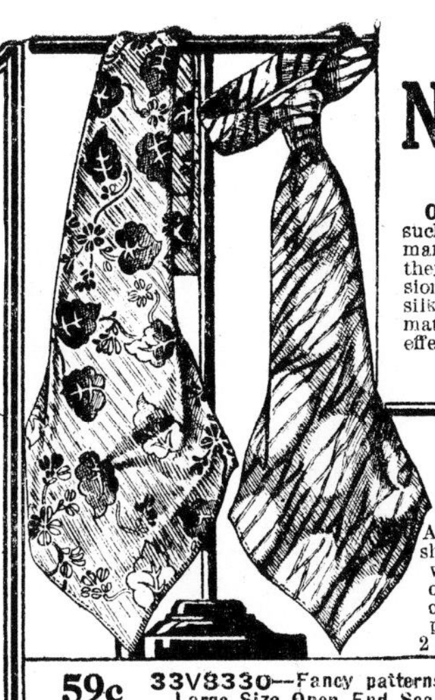

**59c EACH** 33V8330—Fancy patterns. Large Size Open End Scarf made of fancy pattern fabrics. Material is of good quality and the shape and patterns are of the latest. We have been very careful in selecting the patterns and colorings and feel sure that you will be well pleased with them. Colors: Navy blue, light blue, red, brown, purple, gray, lavender or green. State color preferred.

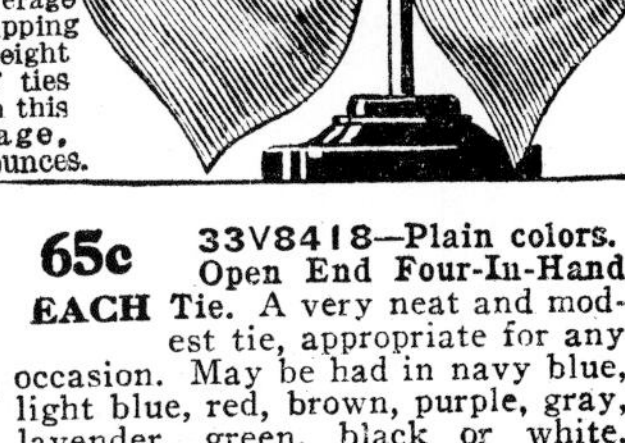

**65c EACH** 33V8418—Plain colors. Open End Four-In-Hand Tie. A very neat and modest tie, appropriate for any occasion. May be had in navy blue, light blue, red, brown, purple, gray, lavender, green, black or white. State color.

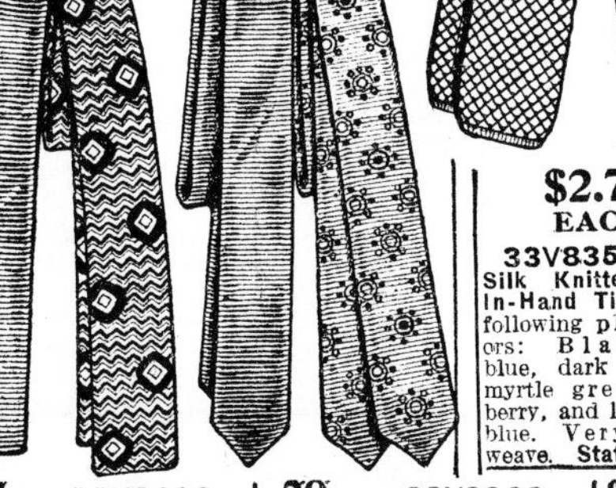

**55c EACH** 33V8406 Fancy patterns. Better quality reversible Four-In-Hand Tie. Gives you double wear. Colors: Navy blue, red, brown, purple, gray, lavender, green, black or white. State color.
33V8398—Same as above, but in plain colors only.

**39c EACH** 33V8366 Fancy patterns. Good quality reversible Four-In-Hand Tie. Gives you double wear. Colors: Navy blue, red, brown, purple, gray, lavender, green, black or white. State color.
33V8390—Same as above, in plain colors only.

**$2.75 EACH** 33V8355—All Silk Knitted Four-In-Hand Ties in the following plain colors: Black, navy blue, dark purple, myrtle green, mulberry, and light royal blue. Very pretty weave. State color.

**$1.39** 33V8343 **EACH** Fancy knit. Tubular Knitted Four-In-Hand Tie. Artificial silk and mercerized cotton. Colors: Navy, purple, lavender, dark green and old rose with colored stripes. Very pretty. State color.

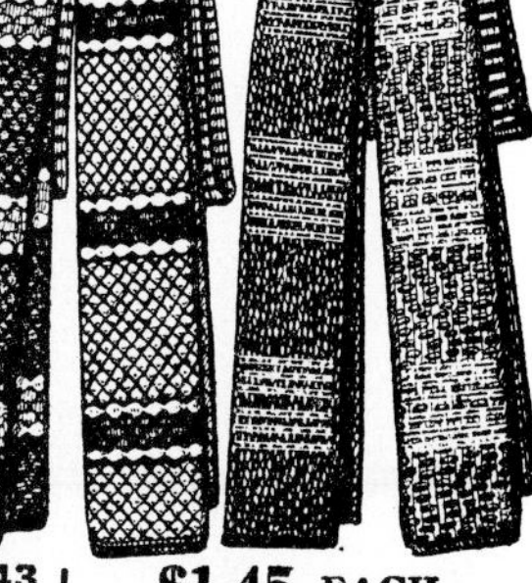

**$1.45 EACH** 33V8375—Knitted Four-In-Hand Tie. Made of artificial silk and cotton with fancy crossbar stripes. Following combination colors: Black and purple; royal and green; brown and myrtle green; mulberry, green and royal blue; purple and emerald; purple and light blue. Very stylish. State color.

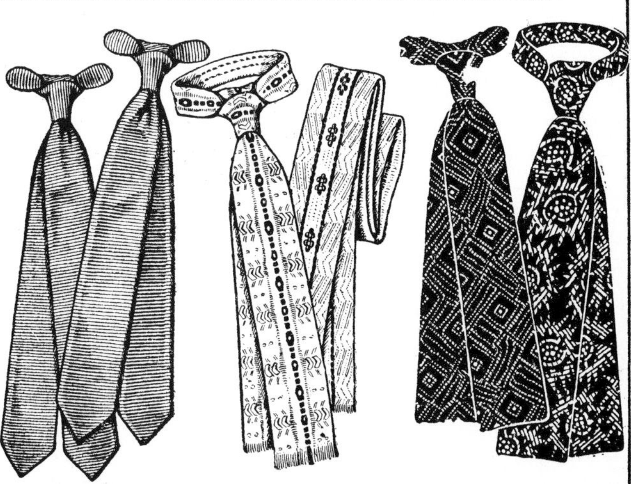

**27c EACH** 33V8310—Shield Teck Tie, made up ready for use with turndown collars. For those who desire a perfect knot without the trouble of tying it themselves. Comes in navy blue, light blue, red, brown, purple, gray, lavender, plain black, plain white, fancy black or green. State color.

**45c EACH** 33V8350—Very pretty Summer wash ties made of artificial silk and mercerized cotton. Fancy contrasting stripes and figures on assorted color backgrounds. We are sure they will please you.

**29c EACH** 33V8306—Fancy patterns. Band Teck Tie of good quality, made up ready for use.
33V8308—Fancy patterns. Same as above, with shield for turndown collars. Colors: Navy blue, light blue, red, brown, purple, gray, lavender, fancy black, plain white, plain black or green. State color.

Be Sure to State Color Wanted

# BOW TIES

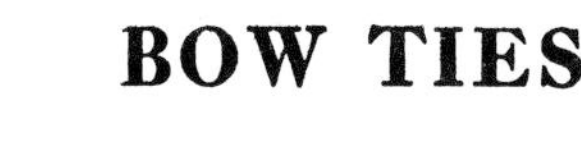

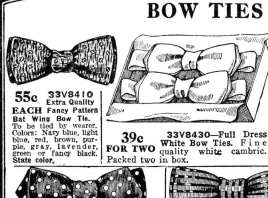

**55c EACH** 33V8410 Extra Quality Fancy Pattern Bat Wing Bow Tie. To be tied by wearer. Colors: Navy blue, light blue, red, brown, purple, gray, lavender, green or fancy black. State color.

**39c FOR TWO** 33V8430—Full Dress White Bow Ties. Fine quality white cambric. Packed two in box.

**55c EACH** 33V8422 Fancy colors. Graduated End Bow Tie in fancy patterns. To be tied by the wearer. Tie is $1\frac{3}{4}$ inches wide at end. Colors: Navy blue, light blue, red, brown, gray, lavender, purple, green or fancy black. State color.

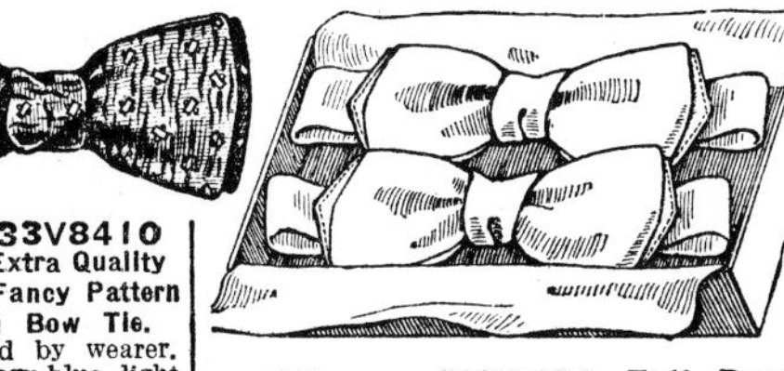

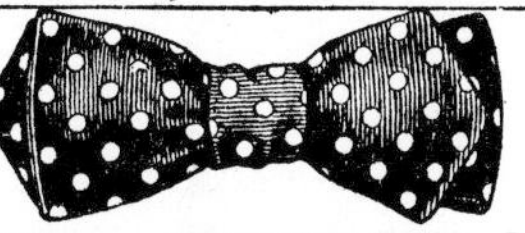

**55c EACH** 33V8425—Polka Dot Bat Wing Bow Tie. Assorted size dots. Very neat and stylish. To be tied by wearer. Navy blue with white dots only.

**35c Each** 33V8412 Plain colors. Bat Wing Bow Tie in plain colors. To be tied by the wearer. Colors: Navy blue, light blue, red, brown, purple, gray, lavender, white or black. State color desired.

**35c EACH** 33V8413—Bat Wing Style Bow Tie in fancy patterns, to be tied by wearer. Colors: Navy blue, light blue, red, brown, gray, purple, lavender, fancy black or green. State color.

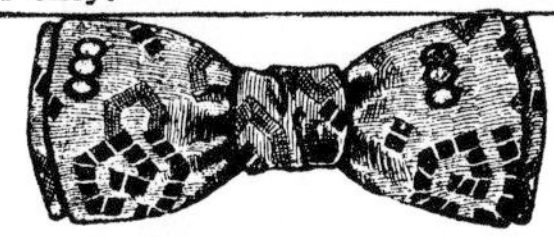

**25c EACH** 33V8420—Made Up Bow Tie with shield on back for turndown collars. Pretty patterns. Colors: Navy blue, light blue, red, brown, purple, gray, lavender, green, fancy black, plain white or plain black. State color.

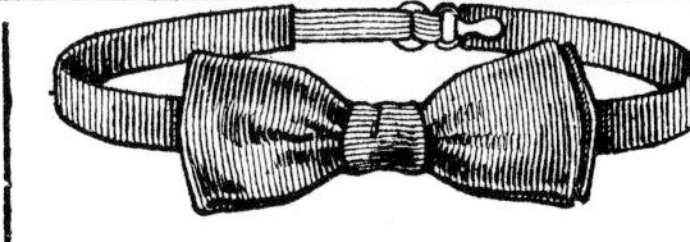

**29c EACH** 33V8429—Made Up Band Bow Tie. Elastic band and hook fastener. Colors: Navy blue, light blue, red, brown, purple, gray, lavender, green, fancy black, plain black or plain white. State color.

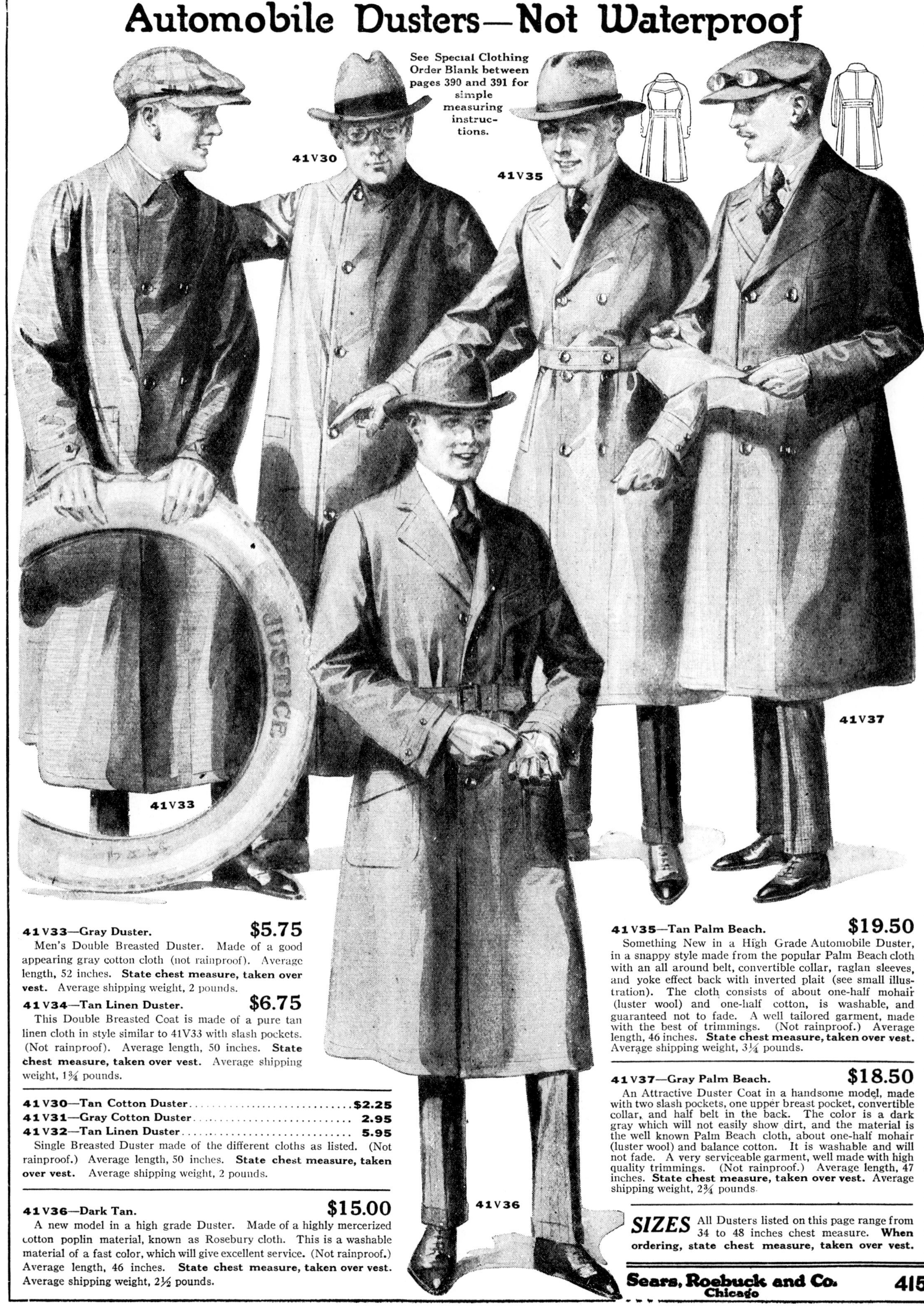

# Automobile Dusters—Not Waterproof

See Special Clothing Order Blank between pages 390 and 391 for simple measuring instructions.

41V30 41V35 41V33 41V37 41V36

**41V33—Gray Duster.** **$5.75**
Men's Double Breasted Duster. Made of a good appearing gray cotton cloth (not rainproof). Average length, 52 inches. **State chest measure, taken over vest.** Average shipping weight, 2 pounds.

**41V34—Tan Linen Duster.** **$6.75**
This Double Breasted Coat is made of a pure tan linen cloth in style similar to 41V33 with slash pockets. (Not rainproof). Average length, 50 inches. **State chest measure, taken over vest.** Average shipping weight, 1¾ pounds.

**41V30—Tan Cotton Duster** ........ **$2.25**
**41V31—Gray Cotton Duster** ........ **2.95**
**41V32—Tan Linen Duster** ........ **5.95**
Single Breasted Duster made of the different cloths as listed. (Not rainproof.) Average length, 50 inches. **State chest measure, taken over vest.** Average shipping weight, 2 pounds.

**41V36—Dark Tan.** **$15.00**
A new model in a high grade Duster. Made of a highly mercerized cotton poplin material, known as Rosebury cloth. This is a washable material of a fast color, which will give excellent service. (Not rainproof.) Average length, 46 inches. **State chest measure, taken over vest.** Average shipping weight, 2½ pounds.

**41V35—Tan Palm Beach.** **$19.50**
Something New in a High Grade Automobile Duster, in a snappy style made from the popular Palm Beach cloth with an all around belt, convertible collar, raglan sleeves, and yoke effect back with inverted plait (see small illustration). The cloth consists of about one-half mohair (luster wool) and one-half cotton, is washable, and guaranteed not to fade. A well tailored garment, made with the best of trimmings. (Not rainproof.) Average length, 46 inches. **State chest measure, taken over vest.** Average shipping weight, 3¼ pounds.

**41V37—Gray Palm Beach.** **$18.50**
An Attractive Duster Coat in a handsome model, made with two slash pockets, one upper breast pocket, convertible collar, and half belt in the back. The color is a dark gray which will not easily show dirt, and the material is the well known Palm Beach cloth, about one-half mohair (luster wool) and balance cotton. It is washable and will not fade. A very serviceable garment, well made with high quality trimmings. (Not rainproof.) Average length, 47 inches. **State chest measure, taken over vest.** Average shipping weight, 2¾ pounds.

***SIZES*** All Dusters listed on this page range from 34 to 48 inches chest measure. **When ordering, state chest measure, taken over vest.**

# Hunting Clothing

41V5162—For 12-gauge shells.
41V5163—For 16-gauge shells.
41V5164—For 20-gauge shells.
Price........... **$3.40**

Automatic Shell Vest. Has been recommended by some of the country's best shooters. Made of khaki color duck front and back. Cut on regular vest pattern. Made with four shell compartments on each side, which are fitted with brass clips at the bottom. Vest holds forty shells, or five to each compartment. Shells are always in position for loading. When a shell is pulled, another automatically drops into place until compartment is empty. **SIZES—34 to 46 inches chest measure. Order by catalog number and give chest measure.** Shipping weight, about 2 pounds.

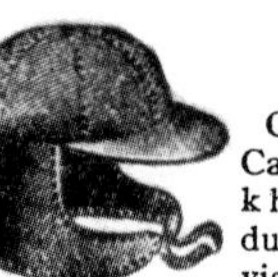

**41V5189**
**$1.25**

Canvas Cape Cap. Made of khaki color duck, single stiff visor, full cape, cotton flannel lined; an excellent rough or cold weather cap. Can also be worn as shown in small illustration above. **SIZES—6¾ to 7¾. State size.** Shipping weight, 9 ounces.

**41V5143**
**$5.25**
**Give chest measure.**

Medium Weight Hunting Coat. Made of 8-ounce khaki color duck with drill lined skirt, three outside cut-in pockets, three inside game pockets; corduroy collar, corduroy lined cuffs. Coat is double stitched. **SIZES—34 to 48 inches chest measure.** Shipping weight, 2⅝ to 3⅛ lbs.

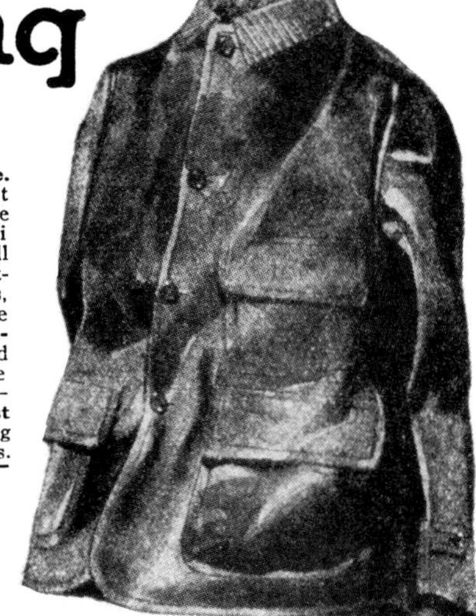

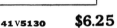

41V5155—For 10 or 12-gauge shells.
41V5156—For 16-gauge shells.
41V5158—For 20-gauge shells.
**$2.15**

Hunting Vest. Khaki color duck in both front and back. Fitted with latest style folding shell loops, made of same material as the vest. Holds 32 to 36 shells. **SIZES—34 to 48 inches chest measure. Order by catalog number and give chest measure.** Shipping weight, 12 ounces to 1¼ pounds.

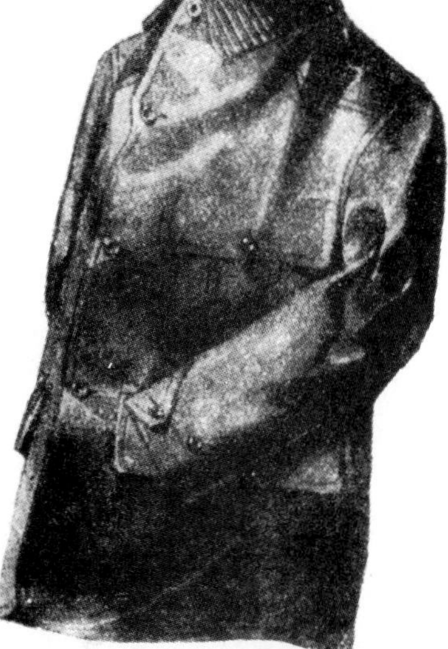

**41V5130** **$6.25**
**Give chest measure.**

Shelter Coat. Made of genuine shelter tent duck, same as used for army purposes; a very fine, closely woven canvas. Very soft and pliable, olive tan shade. Coat is lined with 8-ounce olive tan duck, making it like two coats in one. Corduroy collar, corduroy faced cuffs, gussets under arms, two large shell pockets, one breast and one whistle pocket, all pocket flaps buttoned; three inside game pockets. **SIZES—34 to 48 inches chest measure.** Shipping weight, 3¼ to 3¾ pounds.

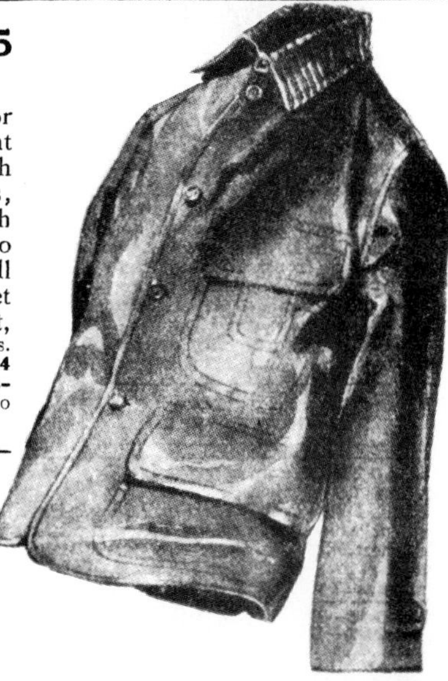

**41V5140** **$5.65**
**Give chest measure.**

Hunting Coat for Men. Medium weight khaki color duck, with reinforced shoulders, three-quarters lined with khaki color drill to match. Two large shell pocket, one breast pocket and one whistle pocket, three inside game pockets. Double stitched. **SIZES—34 to 48 inches chest measure.** Shipping weight, 3 to 3¾ pounds.

**41V5150** **$4.95**
**Give chest measure.**

Boys' Hunting Coat. Made like 41V5140. **SIZES—30, 32 and 34 inches chest measure.** Average shipping weight, 2⅜ to 2½ pounds.

**See order blank between pages 390 and 391 for simple measuring instructions.**

**41V5159** **$3.50**

Heavy Weight Army Duck Hunting Pants, khaki color. Our hunting pants are cut over our improved pattern, full in hips and knees; have two front pockets, two hip pockets with buttoned tab and one watch pocket; belt and tunnel loops. **SIZES—30 to 44 inches waist and 30 to 36 inches inseam measure. Give waist and inseam measures when ordering.** Shipping weight, 2¾ to 3 pounds.

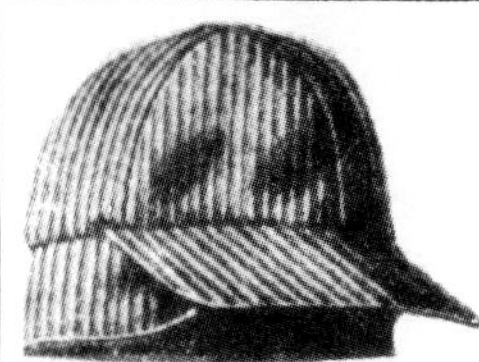

**41V5196** **$1.25**

Reversible Red Lined Cap. Corduroy on the outside and bright red cotton flannel on the inside, with an opening on one side at bottom seam so the top part can be pulled over to cover the corduroy and bring the red side out. Inside turn-down fur lined band. Worn in thick woods and brush and by deer hunters. **SIZES—6¾ to 8. State size.** Shipping weight, 8 ounces.

**41V5198** **$2.25**

Our Hunting and Blizzard Cap. Suitable for any kind of weather. Just the thing for hunters, farmers, teamsters, railroad men, ice cutters and explorers. Material, khaki color duck, serviceable cotton lining. **Has eiderdown lined inside band to pull down, nose piece to cover nose and detachable cape lined with eiderdown.** Can be worn as a regular cap in mild weather or with band over ears in cold weather. **Cape can be readily attached for extremely cold or blizzardy weather. SIZES—6¾ to 8. State size wanted.** Shipping weight, 13 ounces.

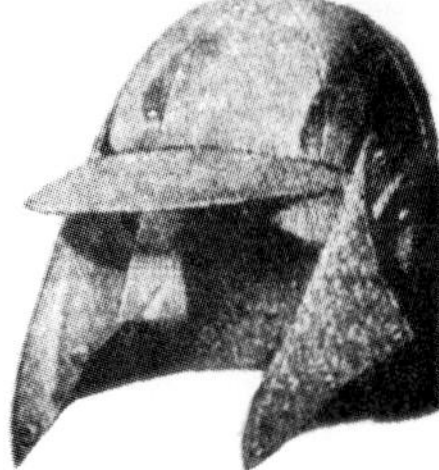

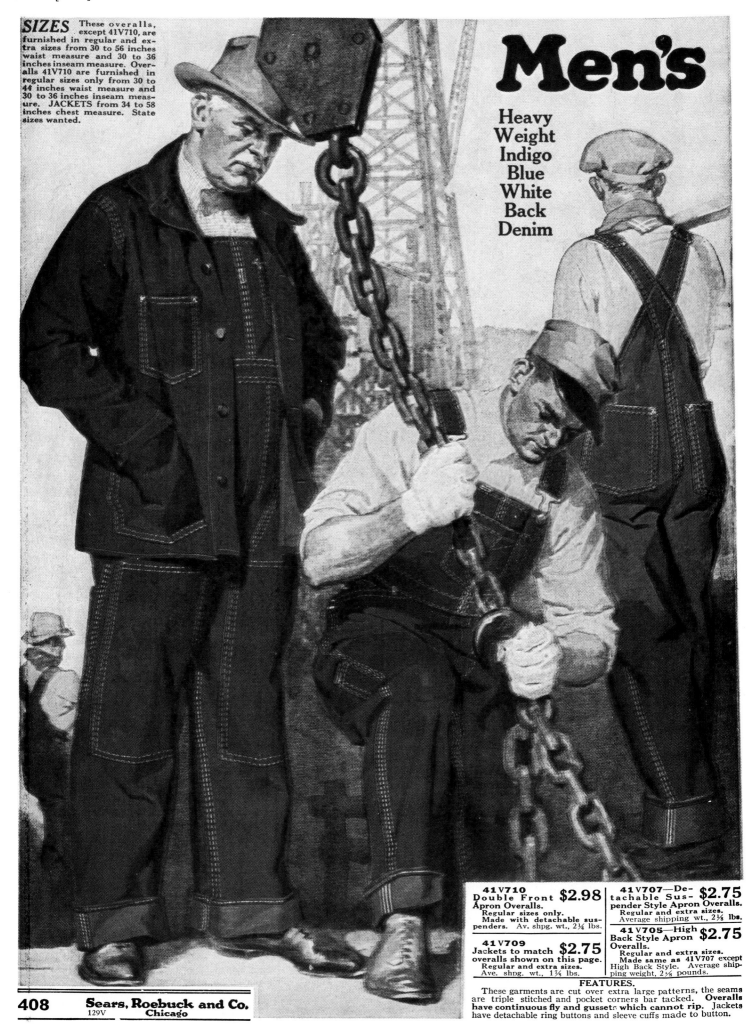

**SIZES** These overalls, except 41V710, are furnished in regular and extra sizes from 30 to 56 inches waist measure and 30 to 36 inches inseam measure. Overalls 41V710 are furnished in regular sizes only from 30 to 44 inches waist measure and 30 to 36 inches inseam measure. JACKETS from 34 to 58 inches chest measure. State sizes wanted.

# Men's

## Heavy Weight Indigo Blue White Back Denim

**41V710** Double Front Apron Overalls. **$2.98**
Regular sizes only.
Made with detachable suspenders. Av. shpg. wt., 2¼ lbs.

**41V709** Jackets to match overalls shown on this page. **$2.75**
Regular and extra sizes.
Ave. shpg. wt., 1⅞ lbs.

**41V707**—Detachable Suspender Style Apron Overalls. **$2.75**
Regular and extra sizes.
Average shipping wt., 2⅛ lbs.

**41V705**—High Back Style Apron Overalls. **$2.75**
Regular and extra sizes.
Made same as 41V707 except High Back Style. Average shipping weight, 2⅛ pounds.

**FEATURES.**

These garments are cut over extra large patterns, the seams are triple stitched and pocket corners bar tacked. **Overalls have continuous fly and gussets which cannot rip.** Jackets have detachable ring buttons and sleeve cuffs made to button.

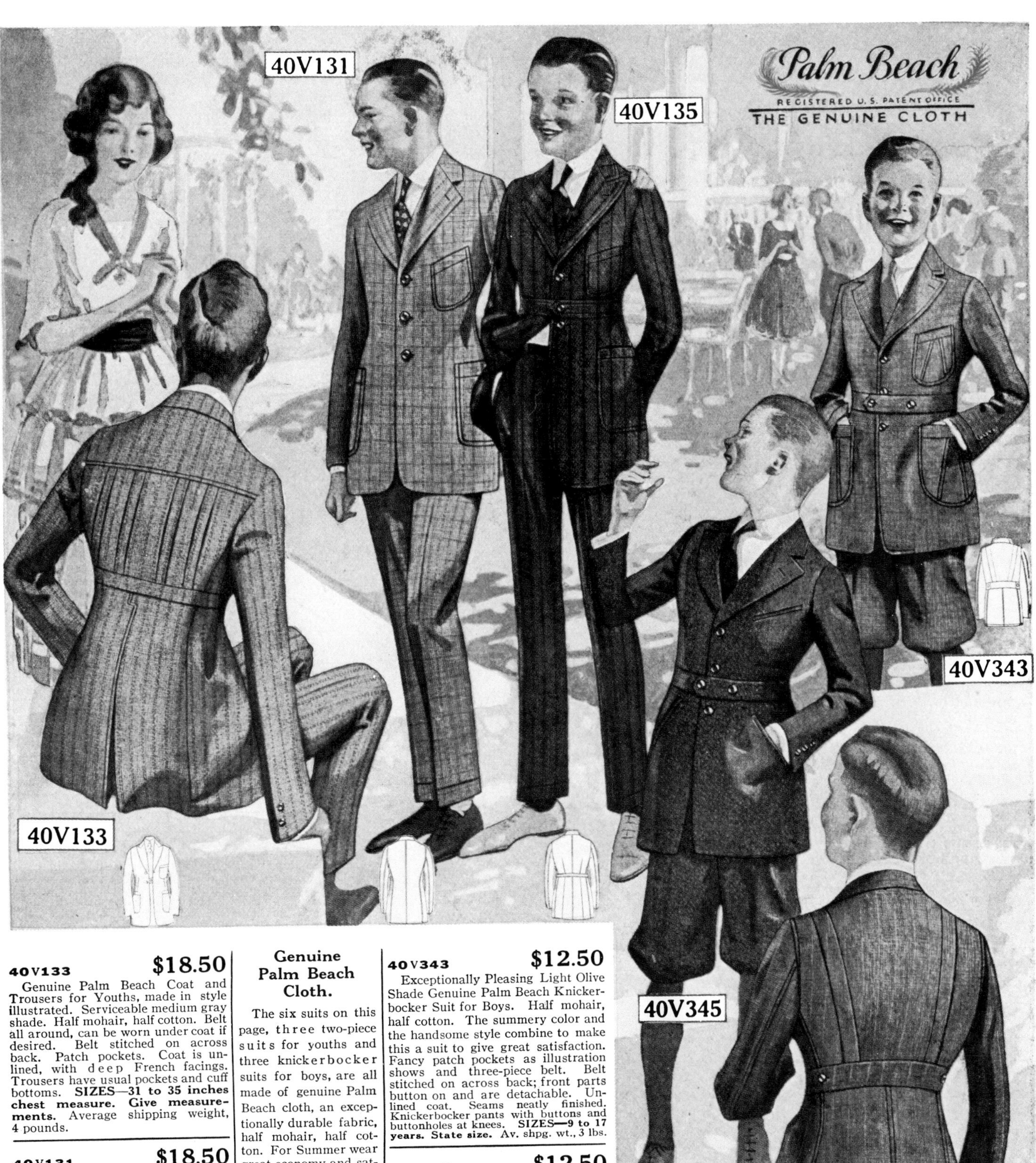


**40V133** **$18.50**

Genuine Palm Beach Coat and Trousers for Youths, made in style illustrated. Serviceable medium gray shade. Half mohair, half cotton. Belt all around, can be worn under coat if desired. Belt stitched on across back. Patch pockets. Coat is unlined, with deep French facings. Trousers have usual pockets and cuff bottoms. **SIZES—31 to 35 inches chest measure. Give measurements.** Average shipping weight, 4 pounds.

**40V131** **$18.50**

A Semi-Conservative Style in Genuine Palm Beach Cloth Coat and Trousers for Youths. Medium tan shade, one of the most popular of Palm Beach colors. Material one-half mohair, balance cotton. Three-button coat with patch pockets. Plain back. Coat is unlined, with deep French facings. Trousers have usual pockets and cuff bottoms. Tunnel belt loops. **SIZES —31 to 35 inches chest measure. Give measurements.** Average shipping weight, 4 pounds.

**40V135** **$20.00**

Exceptionally Attractive Palm Beach Coat and Trousers for Youths, in a dark brown striped pattern. Material half mohair, half cotton. Belt all around, stitched on across back. Patch pockets. Coat is unlined, with deep French facings. Trousers have usual pockets and cuff bottoms. **SIZES—31 to 35 inches chest measure. Give measurements.** Average shpg. wt., 4 lbs.

## Genuine Palm Beach Cloth.

The six suits on this page, three two-piece suits for youths and three knickerbocker suits for boys, are all made of genuine Palm Beach cloth, an exceptionally durable fabric, half mohair, half cotton. For Summer wear great economy and satisfaction will be found in the purchase of these garments—economy especially when the high cost of woolens is considered.

The styles are what youths and boys are wearing for this Spring and Summer. Note the high waisted effect on the belted styles. This is one of the newest style features in boys' and youths' clothes.

**For Special Clothing Order Blank see pages 374A and 374B, or 390A and 390B.**

**40V343** **$12.50**

Exceptionally Pleasing Light Olive Shade Genuine Palm Beach Knickerbocker Suit for Boys. Half mohair, half cotton. The summery color and the handsome style combine to make this a suit to give great satisfaction. Fancy patch pockets as illustration shows and three-piece belt. Belt stitched on across back; front parts button on and are detachable. Unlined coat. Seams neatly finished. Knickerbocker pants with buttons and buttonholes at knees. **SIZES—9 to 17 years. State size.** Av. shpg. wt., 3 lbs.

**40V345** **$12.50**

A Nifty Bronze Green Genuine Palm Beach Cloth Knickerbocker Suit for Boys, in the very attractive style illustrated. Material half mohair, half cotton. The fabric is dark enough not to readily show soil marks and the model is one of the most popular. Belt all around is detachable. Coat unlined, with deep French facings. Knickerbocker pants with buttons and buttonholes at knees. **SIZES —9 to 17 years. State size.** Average shipping weight, 3 pounds.

**40V347** **$12.50**

A Grayish Green Genuine Palm Beach Knickerbocker Suit for Boys, in the very snappy style illustrated at the right. The back view is unusually pleasing, and the front with the pockets concealed under plaits is new and attractive. Belt all around is detachable. Coat unlined, with deep French facings. Knickerbocker pants with buttons and buttonholes at knees. **SIZES—9 to 17 years. State size.** Average shipping weight, 3 pounds.

# Rompers and Wash Suits for Little Fellows

Rah-Rah Hats to wear with wash suits on this page. The blue hat will go especially well with the suit it is illustrated with and the white one can, of course, be worn with any suit. Full lined. Cloth sweatband. **SIZES—6¼ to 6¾. State size.** Average shipping weight, 6 ounces.

**40V903**—Blue Rah-Rah Hat .............................. **85c**
**40V901**—White Rah-Rah Hat .............................. **85c**

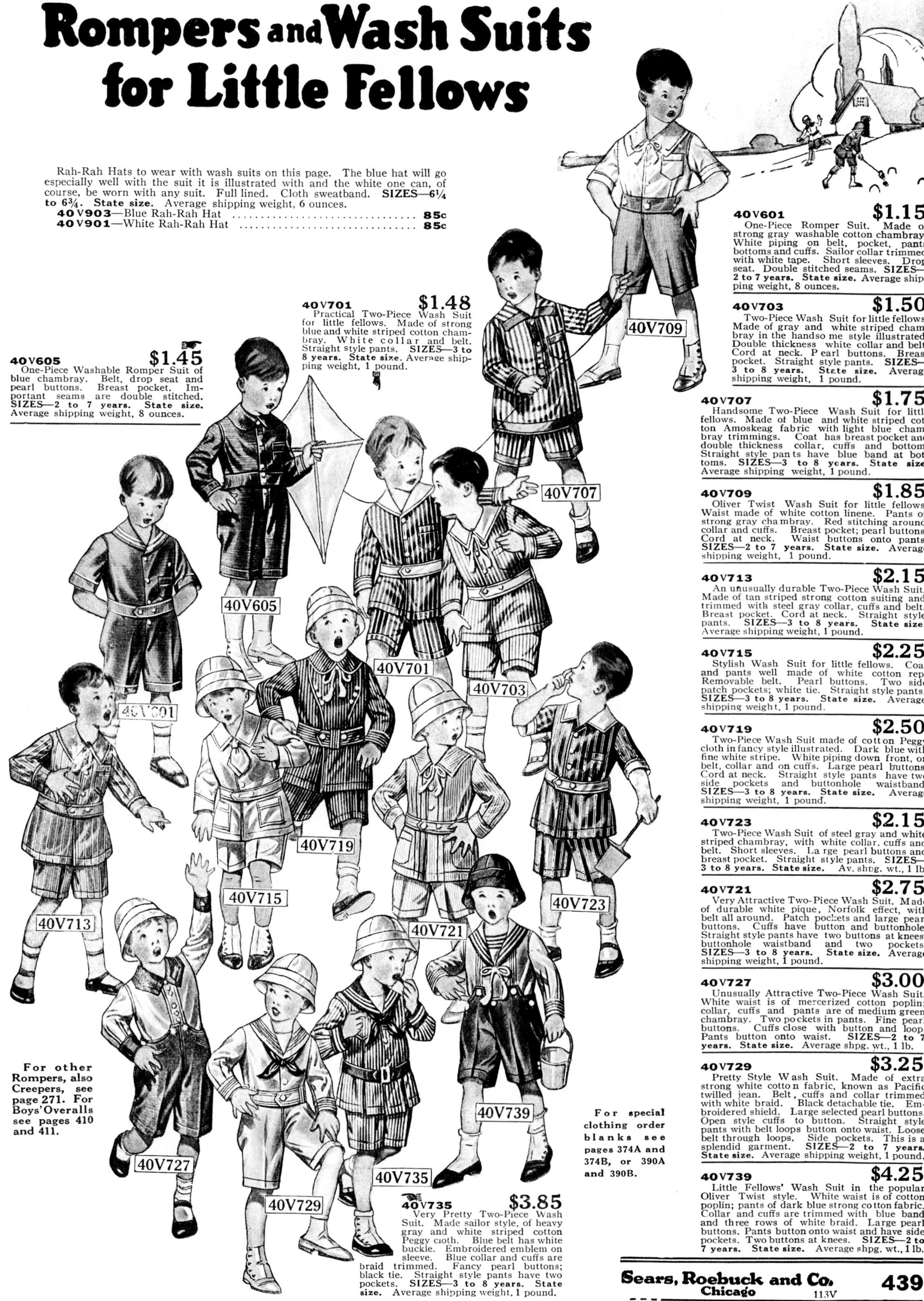


**40V605** **$1.45**
One-Piece Washable Romper Suit of blue chambray. Belt, drop seat and pearl buttons. Breast pocket. Important seams are double stitched. **SIZES—2 to 7 years. State size.** Average shipping weight, 8 ounces.

**40V701** **$1.48**
Practical Two-Piece Wash Suit for little fellows. Made of strong blue and white striped cotton chambray. White collar and belt. Straight style pants. **SIZES—3 to 8 years. State size.** Average shipping weight, 1 pound.

**40V601** **$1.15**
One-Piece Romper Suit. Made of strong gray washable cotton chambray. White piping on belt, pocket, pants bottoms and cuffs. Sailor collar trimmed with white tape. Short sleeves. Drop seat. Double stitched seams. **SIZES—2 to 7 years. State size.** Average shipping weight, 8 ounces.

**40V703** **$1.50**
Two-Piece Wash Suit for little fellows. Made of gray and white striped chambray in the handsome style illustrated. Double thickness white collar and belt. Cord at neck. Pearl buttons. Breast pocket. Straight style pants. **SIZES—3 to 8 years. State size.** Average shipping weight, 1 pound.

**40V707** **$1.75**
Handsome Two-Piece Wash Suit for little fellows. Made of blue and white striped cotton Amoskeag fabric with light blue chambray trimmings. Coat has breast pocket and double thickness collar, cuffs and bottom. Straight style pants have blue band at bottoms. **SIZES—3 to 8 years. State size.** Average shipping weight, 1 pound.

**40V709** **$1.85**
Oliver Twist Wash Suit for little fellows. Waist made of white cotton linene. Pants of strong gray chambray. Red stitching around collar and cuffs. Breast pocket; pearl buttons. Cord at neck. Waist buttons onto pants. **SIZES—2 to 7 years. State size.** Average shipping weight, 1 pound.

**40V713** **$2.15**
An unusually durable Two-Piece Wash Suit. Made of tan striped strong cotton suiting and trimmed with steel gray collar, cuffs and belt. Breast pocket. Cord at neck. Straight style pants. **SIZES—3 to 8 years. State size.** Average shipping weight, 1 pound.

**40V715** **$2.25**
Stylish Wash Suit for little fellows. Coat and pants well made of white cotton rep. Removable belt. Pearl buttons. Two side patch pockets; white tie. Straight style pants. **SIZES—3 to 8 years. State size.** Average shipping weight, 1 pound.

**40V719** **$2.50**
Two-Piece Wash Suit made of cotton Peggy cloth in fancy style illustrated. Dark blue with fine white stripe. White piping down front, on belt, collar and on cuffs. Large pearl buttons. Cord at neck. Straight style pants have two side pockets and buttonhole waistband. **SIZES—3 to 8 years. State size.** Average shipping weight, 1 pound.

**40V723** **$2.15**
Two-Piece Wash Suit of steel gray and white striped chambray, with white collar, cuffs and belt. Short sleeves. Large pearl buttons and breast pocket. Straight style pants. **SIZES—3 to 8 years. State size.** Av. shpg. wt., 1 lb.

**40V721** **$2.75**
Very Attractive Two-Piece Wash Suit. Made of durable white pique, Norfolk effect, with belt all around. Patch pockets and large pearl buttons. Cuffs have button and buttonhole. Straight style pants have two buttons at knees, buttonhole waistband and two pockets. **SIZES—3 to 8 years. State size.** Average shipping weight, 1 pound.

**40V727** **$3.00**
Unusually Attractive Two-Piece Wash Suit. White waist is of mercerized cotton poplin; collar, cuffs and pants are of medium green chambray. Two pockets in pants. Fine pearl buttons. Cuffs close with button and loop. Pants button onto waist. **SIZES—2 to 7 years. State size.** Average shpg. wt., 1 lb.

**40V729** **$3.25**
Pretty Style Wash Suit. Made of extra strong white cotton fabric, known as Pacific twilled jean. Belt, cuffs and collar trimmed with white braid. Black detachable tie. Embroidered shield. Large selected pearl buttons. Open style cuffs to button. Straight style pants with belt loops button onto waist. Loose belt through loops. Side pockets. This is a splendid garment. **SIZES—2 to 7 years. State size.** Average shipping weight, 1 pound.

**40V739** **$4.25**
Little Fellows' Wash Suit in the popular Oliver Twist style. White waist is of cotton poplin; pants of dark blue strong cotton fabric. Collar and cuffs are trimmed with blue band and three rows of white braid. Large pearl buttons. Pants button onto waist and have side pockets. Two buttons at knees. **SIZES—2 to 7 years. State size.** Average shpg. wt., 1 lb.

**40V735** **$3.85**
Very Pretty Two-Piece Wash Suit. Made sailor style, of heavy gray and white striped cotton Peggy cloth. Blue belt has white buckle. Embroidered emblem on sleeve. Blue collar and cuffs are braid trimmed. Fancy pearl buttons; black tie. Straight style pants have two pockets. **SIZES—3 to 8 years. State size.** Average shipping weight, 1 pound.

**For other Rompers, also Creepers, see page 271. For Boys' Overalls see pages 410 and 411.**

**For special clothing order blanks see pages 374A and 374B, or 390A and 390B.**

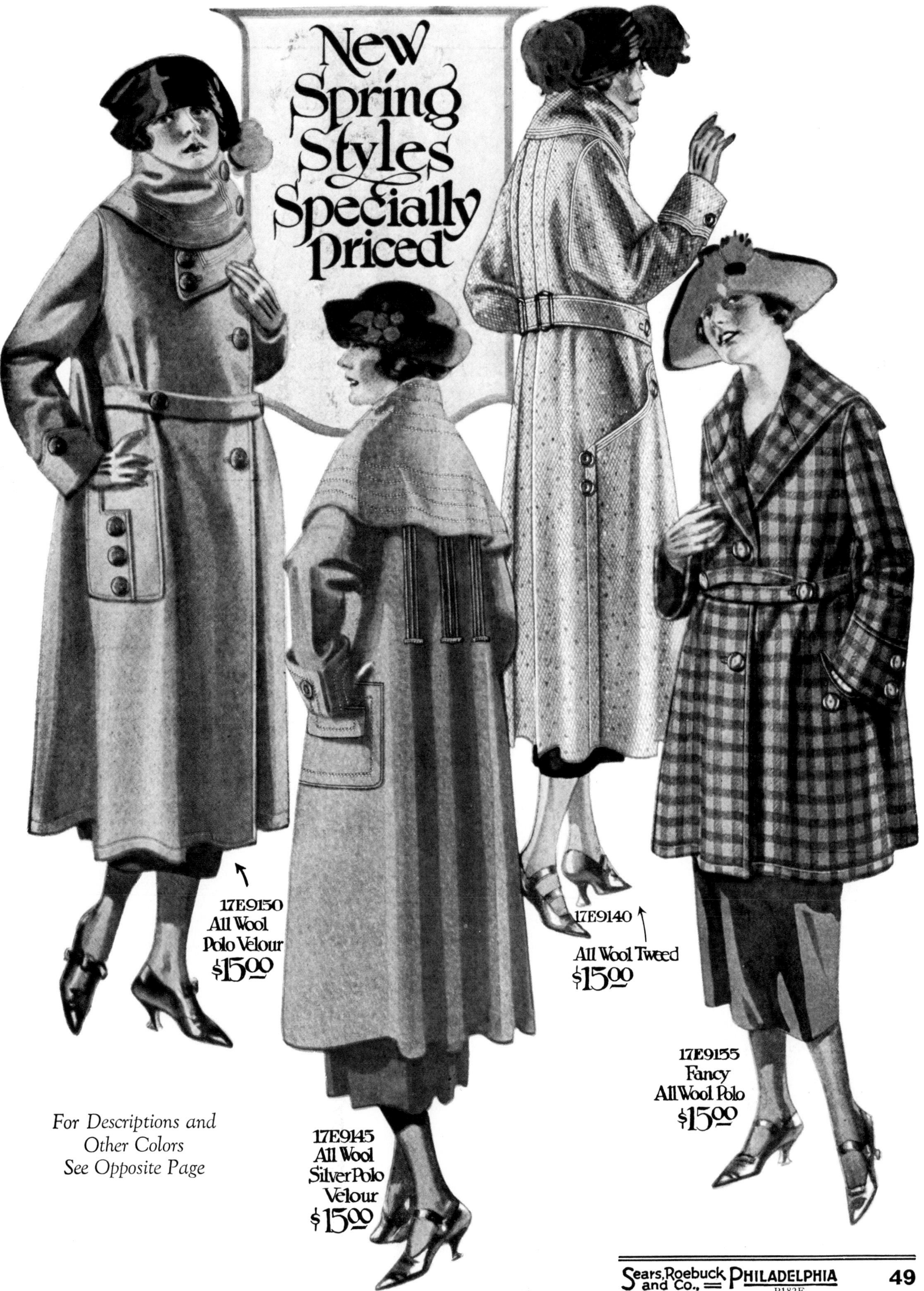
New Spring Styles Specially Priced
17E9150
All Wool
Polo Velour
$15.00
17E9140
All Wool Tweed
$15.00
17E9145
All Wool
Silver Polo
Velour
$15.00
17E9155
Fancy
All Wool Polo
$15.00

*For Descriptions and Other Colors See Opposite Page*

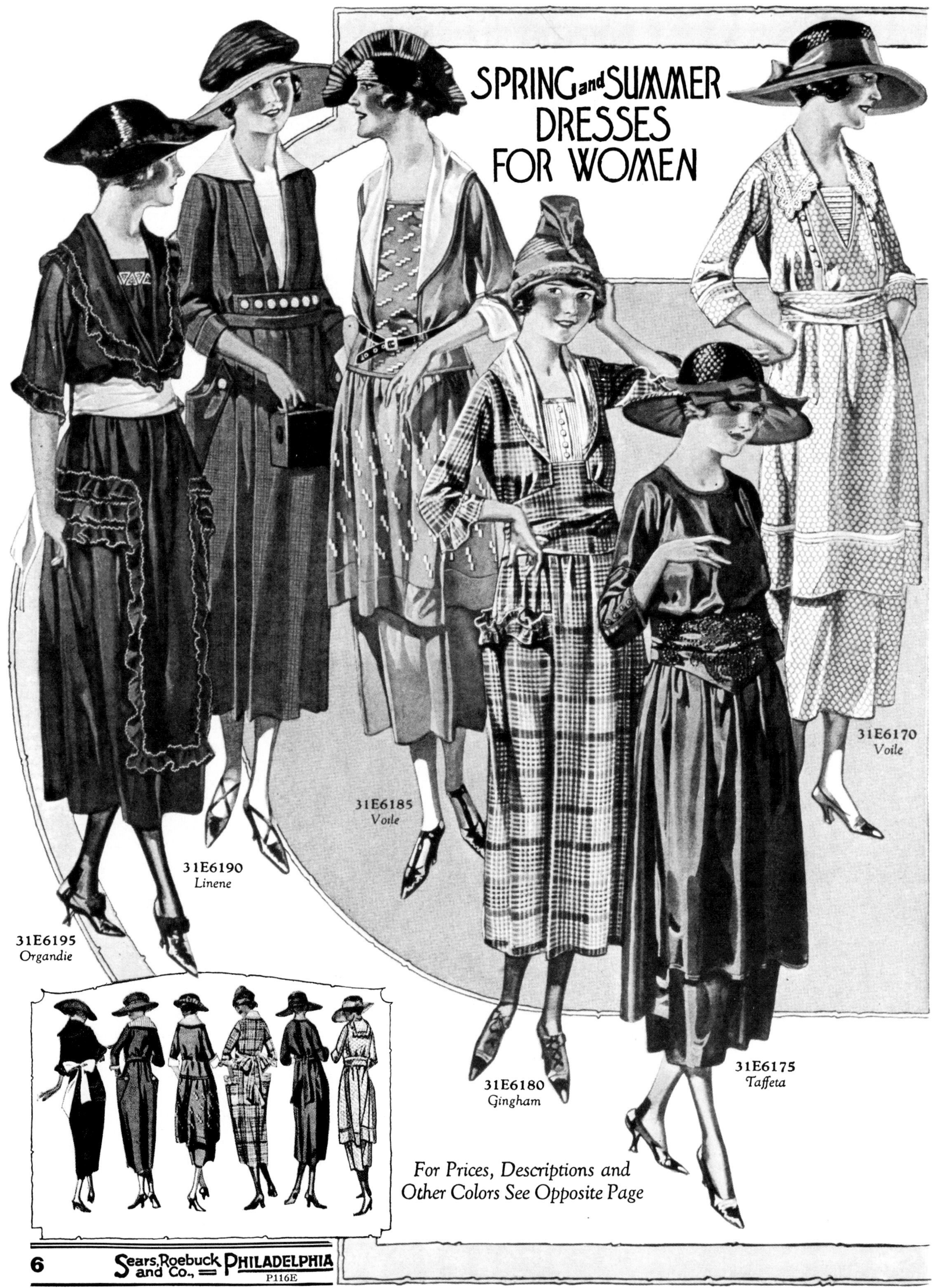
SPRING and SUMMER DRESSES FOR WOMEN
31E6195
Organdie
31E6190
Linene
31E6185
Voile
31E6180
Gingham
31E6175
Taffeta
31E6170
Voile
For Prices, Descriptions and Other Colors See Opposite Page
6
Sears, Roebuck and Co., PHILADELPHIA
P116E

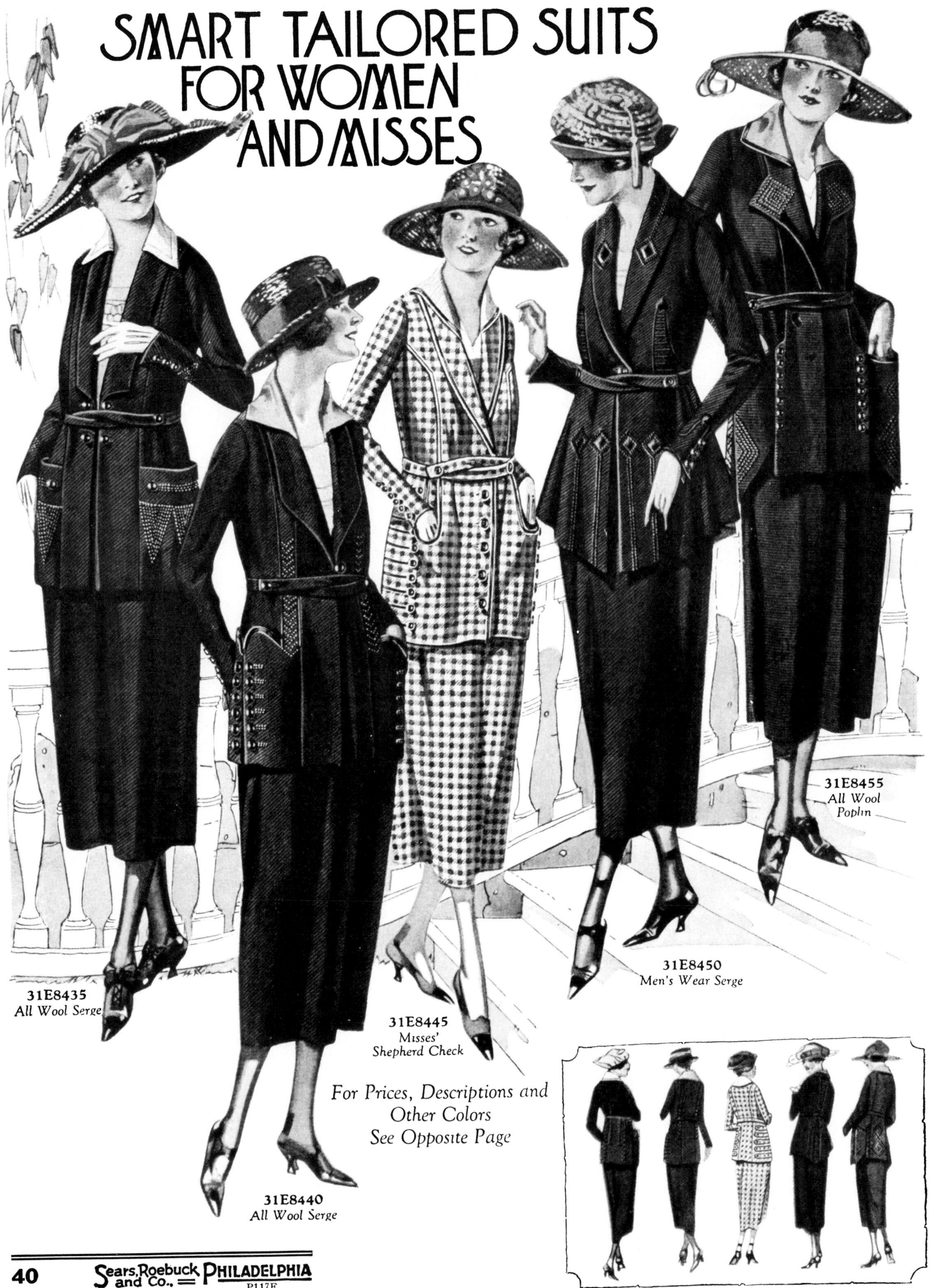
SMART TAILORED SUITS FOR WOMEN AND MISSES
31E8435
All Wool Serge
31E8440
All Wool Serge
31E8445
Misses'
Shepherd Check
31E8450
Men's Wear Serge
31E8455
All Wool
Poplin
For Prices, Descriptions and
Other Colors
See Opposite Page

# NEW STYLES CORRECTLY PRICED

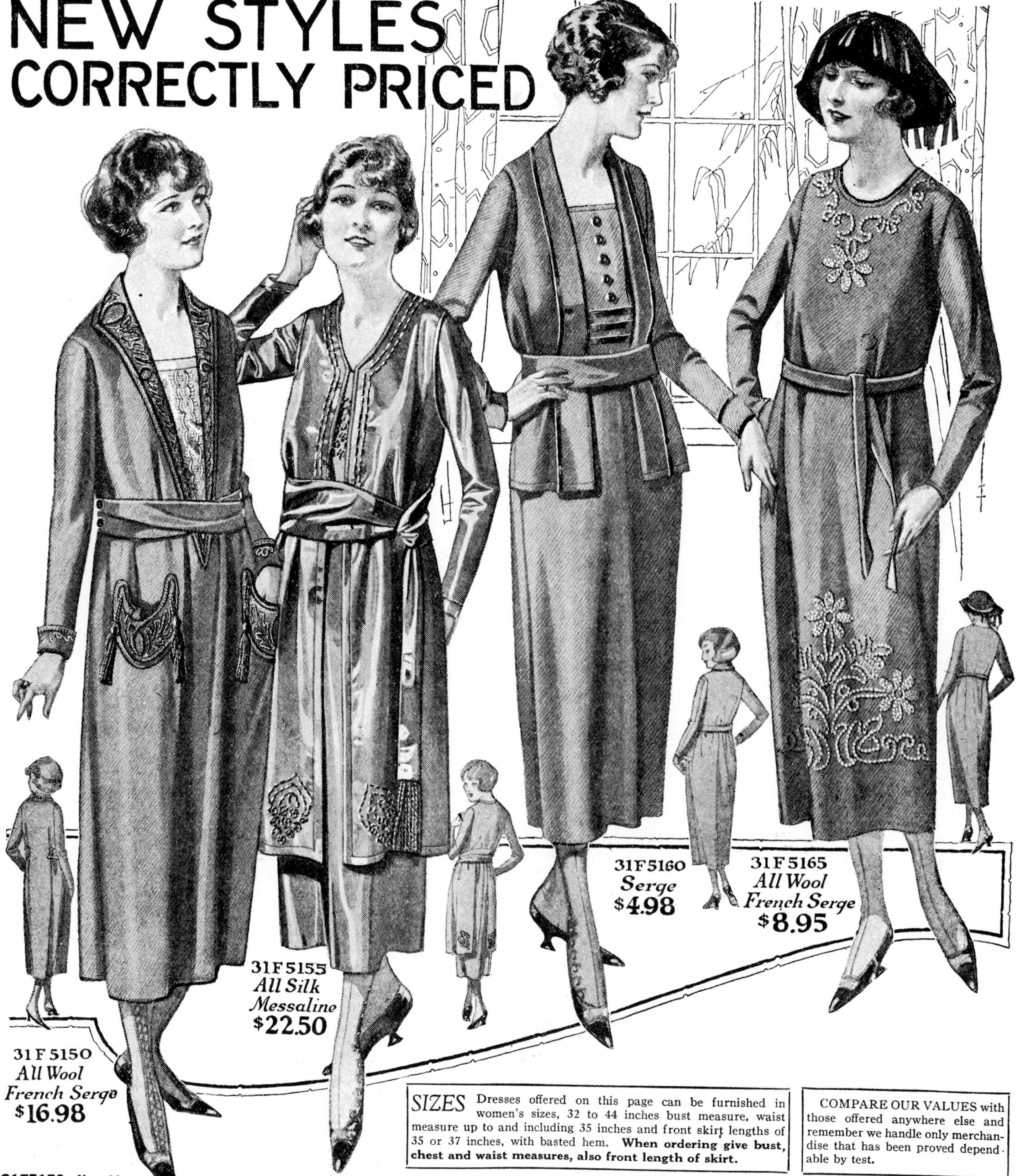


SIZES Dresses offered on this page can be furnished in women's sizes, 32 to 44 inches bust measure, waist measure up to and including 35 inches and front skirt lengths of 35 or 37 inches, with basted hem. **When ordering give bust, chest and waist measures, also front length of skirt.**

COMPARE OUR VALUES with those offered anywhere else and remember we handle only merchandise that has been proved dependable by test.

**31F5150**—Navy blue.
**31F5151**—Dark green.
**31F5152**—Black.
EACH **$16.98**

GOOD TASTE AND SPLENDID EXECUTION OF THE DESIGNER'S IDEA, is evidenced by the handsomely embroidered narrow collar rolling into the deep V tassel trimmed pockets and chic turnback cuffs of this ALL WOOL FRENCH SERGE Dress. The crossover girdle, finished at either side of the back with composition buttons, is lined with contrasting color SATIN, as are the set-on pockets. The vest of embroidered Georgette crepe adds a dainty touch and the lining of batiste may readily be detached to launder. Dress fastens at side. Average skirt sweep, 60 inches. Women's sizes, 32 to 44 inches bust measure. **Give measurements.** Average shipping weight, 2¼ pounds.

**31F5155**—Navy blue.
**31F5156**—Black.
**31F5157**—Taupe.
EACH **$22.50**

ONE MATERIAL THAT EVER FIGURES IN FASHION'S SCHEME OF THINGS, regardless of the season, is ALL SILK SATIN MESSALINE. Youthful grace has been displayed in the lines of the divided panels, so artistically trimmed with iridescent BEAD MOTIFS. The generous girdle is adjusted in a novel way—the long fringe trimmed streamer slips through a loop, having the appearance of a knot. The waist lining of good quality batiste, is neatly finished at the top with a lacy looking edging. Average skirt sweep, 56 inches. Women's sizes, 32 to 44 inches bust measure. **Give measurements.** Average shipping weight, 1¾ pounds.

**31F5160**—Navy blue.
**31F5161**—Dark wine.
**31F5162**—Black.
EACH **$4.98**

BRAID AND BUTTON TRIMMING is ever an appropriate adornment for a cloth dress and when applied as neatly as it is to this very inexpensive model, fashioned of SERGE, nearly half wool, balance cotton, the dress is really an exceptional value which we have arranged for our customers who wish a simple, sensible dress at a low price. The long braid trimmed roll collar is continued below the belt onto the small peplums in a Tuxedo effect, so very becoming to any type. The neat turnback cuffs are also bound with braid and dress closes at side. WITH A HAT TO COMPLETE YOUR OUTFIT, THIS DRESS CAN BE WORN WELL INTO THE FALL MONTHS. Average skirt sweep, 58 inches. Women's sizes, 32 to 44 inches bust measure. **Give measurements.** Average shipping weight, 2 pounds.

**31F5165**—Navy blue.
**31F5166**—Dark brown.
**31F5167**—Black.
EACH **$8.95**

THE ONE-PIECE STRAIGHT LINE FROCKS STILL HOLD SWAY and, when adorned with wool embroidery in a French knot design, the result is decidedly pleasing. Dress is made of excellent quality ALL WOOL FRENCH SERGE and has waist lining of batiste. Neat tailoring is evidenced by the narrow tie belt, suggesting the waistline. Dress closes at side. For everyday wear we highly recommend this selection. A remarkable value. Av. skirt sweep, 58 in. Women's sizes, 32 to 44 inches bust measure. **Give measurements.** Av. shpg. wt., 2¼ lbs.

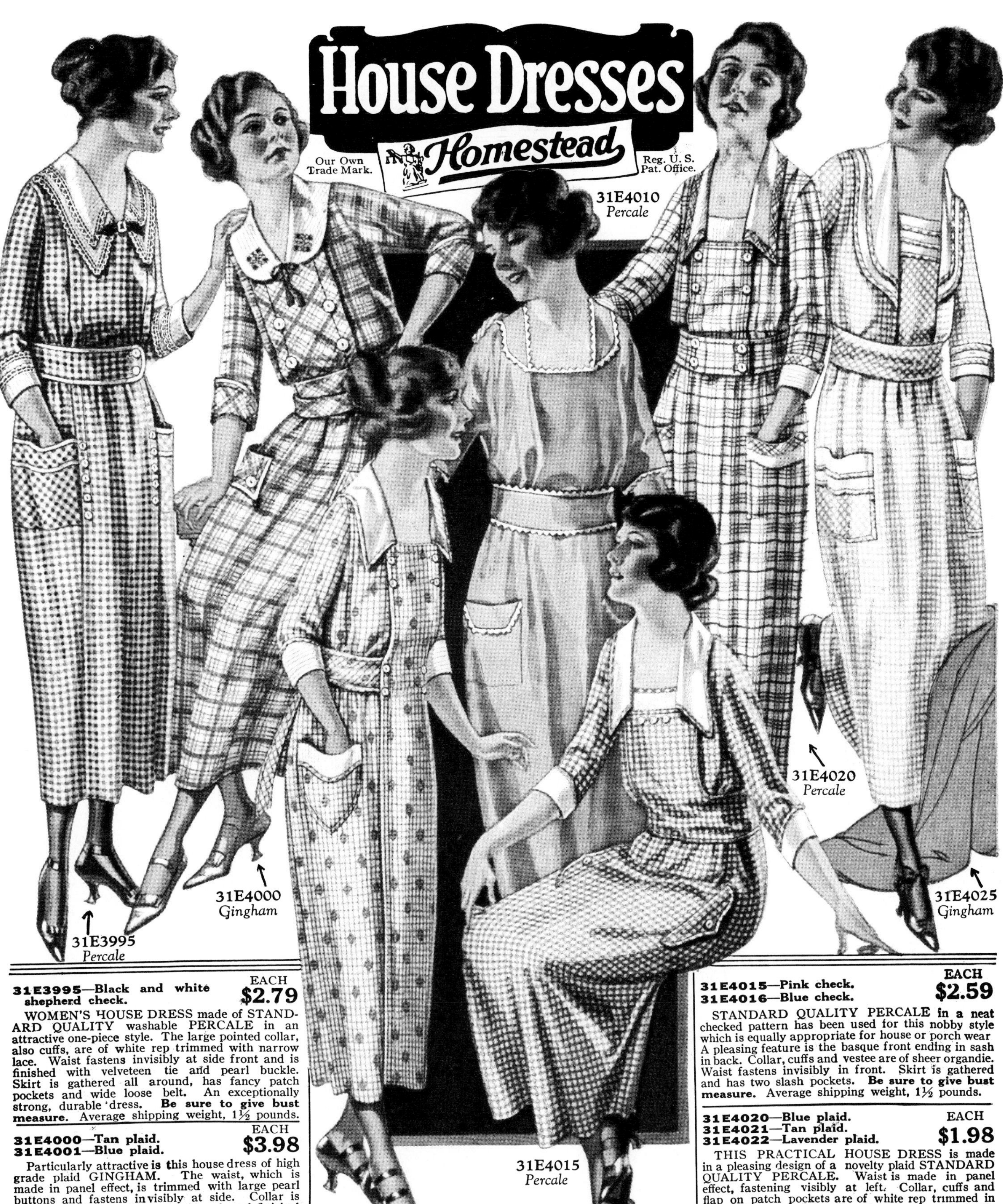


**31E3995—Black and white shepherd check.** EACH **$2.79**

WOMEN'S HOUSE DRESS made of STANDARD QUALITY washable PERCALE in an attractive one-piece style. The large pointed collar, also cuffs, are of white rep trimmed with narrow lace. Waist fastens invisibly at side front and is finished with velveteen tie and pearl buckle. Skirt is gathered all around, has fancy patch pockets and wide loose belt. An exceptionally strong, durable dress. **Be sure to give bust measure.** Average shipping weight, 1½ pounds.

**31E4000—Tan plaid.**
**31E4001—Blue plaid.** EACH **$3.98**

Particularly attractive is this house dress of high grade plaid GINGHAM. The waist, which is made in panel effect, is trimmed with large pearl buttons and fastens invisibly at side. Collar is of white poplin, prettily embroidered, and finished with cord tie. Skirt is gathered, has button trimmed pockets and wide sash tying in back. **Be sure to give bust measure.** Av. shpg. wt., 1½ lbs.

**31E4005—Blue check, green dot.**
**31E4006—Tan check, blue dot.** EACH **$2.39**

A pleasing checked pattern PERCALE of STANDARD QUALITY is used in this nobby panel front house dress. Fastening is at side of panel. The collar, cuffs and tops of pockets are of white poplin, neatly bound in checked material. The wide sash, which extends to panel in front, ties in back. A practical and comfortable dress. **Be sure to give bust measure.** Average shipping weight, 1½ pounds.

When we describe material as "STANDARD QUALITY PERCALE," we refer to a printed cloth which averages 68 threads in the warp and 56 threads in the filling to the inch, or its equivalent. When we say "Better Quality Percale," we mean something better than Standard Quality.

**31E4010—Blue.**
**31E4011—Lavender.** EACH **$1.49**

NOBBY KITCHEN DRESS of STANDARD QUALITY solid color PERCALE. The plaits at belt, on waist and skirt give it the necessary fullness. Effectively trimmed throughout with rickrack braid. Belt is stitched down in front and has the popular sash back (see small illustration). A good looking practical garment. **Be sure to give bust measure.** Average shipping weight, 1½ pounds.

**House dresses on this page are furnished in sizes 34 to 46 inches bust measure. Be sure to give bust measure when ordering.**

**31E4015—Pink check.**
**31E4016—Blue check.** EACH **$2.59**

STANDARD QUALITY PERCALE in a neat checked pattern has been used for this nobby style which is equally appropriate for house or porch wear. A pleasing feature is the basque front ending in sash in back. Collar, cuffs and vestee are of sheer organdie. Waist fastens invisibly in front. Skirt is gathered and has two slash pockets. **Be sure to give bust measure.** Average shipping weight, 1½ pounds.

**31E4020—Blue plaid.**
**31E4021—Tan plaid.**
**31E4022—Lavender plaid.** EACH **$1.98**

THIS PRACTICAL HOUSE DRESS is made in a pleasing design of a novelty plaid STANDARD QUALITY PERCALE. Waist is made in panel effect, fastening visibly at left. Collar, cuffs and flap on patch pockets are of white rep trimmed in plaid. Skirt is gathered and has wide detachable belt. **Be sure to give bust measure.** Average shipping weight, 1½ pounds.

**31E4025—Blue check.**
**31E4026—Pink check.** EACH **$2.98**

The double collar and cuffs of sheer white organdie lend a smart touch to this nobby house dress of STANDARD QUALITY checked GINGHAM. Waist is made with vestee effect front and fastens invisibly. Skirt is gathered and has wide loose sash tying in back. An especially becoming dress. **Be sure to give bust measure.** Average shipping weight, 1½ pounds.

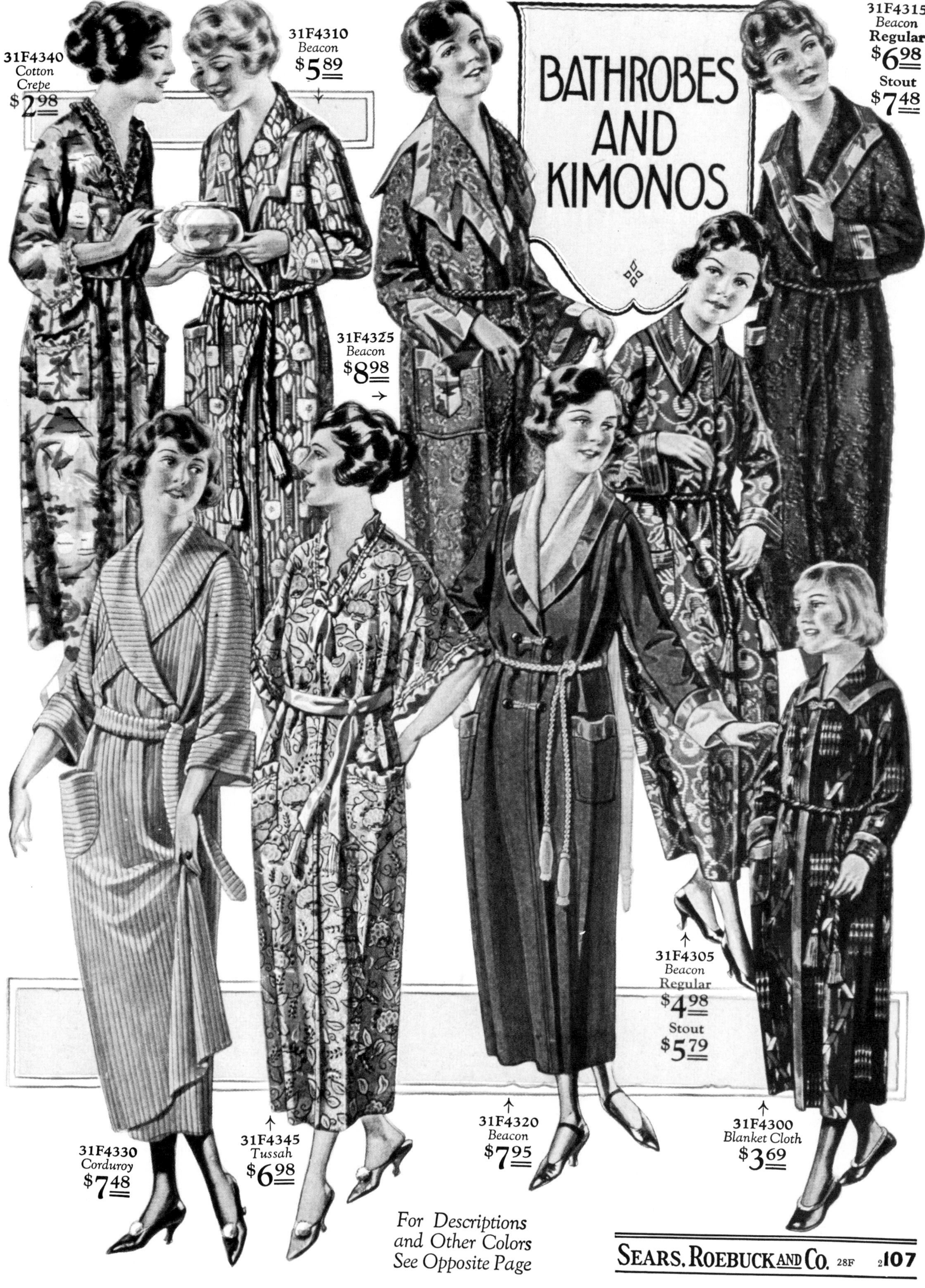
BATHROBES AND KIMONOS
31F4340
Cotton Crepe
$2.98
31F4310
Beacon
$5.89
31F4315
Beacon
Regular
$6.98
Stout
$7.48
31F4325
Beacon
$8.98
31F4305
Beacon
Regular
$4.98
Stout
$5.79
31F4330
Corduroy
$7.48
31F4345
Tussah
$6.98
31F4320
Beacon
$7.95
31F4300
Blanket Cloth
$3.69
For Descriptions
and Other Colors
See Opposite Page
SEARS, ROEBUCK AND CO. 28F 2107

# A Spring and Fall Necessity Rain

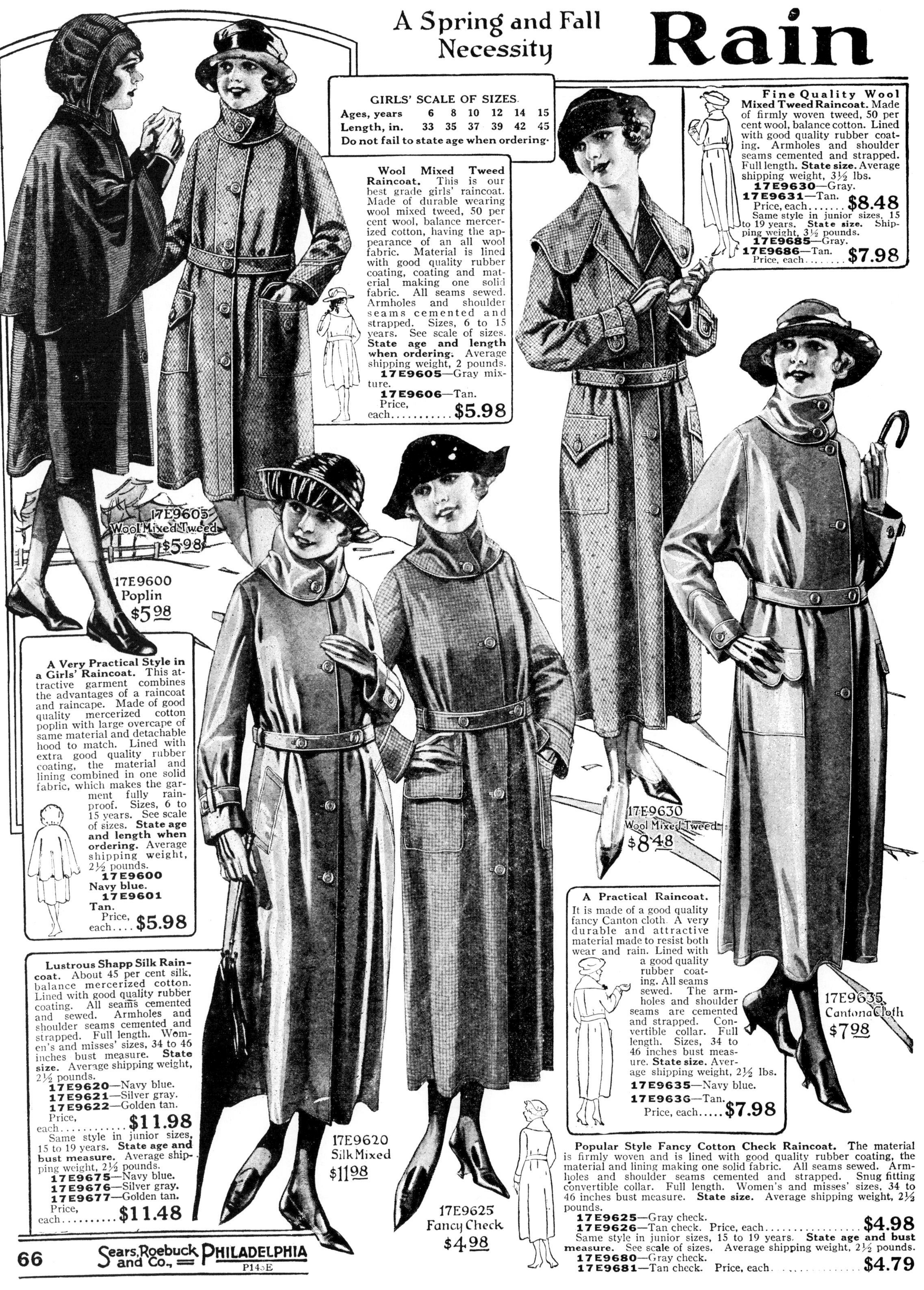


| GIRLS' SCALE OF SIZES | | | | | | |
|---|---|---|---|---|---|---|
| Ages, years | 6 | 8 | 10 | 12 | 14 | 15 |
| Length, in. | 33 | 35 | 37 | 39 | 42 | 45 |

Do not fail to state age when ordering.

**Wool Mixed Tweed Raincoat.** This is our best grade girls' raincoat. Made of durable wearing wool mixed tweed, 50 per cent wool, balance mercerized cotton, having the appearance of an all wool fabric. Material is lined with good quality rubber coating, coating and material making one solid fabric. All seams sewed. Armholes and shoulder seams cemented and strapped. Sizes, 6 to 15 years. See scale of sizes. **State age and length when ordering.** Average shipping weight, 2 pounds.
**17E9605**—Gray mixture.
**17E9606**—Tan. Price, each........... **$5.98**

**Fine Quality Wool Mixed Tweed Raincoat.** Made of firmly woven tweed, 50 per cent wool, balance cotton. Lined with good quality rubber coating. Armholes and shoulder seams cemented and strapped. Full length. **State size.** Average shipping weight, 3½ lbs.
**17E9630**—Gray.
**17E9631**—Tan. Price, each....... **$8.48**
Same style in junior sizes, 15 to 19 years. **State size.** Shipping weight, 3½ pounds.
**17E9685**—Gray.
**17E9686**—Tan. Price, each....... **$7.98**

**A Very Practical Style in a Girls' Raincoat.** This attractive garment combines the advantages of a raincoat and raincape. Made of good quality mercerized cotton poplin with large overcape of same material and detachable hood to match. Lined with extra good quality rubber coating, the material and lining combined in one solid fabric, which makes the garment fully rainproof. Sizes, 6 to 15 years. See scale of sizes. **State age and length when ordering.** Average shipping weight, 2½ pounds.
**17E9600** Navy blue.
**17E9601** Tan. Price, each.... **$5.98**

**Lustrous Shapp Silk Raincoat.** About 45 per cent silk, balance mercerized cotton. Lined with good quality rubber coating. All seams cemented and sewed. Armholes and shoulder seams cemented and strapped. Full length. Women's and misses' sizes, 34 to 46 inches bust measure. **State size.** Average shipping weight, 2½ pounds.
**17E9620**—Navy blue.
**17E9621**—Silver gray.
**17E9622**—Golden tan. Price, each........... **$11.98**
Same style in junior sizes, 15 to 19 years. **State age and bust measure.** Average shipping weight, 2½ pounds.
**17E9675**—Navy blue.
**17E9676**—Silver gray.
**17E9677**—Golden tan. Price, each.......... **$11.48**

**A Practical Raincoat.** It is made of a good quality fancy Canton cloth. A very durable and attractive material made to resist both wear and rain. Lined with a good quality rubber coating. All seams sewed. The armholes and shoulder seams are cemented and strapped. Convertible collar. Full length. Sizes, 34 to 46 inches bust measure. **State size.** Average shipping weight, 2½ lbs.
**17E9635**—Navy blue.
**17E9636**—Tan. Price, each..... **$7.98**

**Popular Style Fancy Cotton Check Raincoat.** The material is firmly woven and is lined with good quality rubber coating, the material and lining making one solid fabric. All seams sewed. Armholes and shoulder seams cemented and strapped. Snug fitting convertible collar. Full length. Women's and misses' sizes, 34 to 46 inches bust measure. **State size.** Average shipping weight, 2½ pounds.
**17E9625**—Gray check.
**17E9626**—Tan check. Price, each................ **$4.98**
Same style in junior sizes, 15 to 19 years. **State age and bust measure.** See scale of sizes. Average shipping weight, 2½ pounds.
**17E9680**—Gray check.
**17E9681**—Tan check. Price, each................ **$4.79**

# OUTDOOR APPAREL

## FOR WORK OR SPORT

These togs will prove very pleasant aids for almost any outdoor sport—horseback, bicycle and auto riding, motorcycling, mountain climbing, etc. The styles are very sensible and appropriate, as they are made to give plenty of freedom for movement, ease and comfort. For country excursions, hiking, climbing, or everyday work on the farm or in the garden, nothing could be more fitting than the divided riding skirts we offer in various materials. To fully enjoy your hours of recreation and sport, you will need one of these suits, dresses or skirts.

***SIZES*** Riding and Outing Apparel shown on this page is furnished in the following sizes: SKIRTS, from 22 to 32 inches waist measure and 34 to 41 inches front length of skirt. **State waist and hip measures and front length of skirt.** RIDING HABITS, DRESSES, SUITS AND OUTFITS, from 32 to 44 inches bust measure, 22 to 32 inches waist measure and 34 to 41 inches front length of skirt. **State bust, waist and hip measures, also front length of skirt.** MIDDY, from 32 to 44 inches bust measure. When ordering 31E8555, 31E8557, 31E8558 and outfits **state calf measure** in addition to other measurements. LEGGINGS, sizes, 12, 13, 14 and 15 inches calf measure. **State calf measure.** All skirts and dresses furnished with open basted hem.

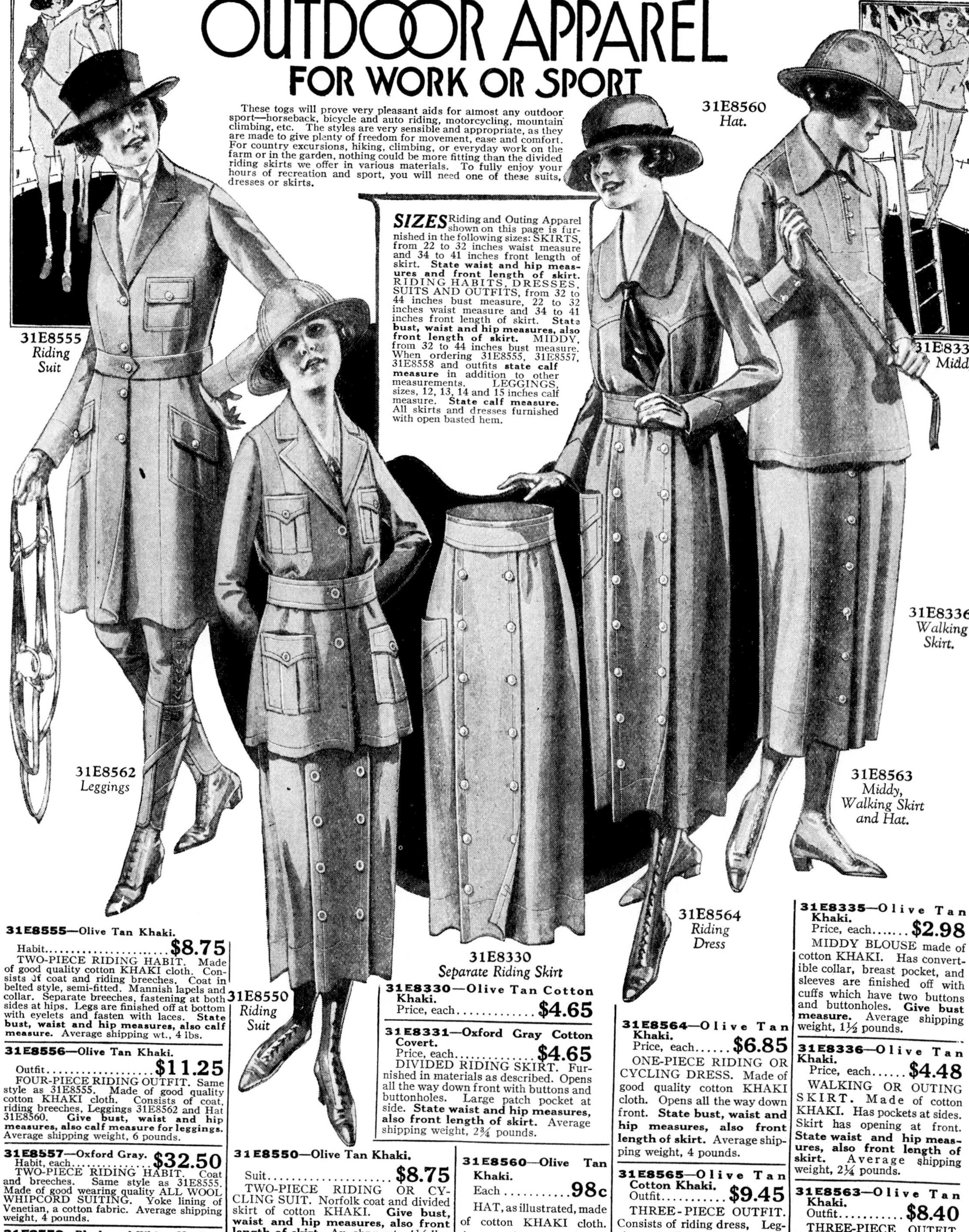

31E8555 *Riding Suit*

31E8560 *Hat.*

31E8335 *Middy.*

31E8336 *Walking Skirt.*

31E8562 *Leggings*

31E8563 *Middy, Walking Skirt and Hat.*

31E8564 *Riding Dress*

31E8330 *Separate Riding Skirt*

31E8550 *Riding Suit*

**31E8555—Olive Tan Khaki.**
Habit.......................... **$8.75**
TWO-PIECE RIDING HABIT. Made of good quality cotton KHAKI cloth. Consists of coat and riding breeches. Coat in belted style, semi-fitted. Mannish lapels and collar. Separate breeches, fastening at both sides at hips. Legs are finished off at bottom with eyelets and fasten with laces. **State bust, waist and hip measures, also calf measure.** Average shipping wt., 4 lbs.

**31E8556—Olive Tan Khaki.**
Outfit.................... **$11.25**
FOUR-PIECE RIDING OUTFIT. Same style as 31E8555. Made of good quality cotton KHAKI cloth. Consists of coat, riding breeches, Leggings 31E8562 and Hat 31E8560. **Give bust, waist and hip measures, also calf measure for leggings.** Average shipping weight, 6 pounds.

**31E8557—Oxford Gray.**
Habit, each................ **$32.50**
TWO-PIECE RIDING HABIT. Coat and breeches. Same style as 31E8555. Made of good wearing quality ALL WOOL WHIPCORD SUITING. Yoke lining of Venetian, a cotton fabric. Average shipping weight, 4 pounds.

**31E8558—Black and White Check.**
Habit, each.................. **$9.58**
TWO-PIECE RIDING HABIT. Made of checked SUITING, about one-half wool and one-half cotton. Consists of coat and riding breeches. Coat in semi-fitted style, with full flare. Patch pocket at each side. Breast pocket. Separate breeches, buttoning at both sides at hips. This style is very similar to Suit 31E8555, but it has no belt and has buttons on the legs instead of lacings. **State bust, waist and hip measures, also calf measure.** Average shipping wt., 4 lbs.

**31E8330—Olive Tan Cotton Khaki.**
Price, each............. **$4.65**

**31E8331—Oxford Gray Cotton Covert.**
Price, each............. **$4.65**
DIVIDED RIDING SKIRT. Furnished in materials as described. Opens all the way down front with buttons and buttonholes. Large patch pocket at side. **State waist and hip measures, also front length of skirt.** Average shipping weight, 2¾ pounds.

**31E8550—Olive Tan Khaki.**
Suit.................... **$8.75**
TWO-PIECE RIDING OR CYCLING SUIT. Norfolk coat and divided skirt of cotton KHAKI. **Give bust, waist and hip measures, also front length of skirt.** Av. shpg. wt., 4½ lbs.

**31E8551—Olive Tan Khaki.**
Outfit................. **$11.25**
FOUR-PIECE OUTFIT. Norfolk coat, divided skirt, Leggings 31E8562 and Hat 31E8560 to match. Made of cotton KHAKI. **Give bust, waist and hip measures, also front length of skirt and calf measure for leggings.** Average shipping weight, 7½ pounds.

**31E8560—Olive Tan Khaki.**
Each........... **98c**
HAT, as illustrated, made of cotton KHAKI cloth. Average shpg. wt., 1 lb.

**31E8562—Olive Tan Cotton Khaki.**
Per pair..... **$1.65**
LEGGINGS, as illustrated. See size paragraph. **Average shpg. wt., 1½ lbs.**

**31E8564—Olive Tan Khaki.**
Price, each...... **$6.85**
ONE-PIECE RIDING OR CYCLING DRESS. Made of good quality cotton KHAKI cloth. Opens all the way down front. **State bust, waist and hip measures, also front length of skirt.** Average shipping weight, 4 pounds.

**31E8565—Olive Tan Cotton Khaki.**
Outfit.......... **$9.45**
THREE-PIECE OUTFIT. Consists of riding dress, Leggings 31E8562 and Hat 31E8560 to match. **Give bust, waist and hip measures, front length of skirt, also calf measure for leggings.** Average shipping weight, 6 pounds.

**31E8335—Olive Tan Khaki.**
Price, each....... **$2.98**
MIDDY BLOUSE made of cotton KHAKI. Has convertible collar, breast pocket, and sleeves are finished off with cuffs which have two buttons and buttonholes. **Give bust measure.** Average shipping weight, 1½ pounds.

**31E8336—Olive Tan Khaki.**
Price, each...... **$4.48**
WALKING OR OUTING SKIRT. Made of cotton KHAKI. Has pockets at sides. Skirt has opening at front. **State waist and hip measures, also front length of skirt.** Average shipping weight, 2¼ pounds.

**31E8563—Olive Tan Khaki.**
Outfit.......... **$8.40**
THREE-PIECE OUTFIT, consisting of Middy 31E8335, Walking Skirt 31E8336 and Hat 31E8560. Made of cotton KHAKI. **Give bust, waist and hip measures, also front length of skirt.** Average shipping weight, 4¼ pounds.

# SILK UNDERWEAR

In our silk underwear, we aim to give our customers the wearing qualities expected by the wearer of this class of underwear. High grade silks are always the most satisfactory, not only in beauty but in the longer service they will give. Our prices are reasonably lower than you can find elsewhere for the same quality merchandise. You will find the workmanship the very best, and absolutely guaranteed to give you satisfaction.

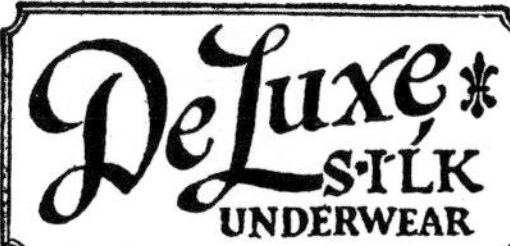


**Price, Each, $2.98**
**38E9744**—Flesh.
**Women's Silk Crepe de Chine Envelope Chemise.** Step-in style. Neatly trimmed in front with rows of lace insertion. Top and bottom edged with lace to match. Set off with rosettes. Has silk ribbon shoulder straps and draw string. Sizes, 34 to 44 inches bust measure. **State size.** Shipping weight, 12 oz. →

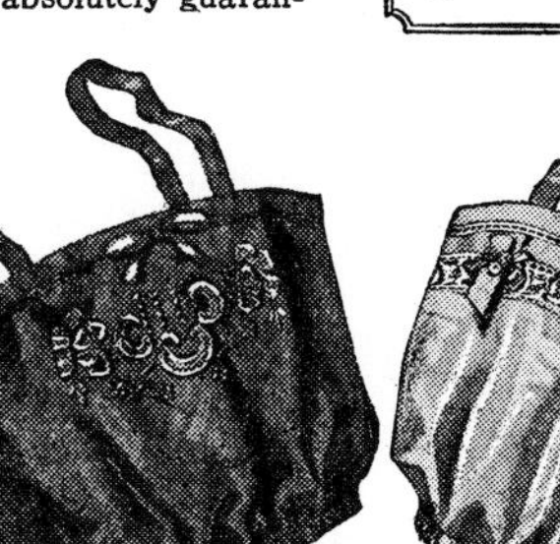

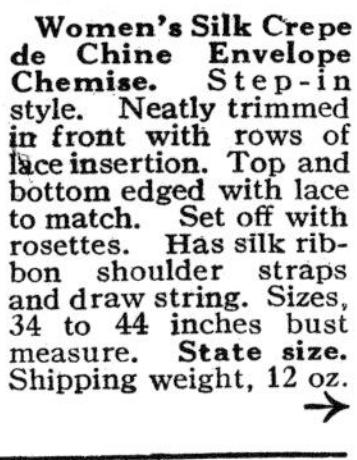

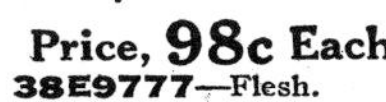

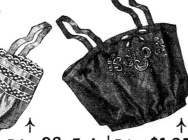

**Price, 98c Each**
**38E9777**—Flesh.
**Women's Slipover Style Camisole.** Made of good quality washable satin. Front and back trimmed with Valenciennes lace insertion and edge. Has ribbon shoulder straps and draw string. Elastic at waist. A good value. Sizes, 34 to 44 inches bust measure. **State size.** Shipping weight, 10 ounces.

**Price, $1.85 Each**
**38E9778**—Navy blue.
**38E9775**—Dark brown.
**Women's Camisole.** Slipover style. Made of good quality washable satin. Front is attractively trimmed with fancy embroidery work in beautiful colors. A very popular style. Finished at top with hemstitching. Has ribbon shoulder straps and draw string. Elastic at waist. Sizes, 34 to 44 inches bust measure. **State size.** Shipping weight, 10 oz.

**Price, $1.58 Each**
**38E9779**—Flesh.
**Women's Slipover Style Camisole.** Body made of washable satin. Top of Georgette crepe and attractive lace insertion, neatly hemstitched and set off with rosettes. Silk ribbon shoulder straps and draw string. Elastic at waist. Sizes, 34 to 44 inches bust measure. **State size.** Shipping weight, 10 ounces.

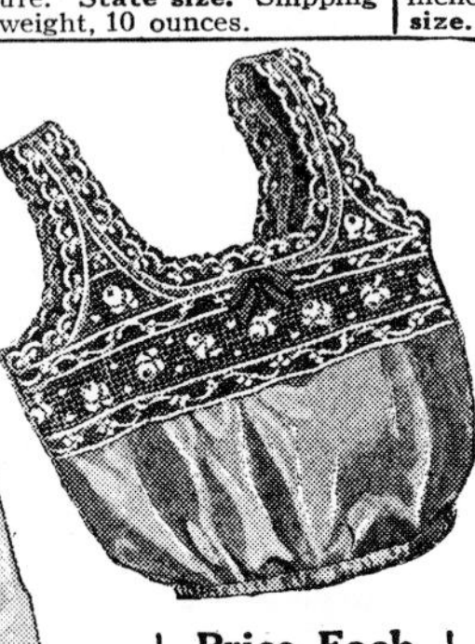

**Price, Each, $1.89**
**38E9780**
Flesh.
**Women's Washable Satin Slipover Style Corset Cover.** Front and back made of good quality lace insertion. Lace shoulder straps to match. Has ribbon draw. Elastic at waist. Sizes, 34 to 44 inches bust measure. **State size.** Shipping weight, 10 ounces.

**Price, Each, $1.78**
**38E9781**
Flesh.
**Women's Good Quality Crepe de Chine Corset Cover.** Front and back trimmed with good quality Valenciennes lace insertion and edge. Front also set off with fancy embroidery work in light colors. Has ribbon draw. Elastic at waist. Sizes, 34 to 44 inches bust measure. **State size.** Shipping weight, 10 ounces.

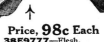

**Price, Each, $3.48**
**38E9742**—Flesh.
**Women's Envelope Chemise.** Top made of good quality washable satin, bottom of high grade crepe de chine. Front and back neatly finished with hemstitching and Valenciennes lace. This chemise is attractively set off with rosettes, pearl buttons and silk ribbon. Has silk ribbon shoulder straps which will not slip. Ribbon draw. Bottom is neatly hemstitched and edged with Valenciennes lace. Sizes, 34 to 44 inches bust measure. **State size.** Shipping weight, 12 ounces

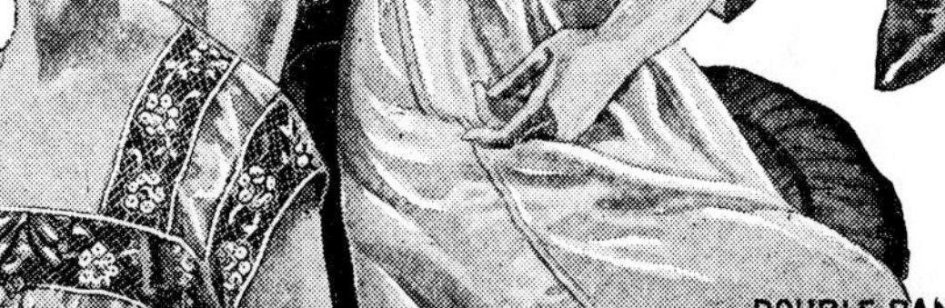


Every garment on this page is packed in an individual box.

Our Glove Silk Underwear and Kool-Est Brand are shown on page 170.

THE MORE YOU CONSIDER THE QUALITY of our goods the more impressed you will be with the fact that our prices are low. On another page of this catalog we explain what we do to make sure that the goods you buy will be right in quality.

**Price, $4.98 Each**
**38E9745**—Flesh.
**Women's Sleeveless Silk Crepe de Chine Nightgown.** Slipover style. Front and back attractively finished with assorted patterns Valenciennes lace, set off in front with rosette and shirred with hemstitching. Has ribbon draw. Sizes, 34 to 44 inches bust measure. **State size.** Shipping weight, 1 pound.

**Price, $4.98 Each**
**38E9746**—White.
**Women's Silk Underskirt.** Made of high grade washable satin. Flounce is neatly finished with shirring, hemstitching and tuck. Has double panel in front and back which makes this garment shadow-proof. An ideal garment for Spring and Summer wear. Elastic at waist. Lengths, 34 to 42 inches. **State length.** Shipping weight, 1 pound.

# AND SLEEPING SUITS

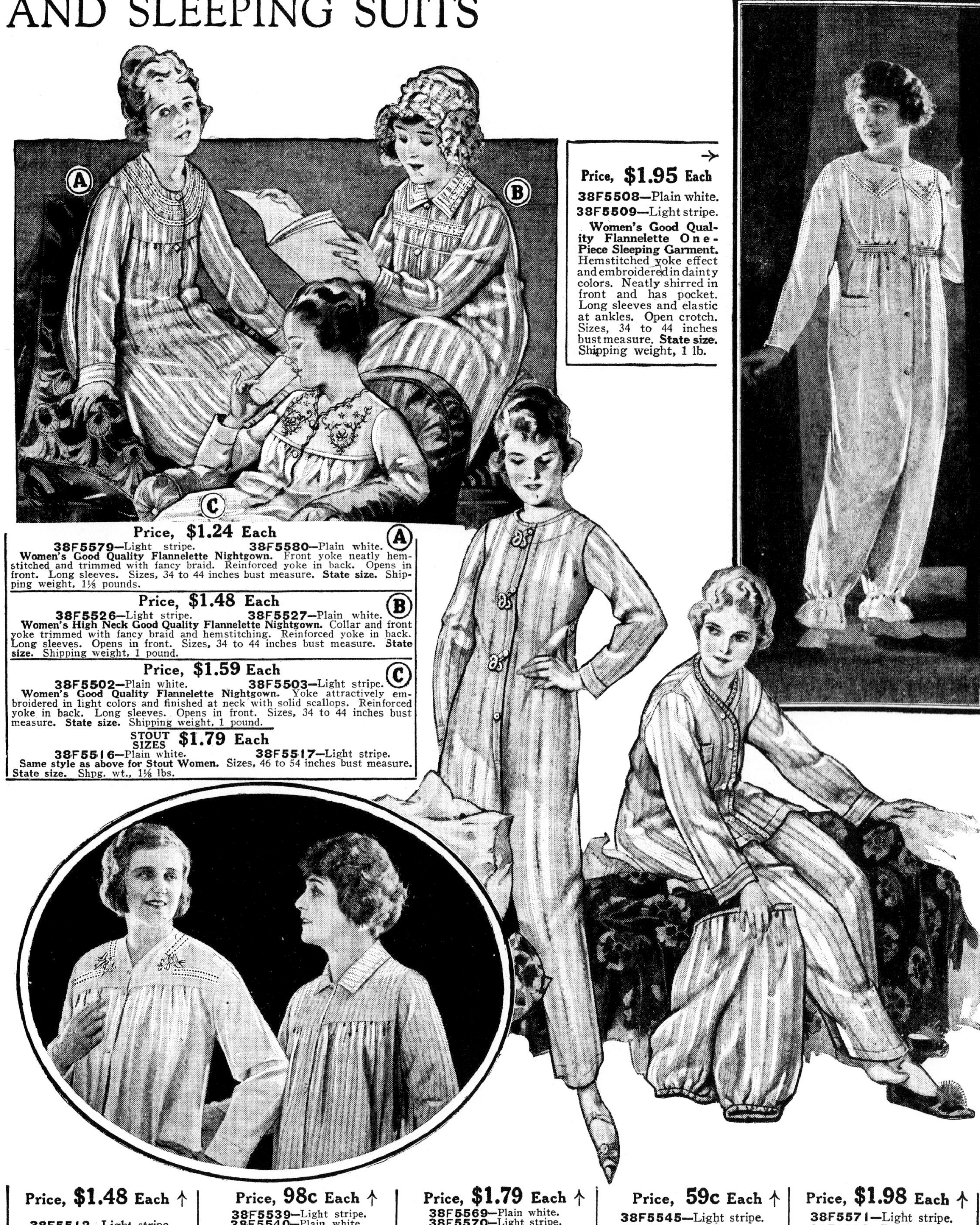

**Price, $1.95 Each** →

**38F5508**—Plain white.
**38F5509**—Light stripe.

**Women's Good Quality Flannelette One-Piece Sleeping Garment.** Hemstitched yoke effect and embroidered in dainty colors. Neatly shirred in front and has pocket. Long sleeves and elastic at ankles. Open crotch. Sizes, 34 to 44 inches bust measure. **State size.** Shipping weight, 1 lb.

**Price, $1.24 Each** (A)

**38F5579**—Light stripe. **38F5580**—Plain white.
**Women's Good Quality Flannelette Nightgown.** Front yoke neatly hemstitched and trimmed with fancy braid. Reinforced yoke in back. Opens in front. Long sleeves. Sizes, 34 to 44 inches bust measure. **State size.** Shipping weight, 1⅛ pounds.

**Price, $1.48 Each** (B)

**38F5526**—Light stripe. **38F5527**—Plain white.
**Women's High Neck Good Quality Flannelette Nightgown.** Collar and front yoke trimmed with fancy braid and hemstitching. Reinforced yoke in back. Long sleeves. Opens in front. Sizes, 34 to 44 inches bust measure. **State size.** Shipping weight, 1 pound.

**Price, $1.59 Each** (C)

**38F5502**—Plain white. **38F5503**—Light stripe.
**Women's Good Quality Flannelette Nightgown.** Yoke attractively embroidered in light colors and finished at neck with solid scallops. Reinforced yoke in back. Long sleeves. Opens in front. Sizes, 34 to 44 inches bust measure. **State size.** Shipping weight, 1 pound.

**STOUT SIZES $1.79 Each**

**38F5516**—Plain white. **38F5517**—Light stripe.
**Same style as above for Stout Women.** Sizes, 46 to 54 inches bust measure. **State size.** Shpg. wt., 1⅛ lbs.

**Price, $1.48 Each** ↑

**38F5512**—Light stripe.
**38F5513**—Plain white.

**Women's Good Quality Flannelette Nightgown.** Front yoke attractively embroidered and hemstitched in light colors. Reinforced yoke in back. Has long sleeves. Sizes, 34 to 44 inches bust measure. **State size.** Shipping weight, 1 lb.

**Price, 98c Each** ↑

**38F5539**—Light stripe.
**38F5540**—Plain white.
**Women's High Neck Good Quality Flannelette Nightgown With Collar.** Reinforced yoke in back. Long sleeves and opens in front. Sizes, 34 to 44 inches bust measure. **State size.** Shpg. wt., 1 lb.

STOUT SIZES.
**Price, $1.18 Each**

**38F5573**—Light stripe.
**38F5574**—Plain white.
**Same as above for Stout Women.** Sizes, 46 to 54 inches bust measure. **State size.** Shpg. wt., 1¼ lbs.

**Price, $1.79 Each** ↑

**38F5569**—Plain white.
**38F5570**—Light stripe.
**Women's Good Quality Flannelette One-Piece Sleeping Garment.** Long sleeves. Has drop seat and buttons down front. Trimmed with frogs. Sizes, 34 to 44 inches bust measure. **State size.** Shipping weight, 1⅛ pounds.

STOUT SIZES.
**Price, $1.98 Each**

**38F5541**—Light stripe.
**38F5542**—Plain white.
**Same as above for Stout Women.** Sizes, 46 to 54 inches bust measure. **State size.** Shpg. wt., 1¼ lbs.

**Price, 59c Each** ↑

**38F5545**—Light stripe.
**38F5546**—Plain white.

**Women's Good Quality Flannelette Bloomers.** Well made and cut over full size pattern. Elastic at waist and knees. Sizes: Small, medium and large. **State size.** Shipping weight, 10 ounces.

**Price, $1.98 Each** ↑

**38F5571**—Light stripe.
**38F5572**—Plain white.

**Women's Two-Piece Pajama Suit.** Made of good quality flannelette and trimmed with braid. Draw string at waist of trousers. Has long sleeves and pocket. Sizes, 34 to 44 inches bust measure. **State size.** Shipping weight, 1¼ lbs.

# Carefully Selected Layettes

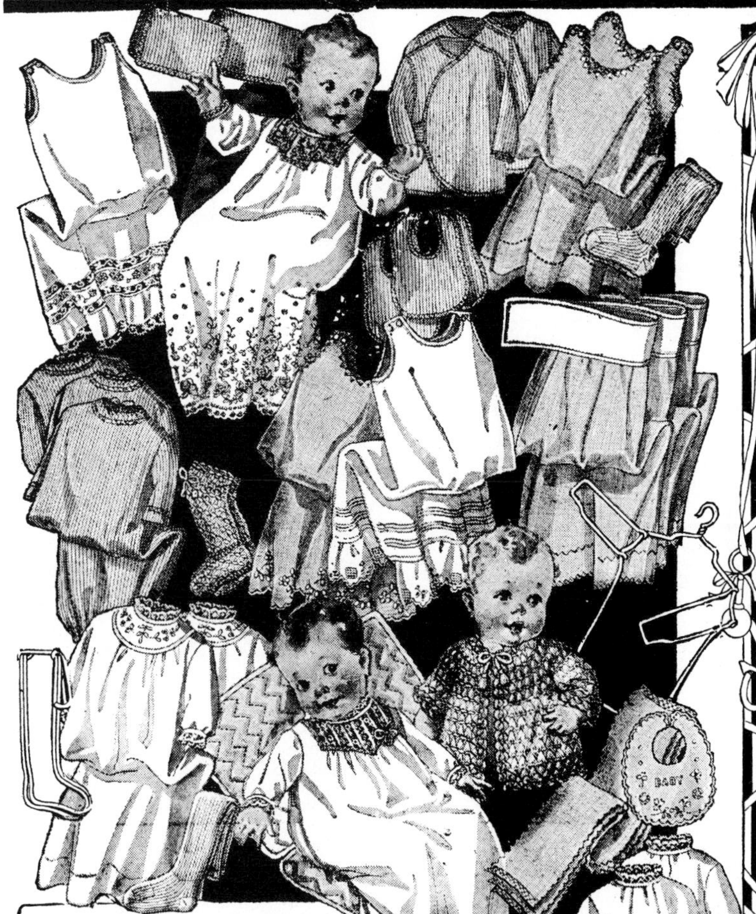

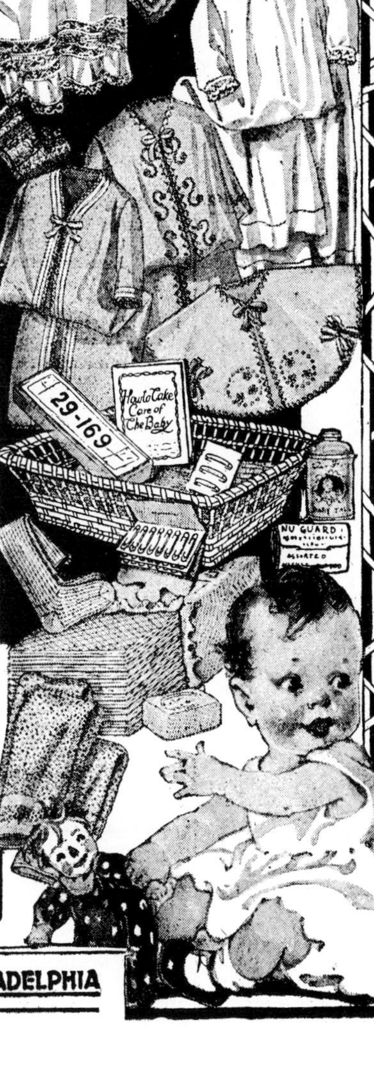

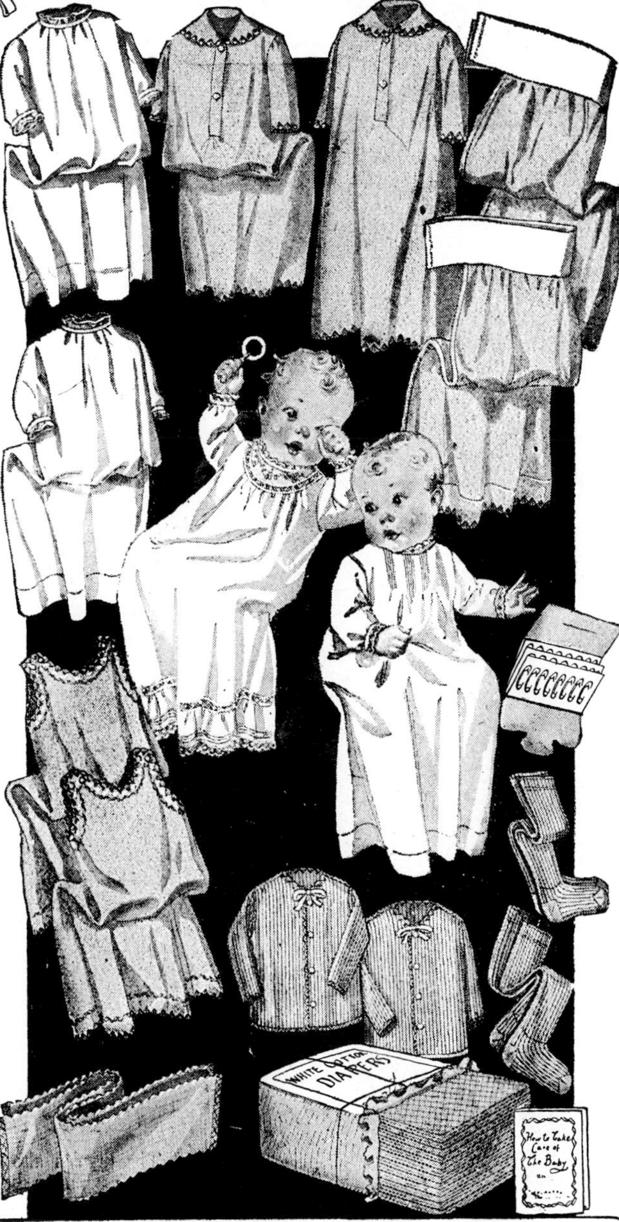

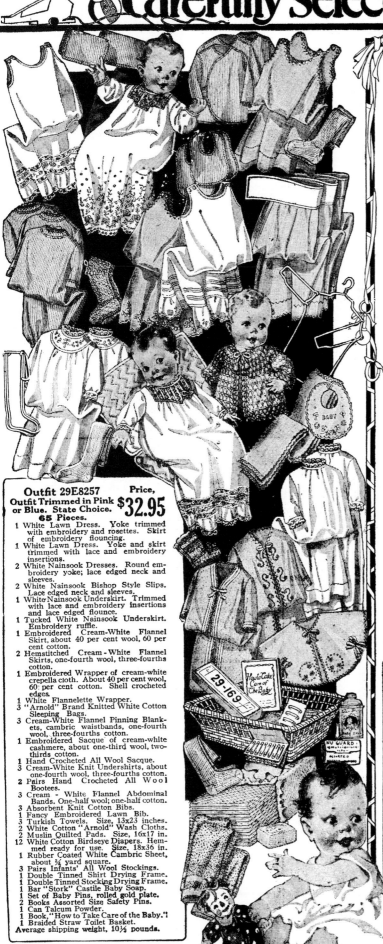

**Outfit 29E8257**

**Outfit Trimmed in Pink or Blue. State Choice.**

**Price, $32.95**

**65 Pieces.**

1 White Lawn Dress. Yoke trimmed with embroidery and rosettes. Skirt of embroidery flouncing.
1 White Lawn Dress. Yoke and skirt trimmed with lace and embroidery insertions.
2 White Nainsook Dresses. Round embroidery yoke; lace edged neck and sleeves.
2 White Nainsook Bishop Style Slips. Lace edged neck and sleeves.
1 White Nainsook Underskirt. Trimmed with lace and embroidery insertions and lace edged flounce.
1 Tucked White Nainsook Underskirt. Embroidery ruffle.
1 Embroidered Cream-White Flannel Skirt, about 40 per cent wool, 60 per cent cotton.
2 Hemstitched Cream-White Flannel Skirts, one-fourth wool, three-fourths cotton.
1 Embroidered Wrapper of cream-white crepella cloth. About 40 per cent wool, 60 per cent cotton. Shell crocheted edges.
1 White Flannelette Wrapper.
3 "Arnold" Brand Knitted White Cotton Sleeping Bags.
3 Cream-White Flannel Pinning Blankets, cambric waistbands, one-fourth wool, three-fourths cotton.
1 Embroidered Sacque of cream-white cashmere, about one-third wool, two-thirds cotton.
1 Hand Crocheted All Wool Sacque.
3 Cream-White Knit Undershirts, about one-fourth wool, three-fourths cotton.
2 Pairs Hand Crocheted All Wool Bootees.
3 Cream - White Flannel Abdominal Bands. One-half wool; one-half cotton.
3 Absorbent Knit Cotton Bibs.
1 Fancy Embroidered Lawn Bib.
3 Turkish Towels. Size, 13x23 inches.
2 White Cotton "Arnold" Wash Cloths.
2 Muslin Quilted Pads. Size, 16x17 in.
12 White Cotton Birdseye Diapers. Hemmed ready for use. Size, 18x36 in.
1 Rubber Coated White Cambric Sheet, about ¾ yard square.
3 Pairs Infants' All Wool Stockings.
1 Double Tinned Shirt Drying Frame.
1 Double Tinned Stocking Drying Frame.
1 Bar "Stork" Castile Baby Soap.
1 Set of Baby Pins, rolled gold plate.
2 Books Assorted Size Safety Pins.
1 Can Talcum Powder.
1 Book, "How to Take Care of the Baby."
1 Braided Straw Toilet Basket.

Average shipping weight, 10½ pounds.

## Our Smallest Complete Outfit

**30 Pieces** **Outfit 29E8251** **Price, $9.65**

Though made up of a smaller number of pieces, this outfit contains all the garments necessary for baby's first wardrobe. The workmanship and quality of materials are the same high standard as contained in our larger, more expensive layettes.

1 White Nainsook Dress. Round embroidered front yoke. Skirt trimmed with lace insertion and finished with lace edged tucked ruffle. Lace edge in neck and sleeves.
1 White Nainsook Dress. Tucked front. Lace edge in neck and sleeves.
2 White Nainsook Bishop Style Slips. Frill in neck and sleeves.
2 White Flannelette Gertrude Style Underskirts. Trimmed with shell crocheted edges and featherstitching. Buttons at shoulders.
2 White Flannelette Nightgowns. Shell crocheted edges.
2 White Flannelette Pinning Blankets on cambric waistband. Shell crocheted edges.
2 Knitted Cream-White Undershirts, about one-fourth wool and three-fourths cotton.
2 Cream-White Flannel Bands, one-half wool and one-half cotton.
2 Pairs All Wool Cream-White Cashmere Stockings.
12 White Cotton Birdseye Diapers. Hemmed ready for use. Size, about 20x20 inches.
1 Book Assorted Size Safety Pins.
1 Book, "How to Take Care of the Baby."

Average shipping weight, 6 pounds.

# Young Men's Stylish Overcoats

In every community you will find young men who stand apart from the crowd—well dressed young fellows who, because of the sensible originality or individuality of their wearing apparel, fairly radiate success. Those are the chaps who make a visible and forceful impression when entering business life—the kind that appeal to and attract substantial business men.

On this page we offer overcoats of character especially fitting for young men's needs of the present day. We also call your attention to the wide range of our entire overcoat and raincoat line as shown on pages 387 to 399 inclusive. From these pages we feel confident you can easily make a satisfactory selection. Simple measuring instructions are on order blanks in back of this catalog.

*TESTED MERCHANDISE IS DEPENDABLE MERCHANDISE. By testing, we can guarantee QUALITY and service. Every price we quote means unusual value.*

ALL WOOL

Overcoats on this page are ALL WOOL, except 45F4744 and 45F4745 which are 97 per cent wool.

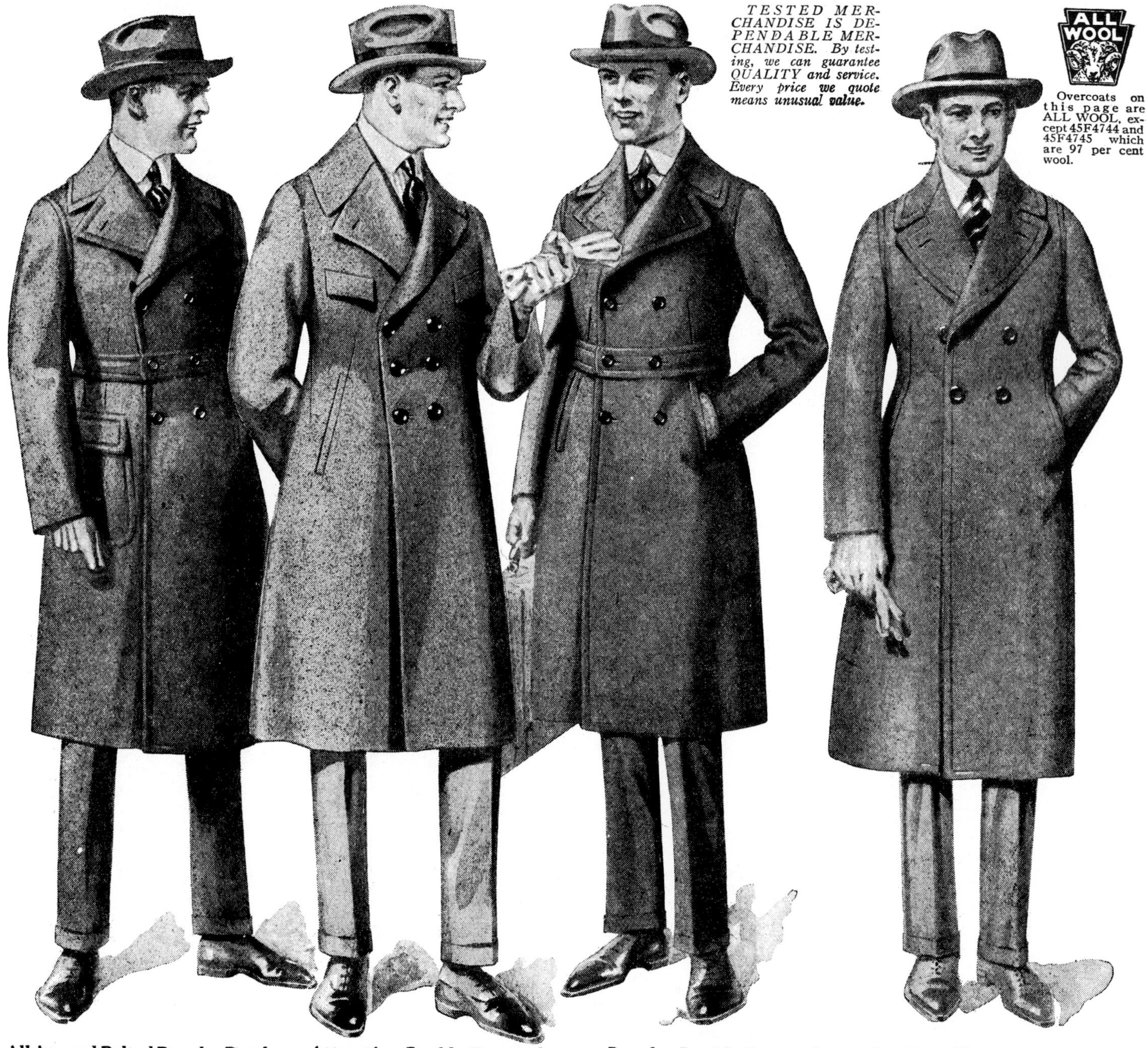

### All Around Belted Popular Patch Pocket Ulsterette.

**45F4734**—Oxford Gray.
**45F4735**—Autumn Brown. **$19.95**

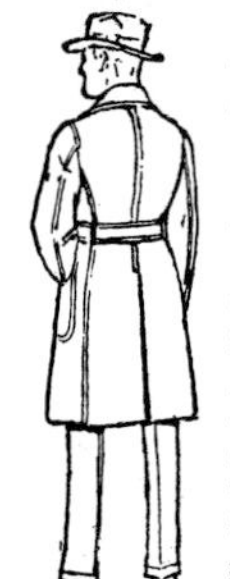

Double Breasted Ulsterette with all around belt, a fashionable model which promises to be very popular. Note the large patch pockets with flap and the convertible collar. Double stitched edges give added strength. Can be had in either the standard oxford gray or the pleasing shade of Autumn brown. Material is a very good quality heavy weight ALL WOOL overcoating, insuring warmth as well as style distinctiveness. Length, 42 inches—the length most young men wear. **SIZES—34 to 42 inches chest measure. State chest measure taken over vest.** Av. shpg. wt., 6½ lbs.

### Attractive Double Breasted Ulsterette.

**45F4732**—Brown and Blue Heather.
**45F4733**—Green Heather. **$28.50**

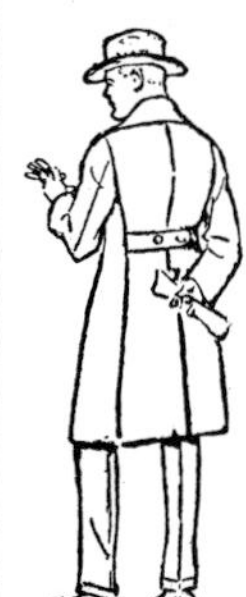

Snappy Three-Button Double Breasted Ulsterette much in favor with young men as well as older men who like youthful lines. Colorings, as noted above, are exceptionally good. The cloth is a heavy weight ALL WOOL specially woven overcoating, soft and warm. Convertible collar, two upper pockets with flap and two lower slash pockets. Venetian yoke and sleeve lining. Just the coat for wide awake young men. Length, 42 inches. **SIZES—34 to 42 inches chest measure. Give chest measure taken over vest.** Av. shpg. wt., 7½ lbs.

### Popular Double Breasted Belted Ulsterette.

**45F4744**—Brown Heather.
**45F4745**—Green Heather. **$18.50**

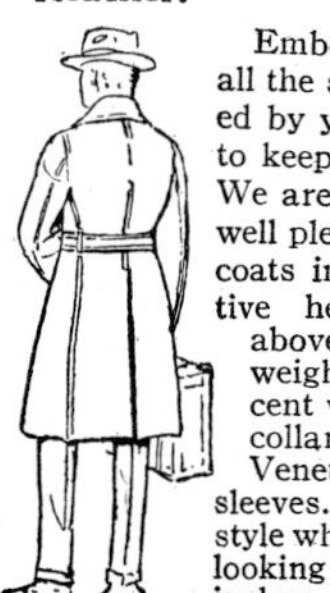

Embodied in this coat are all the style features demanded by young men who desire to keep abreast of the times. We are sure that you will be well pleased with one of these coats in either of the attractive heather shades listed above. Made from heavy weight overcoating, 97 per cent wool. Has convertible collar and slash pockets. Venetian lined in yoke and sleeves. You're sure to be in style when wearing this nobby looking "Belter." Length, 42 inches. **SIZES—34 to 42 inches chest measure. State chest measure taken over vest.** Average shipping weight, 7 pounds.

### Our Best Ulsterette—Favorite Form Fitting Model.

**45F4728**—Brown Heather.
**45F4729**—Green Heather.
**45F4730**—Dark Gray. **$36.50**

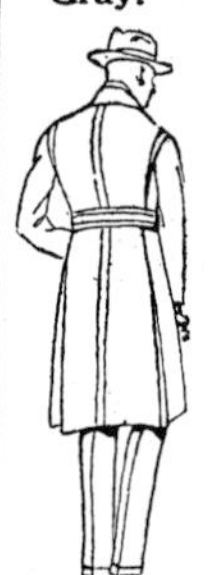

Note the smart, vigorous style of this Double Breasted Ulsterette. Made from an excellent quality good weight ALL WOOL overcoating and hand tailored throughout. Satin yoke and sleeve lining. Fashioned along rather snug fitting lines with belted back and inverted side plaits as illustrated. Convertible collar and slash pockets. Length, 42 inches. **SIZES—34 to 42 inches chest measure. Give chest measure taken over vest.** Average shipping weight, 7⅛ lbs.

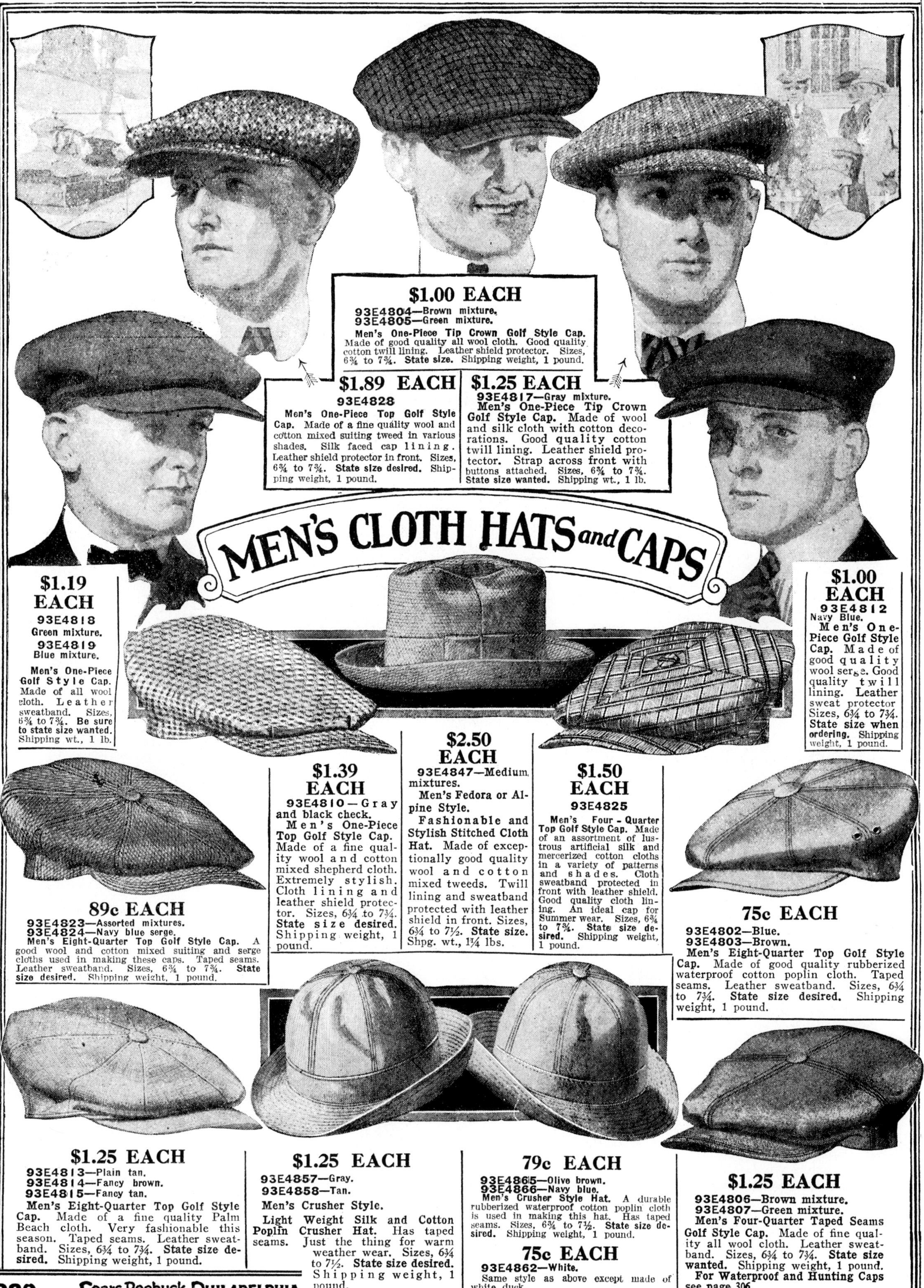

**$1.00 EACH**
93E4804—Brown mixture.
93E4805—Green mixture.
**Men's One-Piece Tip Crown Golf Style Cap.** Made of good quality all wool cloth. Good quality cotton twill lining. Leather shield protector. Sizes, 6¾ to 7¾. **State size.** Shipping weight, 1 pound.

**$1.89 EACH**
93E4828
**Men's One-Piece Top Golf Style Cap.** Made of a fine quality wool and cotton mixed suiting tweed in various shades. Silk faced cap lining. Leather shield protector in front. Sizes, 6¾ to 7¾. **State size desired.** Shipping weight, 1 pound.

**$1.25 EACH**
93E4817—Gray mixture.
**Men's One-Piece Tip Crown Golf Style Cap.** Made of wool and silk cloth with cotton decorations. Good quality cotton twill lining. Leather shield protector. Strap across front with buttons attached. Sizes, 6¾ to 7¾. **State size wanted.** Shipping wt., 1 lb.

# MEN'S CLOTH HATS and CAPS

**$1.19 EACH**
93E4818
Green mixture.
93E4819
Blue mixture.
**Men's One-Piece Golf Style Cap.** Made of all wool cloth. Leather sweatband. Sizes, 6¾ to 7¾. **Be sure to state size wanted.** Shipping wt., 1 lb.

**$1.00 EACH**
93E4812
Navy Blue.
**Men's One-Piece Golf Style Cap.** Made of good quality wool serge. Good quality twill lining. Leather sweat protector Sizes, 6¾ to 7¾. **State size when ordering.** Shipping weight, 1 pound.

**89c EACH**
93E4823—Assorted mixtures.
93E4824—Navy blue serge.
**Men's Eight-Quarter Top Golf Style Cap.** A good wool and cotton mixed suiting and serge cloths used in making these caps. Taped seams. Leather sweatband. Sizes, 6¾ to 7¾. **State size desired.** Shipping weight, 1 pound.

**$1.39 EACH**
93E4810—Gray and black check.
**Men's One-Piece Top Golf Style Cap.** Made of a fine quality wool and cotton mixed shepherd cloth. Extremely stylish. Cloth lining and leather shield protector. Sizes, 6¾ to 7¾. **State size desired.** Shipping weight, 1 pound.

**$2.50 EACH**
93E4847—Medium mixtures.
**Men's Fedora or Alpine Style.**
**Fashionable and Stylish Stitched Cloth Hat.** Made of exceptionally good quality wool and cotton mixed tweeds. Twill lining and sweatband protected with leather shield in front. Sizes, 6¾ to 7½. **State size.** Shpg. wt., 1¼ lbs.

**$1.50 EACH**
93E4825
**Men's Four-Quarter Top Golf Style Cap.** Made of an assortment of lustrous artificial silk and mercerized cotton cloths in a variety of patterns and shades. Cloth sweatband protected in front with leather shield. Good quality cloth lining. An ideal cap for Summer wear. Sizes, 6¾ to 7¾. **State size desired.** Shipping weight, 1 pound.

**75c EACH**
93E4802—Blue.
93E4803—Brown.
**Men's Eight-Quarter Top Golf Style Cap.** Made of good quality rubberized waterproof cotton poplin cloth. Taped seams. Leather sweatband. Sizes, 6¾ to 7¾. **State size desired.** Shipping weight, 1 pound.

**$1.25 EACH**
93E4813—Plain tan.
93E4814—Fancy brown.
93E4815—Fancy tan.
**Men's Eight-Quarter Top Golf Style Cap.** Made of a fine quality Palm Beach cloth. Very fashionable this season. Taped seams. Leather sweatband. Sizes, 6¾ to 7¾. **State size desired.** Shipping weight, 1 pound.

**$1.25 EACH**
93E4857—Gray.
93E4858—Tan.
**Men's Crusher Style.**
**Light Weight Silk and Cotton Poplin Crusher Hat.** Has taped seams. Just the thing for warm weather wear. Sizes, 6¾ to 7½. **State size desired.** Shipping weight, 1 pound.

**79c EACH**
93E4865—Olive brown.
93E4866—Navy blue.
**Men's Crusher Style Hat.** A durable rubberized waterproof cotton poplin cloth is used in making this hat. Has taped seams. Sizes, 6¾ to 7½. **State size desired.** Shipping weight, 1 pound.

**75c EACH**
93E4862—White.
Same style as above except made of white duck.

**$1.25 EACH**
93E4806—Brown mixture.
93E4807—Green mixture.
**Men's Four-Quarter Taped Seams Golf Style Cap.** Made of fine quality all wool cloth. Leather sweatband. Sizes, 6¾ to 7¾. **State size wanted.** Shipping weight, 1 pound.
**For Waterproof and Hunting Caps see page 306.**

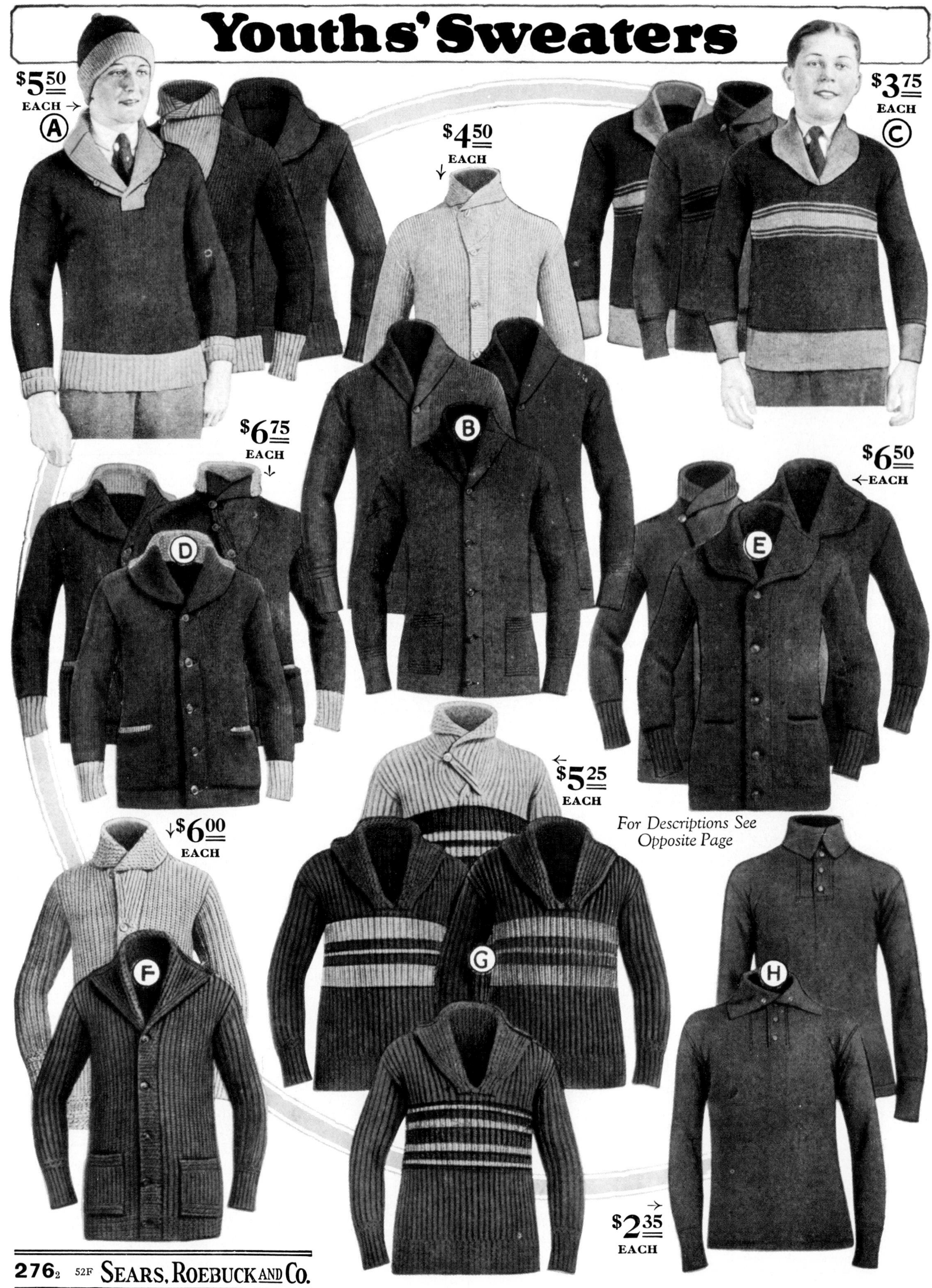
Youths' Sweaters
$5.50 EACH
A
$4.50 EACH
$3.75 EACH
C
$6.75 EACH
B
$6.50 EACH
D
E
$5.25 EACH
For Descriptions See Opposite Page
$6.00 EACH
F
G
H
$2.35 EACH

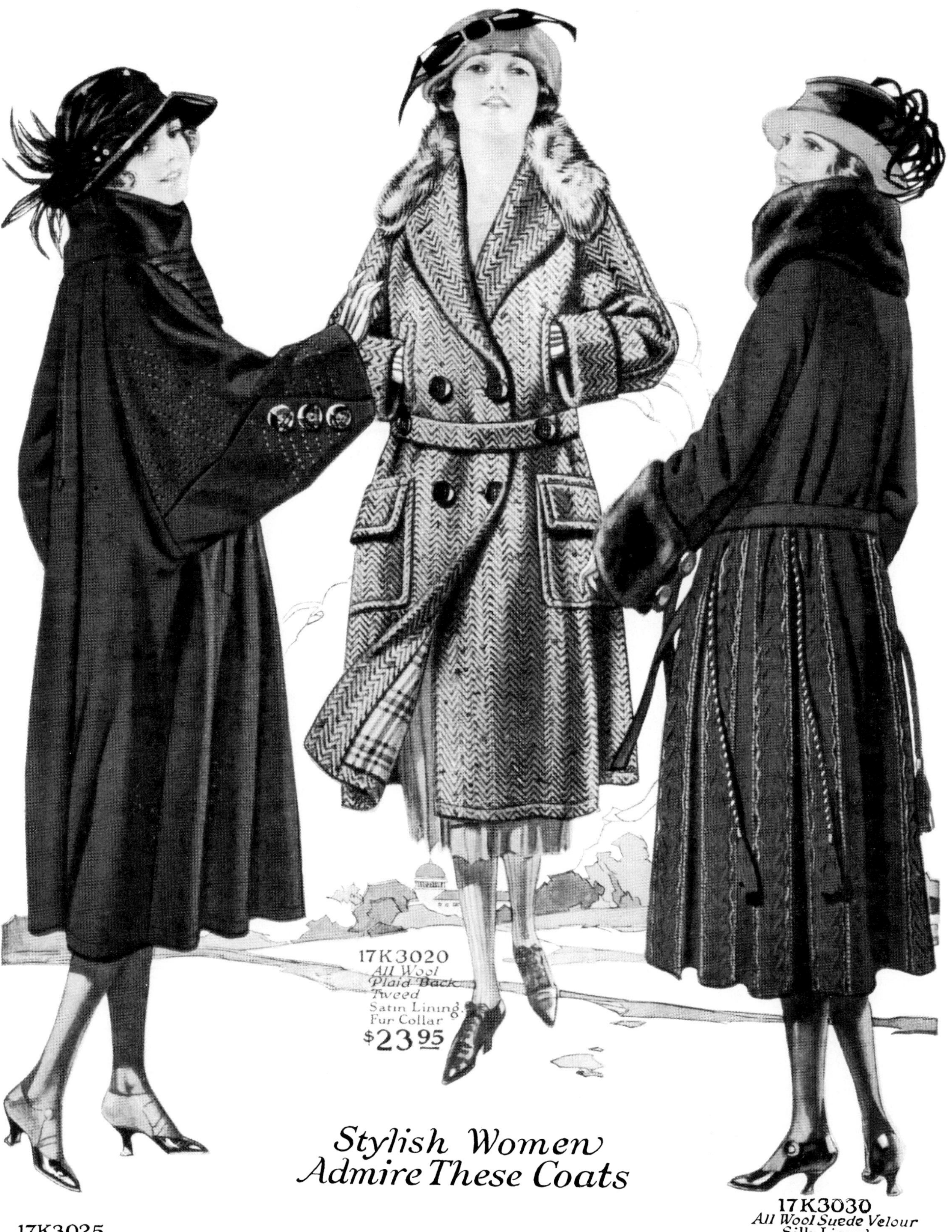
17K3020
All Wool
Plaid Back
Tweed
Satin Lining
Fur Collar
$23.95

*Stylish Women Admire These Coats*

17K3025
*All Wool Velour*
Silk Lining
$19.75

17K3030
*All Wool Suede Velour*
Silk Lining
$24.98

*For Descriptions and Other Colors See Opposite Page*

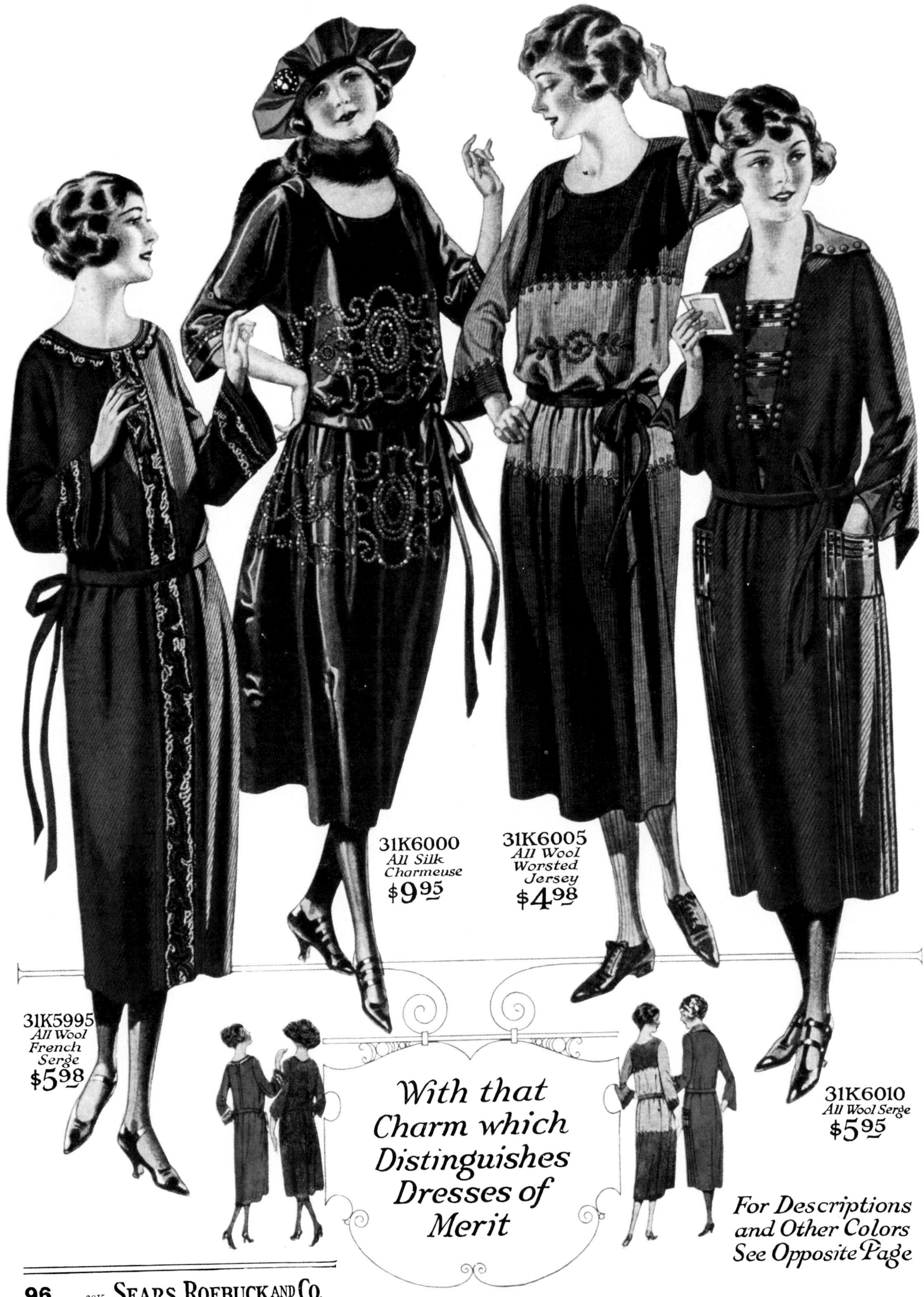
31K6000
All Silk
Charmeuse
$9.95
31K6005
All Wool
Worsted
Jersey
$4.98
31K5995
All Wool
French
Serge
$5.98
With that
Charm which
Distinguishes
Dresses of
Merit
31K6010
All Wool Serge
$5.95
For Descriptions
and Other Colors
See Opposite Page

# Surprisingly Low in Price

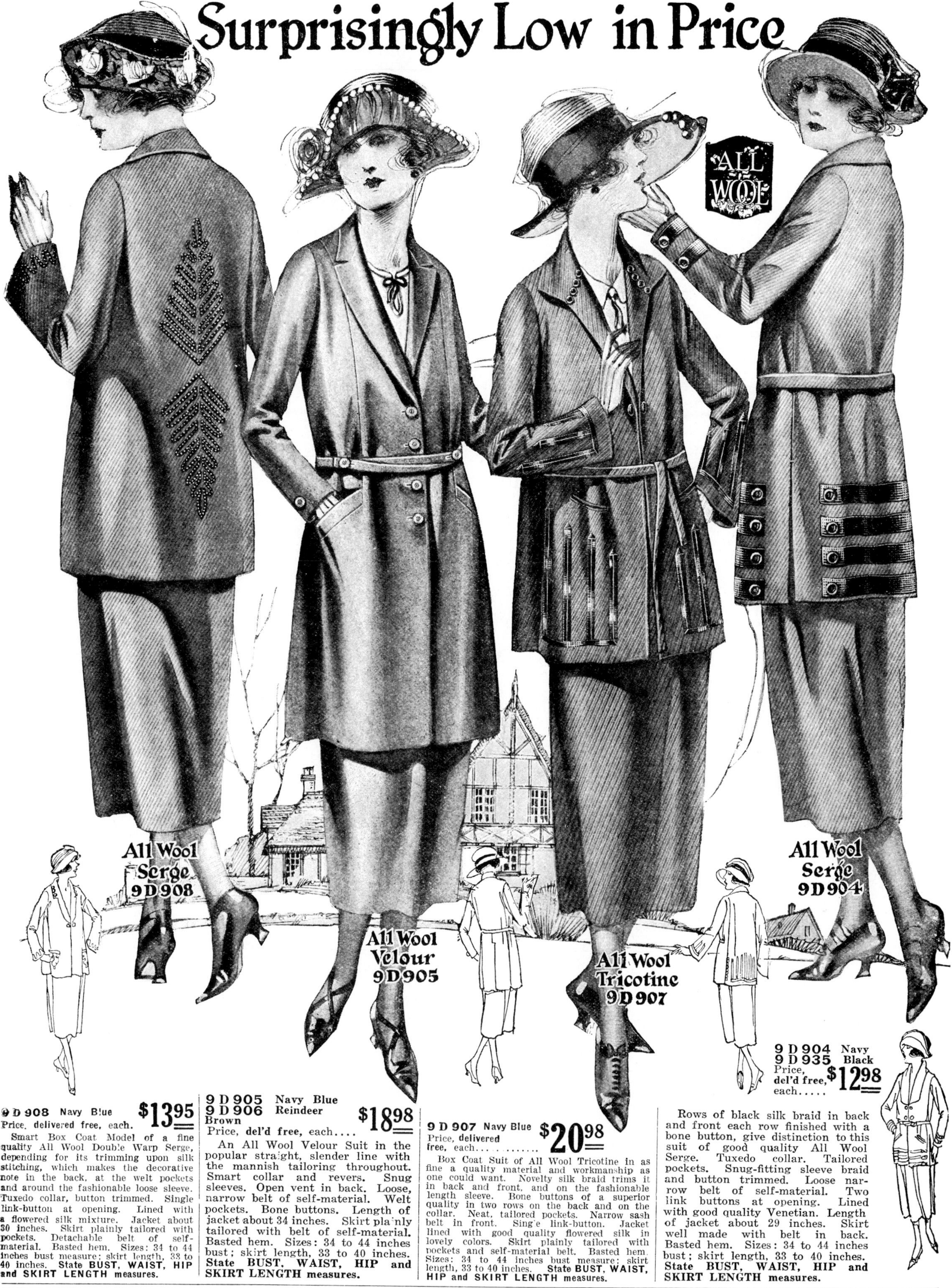


**9 D 908** Navy Blue
Price, delivered free, each. **$13.95**

Smart Box Coat Model of a fine quality All Wool Double Warp Serge, depending for its trimming upon silk stitching, which makes the decorative note in the back, at the welt pockets and around the fashionable loose sleeve. Tuxedo collar, button trimmed. Single link-button at opening. Lined with a flowered silk mixture. Jacket about 30 inches. Skirt plainly tailored with pockets. Detachable belt of self-material. Basted hem. Sizes: 34 to 44 inches bust measure; skirt length, 33 to 40 inches. **State BUST, WAIST, HIP and SKIRT LENGTH measures.**

**9 D 905** Navy Blue
**9 D 906** Reindeer Brown
Price, **del'd free,** each.... **$18.98**

An All Wool Velour Suit in the popular straight, slender line with the mannish tailoring throughout. Smart collar and revers. Snug sleeves. Open vent in back. Loose, narrow belt of self-material. Welt pockets. Bone buttons. Length of jacket about 34 inches. Skirt plainly tailored with belt of self-material. Basted hem. Sizes: 34 to 44 inches bust; skirt length, 33 to 40 inches. **State BUST, WAIST, HIP and SKIRT LENGTH measures.**

**9 D 907** Navy Blue
Price, **delivered free,** each.............. **$20.98**

Box Coat Suit of All Wool Tricotine in as fine a quality material and workmanship as one could want. Novelty silk braid trims it in back and front, and on the fashionable length sleeve. Bone buttons of a superior quality in two rows on the back and on the collar. Neat, tailored pockets. Narrow sash belt in front. Single link-button. Jacket lined with good quality flowered silk in lovely colors. Skirt plainly tailored with pockets and self-material belt. Basted hem. Sizes: 34 to 44 inches bust measure; skirt length, 33 to 40 inches. **State BUST, WAIST, HIP and SKIRT LENGTH measures.**

**9 D 904** Navy
**9 D 935** Black
Price, **del'd free,** each..... **$12.98**

Rows of black silk braid in back and front each row finished with a bone button, give distinction to this suit of good quality All Wool Serge. Tuxedo collar. Tailored pockets. Snug-fitting sleeve braid and button trimmed. Loose narrow belt of self-material. Two link buttons at opening. Lined with good quality Venetian. Length of jacket about 29 inches. Skirt well made with belt in back. Basted hem. Sizes: 34 to 44 inches bust; skirt length, 33 to 40 inches. **State BUST, WAIST, HIP and SKIRT LENGTH measures.**



***We Pay Delivery Charges on Every Article on This Page***

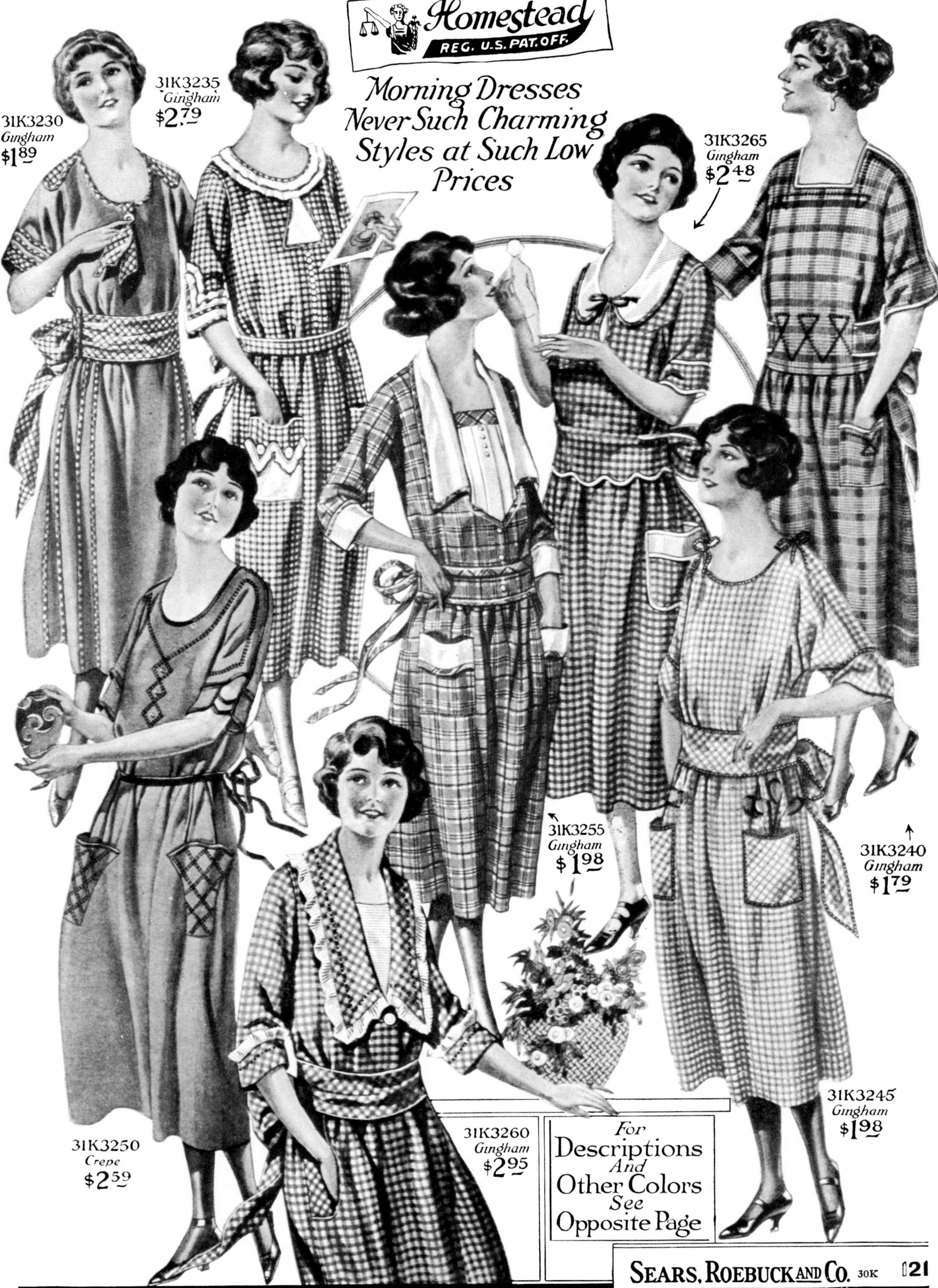
Homestead
REG. U.S. PAT. OFF.
Morning Dresses
Never Such Charming
Styles at Such Low
Prices
31K3230
Gingham
$1.89
31K3235
Gingham
$2.79
31K3265
Gingham
$2.48
31K3255
Gingham
$1.98
31K3240
Gingham
$1.79
31K3250
Crepe
$2.59
31K3260
Gingham
$2.95
31K3245
Gingham
$1.98
For
Descriptions
And
Other Colors
See
Opposite Page
SEARS, ROEBUCK AND CO. 30K 121

# Skirts for Sport

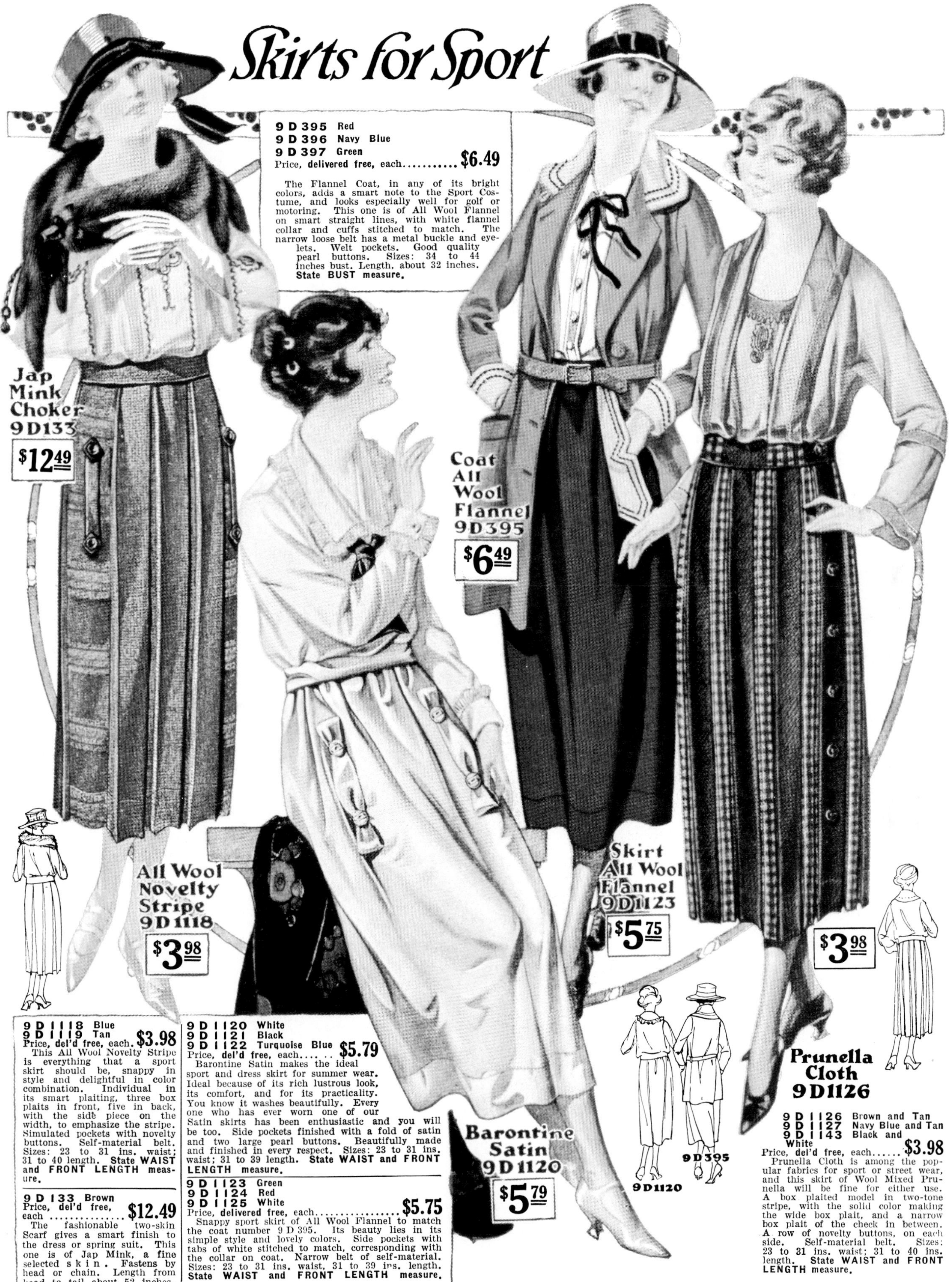


**9 D 395** Red
**9 D 396** Navy Blue
**9 D 397** Green
Price, **delivered free, each**........... **$6.49**

The Flannel Coat, in any of its bright colors, adds a smart note to the Sport Costume, and looks especially well for golf or motoring. This one is of All Wool Flannel on smart straight lines, with white flannel collar and cuffs stitched to match. The narrow loose belt has a metal buckle and eyelets. Welt pockets. Good quality pearl buttons. Sizes: 34 to 44 inches bust. Length, about 32 inches. **State BUST measure.**

**9 D 1118** Blue
**9 D 1119** Tan
**Price, del'd free, each.** **$3.98**

This All Wool Novelty Stripe is everything that a sport skirt should be, snappy in style and delightful in color combination. Individual in its smart plaiting, three box plaits in front, five in back, with the side piece on the width, to emphasize the stripe. Simulated pockets with novelty buttons. Self-material belt. Sizes: 23 to 31 ins. waist; 31 to 40 length. **State WAIST and FRONT LENGTH measure.**

**9 D 133** Brown
**Price, del'd free, each** .............. **$12.49**

The fashionable two-skin Scarf gives a smart finish to the dress or spring suit. This one is of Jap Mink, a fine selected skin. Fastens by head or chain. Length from head to tail about 52 inches.

**9 D 1120** White
**9 D 1121** Black
**9 D 1122** Turquoise Blue
**Price, del'd free, each**...... **$5.79**

Barontine Satin makes the ideal sport and dress skirt for summer wear. Ideal because of its rich lustrous look, its comfort, and for its practicality. You know it washes beautifully. Every one who has ever worn one of our Satin skirts has been enthusiastic and you will be too. Side pockets finished with a fold of satin and two large pearl buttons. Beautifully made and finished in every respect. Sizes: 23 to 31 ins. waist; 31 to 39 length. **State WAIST and FRONT LENGTH measure.**

**9 D 1123** Green
**9 D 1124** Red
**9 D 1125** White
Price, **delivered free, each**................ **$5.75**

Snappy sport skirt of All Wool Flannel to match the coat number 9 D 395. Its beauty lies in its simple style and lovely colors. Side pockets with tabs of white stitched to match, corresponding with the collar on coat. Narrow belt of self-material. Sizes: 23 to 31 ins. waist, 31 to 39 ins. length. **State WAIST and FRONT LENGTH measure.**

**9 D 1126** Brown and Tan
**9 D 1127** Navy Blue and Tan
**9 D 1143** Black and White
**Price, del'd free, each**...... **$3.98**

Prunella Cloth is among the popular fabrics for sport or street wear, and this skirt of Wool Mixed Prunella will be fine for either use. A box plaited model in two-tone stripe, with the solid color making the wide box plait, and a narrow box plait of the check in between. A row of novelty buttons, on each side. Self-material belt. Sizes: 23 to 31 ins. waist; 31 to 40 ins. length. **State WAIST and FRONT LENGTH measure.**

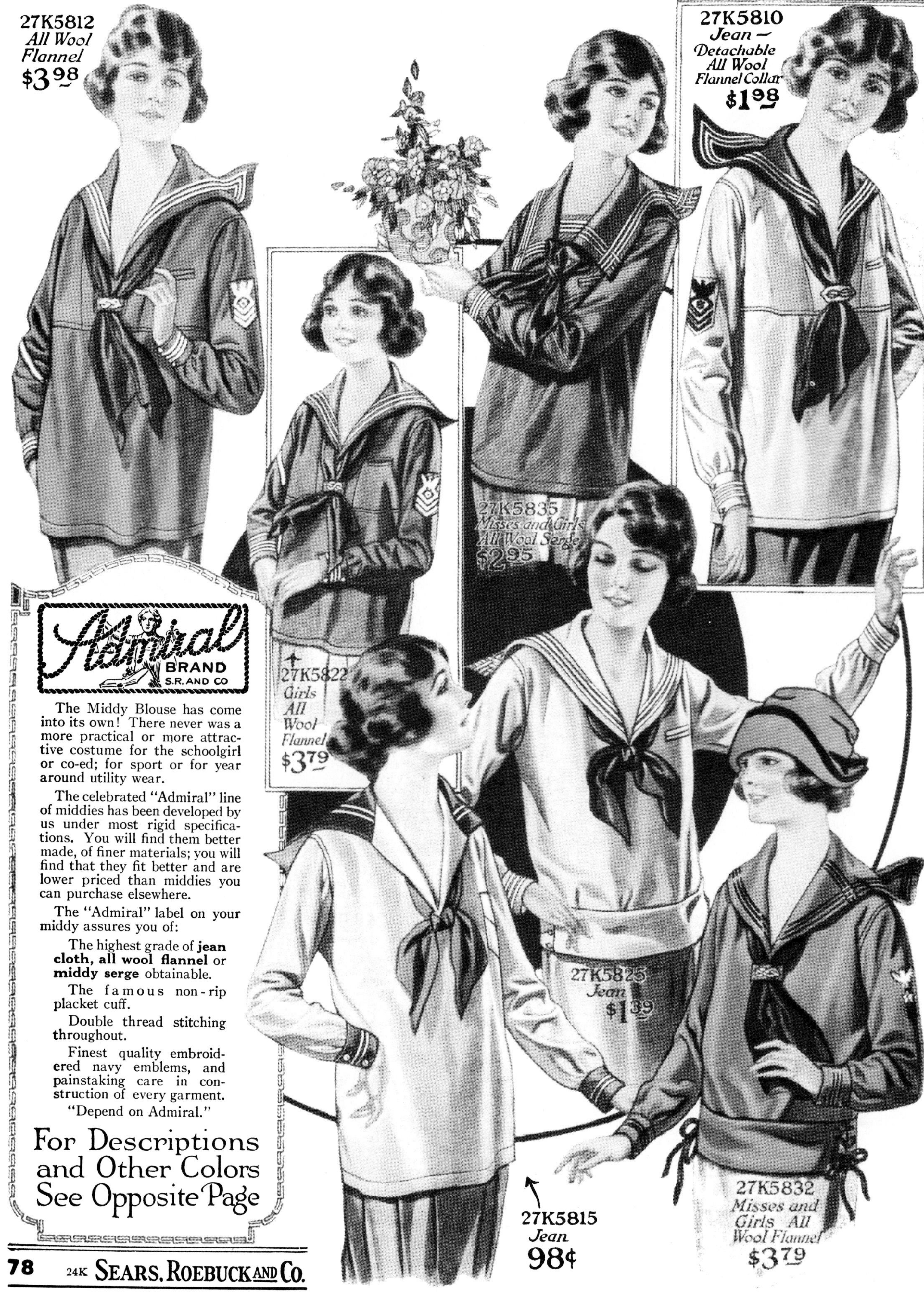
27K5812
All Wool
Flannel
$3.98
27K5810
Jean—
Detachable
All Wool
Flannel Collar
$1.98
27K5835
Misses and Girls
All Wool Serge
$2.95
27K5822
Girls
All
Wool
Flannel
$3.79
Admiral
BRAND
S.R. AND CO
The Middy Blouse has come into its own! There never was a more practical or more attractive costume for the schoolgirl or co-ed; for sport or for year around utility wear.
The celebrated "Admiral" line of middies has been developed by us under most rigid specifications. You will find them better made, of finer materials; you will find that they fit better and are lower priced than middies you can purchase elsewhere.
The "Admiral" label on your middy assures you of:
The highest grade of jean cloth, all wool flannel or middy serge obtainable.
The famous non-rip placket cuff.
Double thread stitching throughout.
Finest quality embroidered navy emblems, and painstaking care in construction of every garment.
"Depend on Admiral."
For Descriptions and Other Colors See Opposite Page
27K5825
Jean
$1.39
27K5815
Jean
98¢
27K5832
Misses and
Girls All
Wool Flannel
$3.79

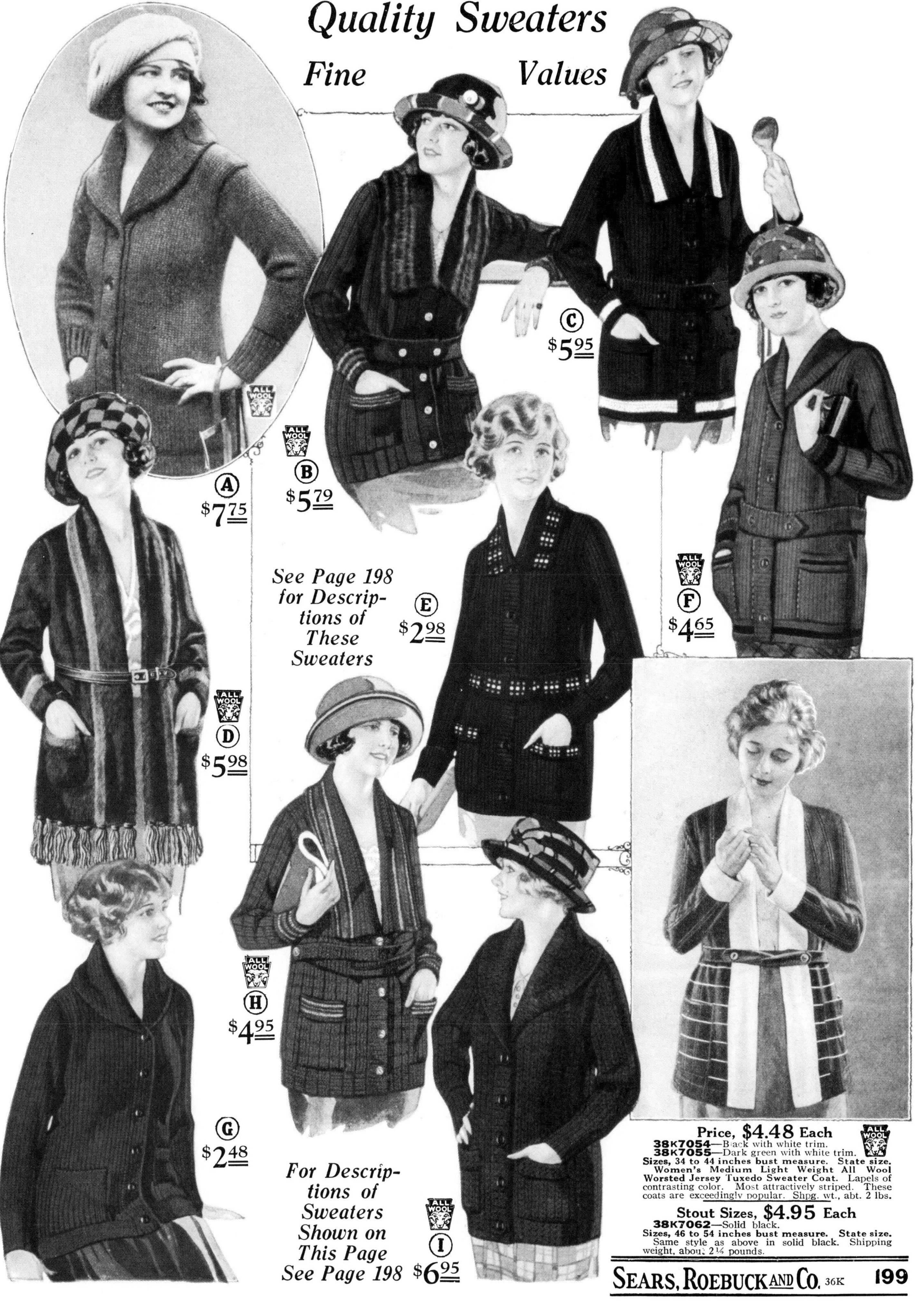

# *Quality Sweaters*

*Fine Values*

A $7.75

ALL WOOL

B $5.79

C $5.95

*See Page 198 for Descriptions of These Sweaters*

E $2.98

ALL WOOL

F $4.65

ALL WOOL

D $5.98

ALL WOOL

H $4.95

G $2.48

*For Descriptions of Sweaters Shown on This Page See Page 198*

ALL WOOL

I $6.95

**Price, $4.48 Each**

ALL WOOL

**38K7054**—Black with white trim.
**38K7055**—Dark green with white trim.
**Sizes, 34 to 44 inches bust measure. State size.**
**Women's Medium Light Weight All Wool Worsted Jersey Tuxedo Sweater Coat.** Lapels of contrasting color. Most attractively striped. These coats are exceedingly popular. Shpg. wt., abt. 2 lbs.

**Stout Sizes, $4.95 Each**

**38K7062**—Solid black.
**Sizes, 46 to 54 inches bust measure. State size.**
Same style as above in solid black. Shipping weight, about 2⅙ pounds.

SEARS, ROEBUCK AND CO. 36K 199

# The Fashion Center of America

Posed by MISS GLORIA SWANSON Famous Paramount Star

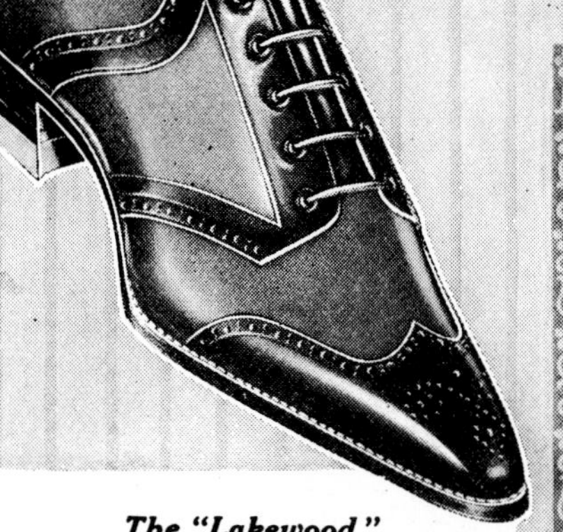

### The "Lakewood."

**15K2847** **The Pair, $4.48**

Even in the great style centers of America you'll see no smarter sport models than this charming Goodyear Welt Oxford. The combination of genuine mahogany and light tan calfskin is unusually striking, and the blucher style is a new feature that gives this pattern real distinction. Remember that it is of Goodyear Welt construction. That, you know, means quality. The woman who knows and demands real character in her footwear will select this pattern.

**Be sure to state size.**

*Sizes, 2½ to 8. Wide widths only. Shipping wt., 1⅛ lbs.*

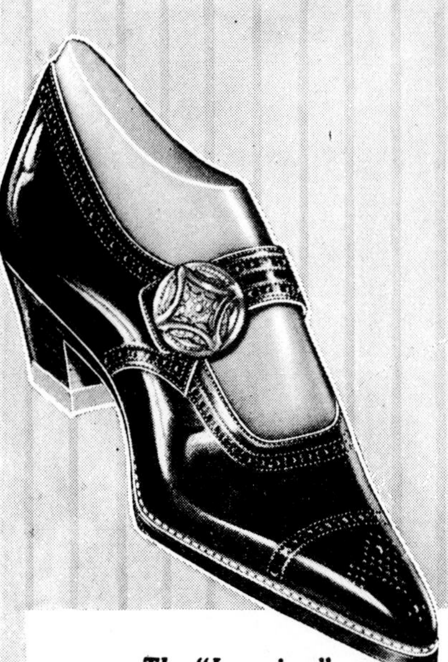

### The "Lorraine."

**15K2848** **The Pair, $3.98**

This is a "patent leather" season, and here is the model Dame Fashion has selected for the greatest popularity. No doubt the quiet beauty of design accounts for her decision. But, of course, there's just enough "dash" to the "Lorraine" to make it distinctive in appearance. Quality is reflected here, too, for this is a Goodyear Welt, the quality kind.

**Be sure to state size.**

*Sizes, 2½ to 8. Wide widths only. Shipping wt., 1½ lbs.*

## Direct From Style Centers of the World to Our Customers.

We aim to be the leading and foremost "Fashion" footwear house in the country. In order to live up to our reputation we maintain a staff of experts who keep in constant contact with the leading style artists of Paris and New York.

The footwear we have selected this season has such matchless beauty and alluring grace that leading authorities have proclaimed our preeminence in the fashions of the day.

Another noteworthy feature besides the style and quality of our footwear is the unbelievably low prices.

Not only our customers, but many outside manufacturers say "How do they do it?"

The answer is simple.

We sell more shoes than any other mail order house. We not only manufacture tremendous quantities of shoes in our own factories but also buy from the largest, best and most successful shoe manufacturers in the country. The enormous quantities we make and purchase mean "Rock Bottom Prices."

We operate on a very small margin of profit and can do so because of the tremendous volume of merchandise we sell.

We advertise merchandise just as it really is and this policy has made millions of customers for us.

We guarantee you the newest styles and best values obtainable. Millions of contented customers are our best recommendation.

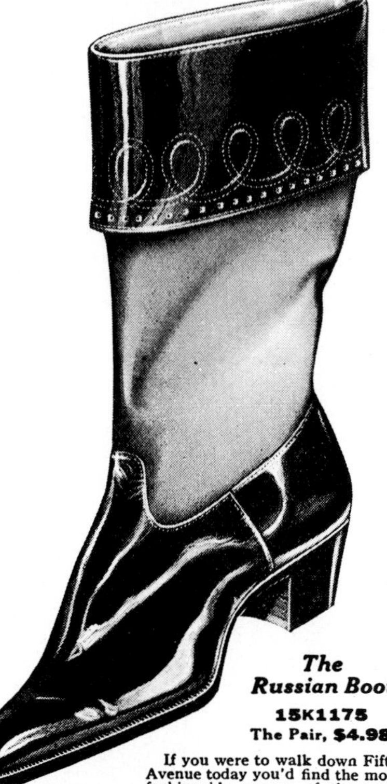

### The Russian Boot

**15K1175**

**The Pair, $4.98**

If you were to walk down Fifth Avenue today you'd find the most fashionable women of the most fashionable city wearing the beautiful new Russian Boot. It's the "last word" in footwear style, and the model we have selected is an unusually charming one. Note the graceful lines and see how striking is the contrast between the patent leather and gray suede. All the stitching is in red and that, of course, adds to the "chic" appearance of this boot. Picture at right shows beautiful Gloria Swanson, famous Paramount star, posing in a pair of these boots.

**Be sure to state size.**

*Sizes, 2½ to 8. Wide widths only. Shipping wt., 1¾ lbs.*

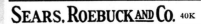

# Girls' Dresses
## 7 to 14 Years

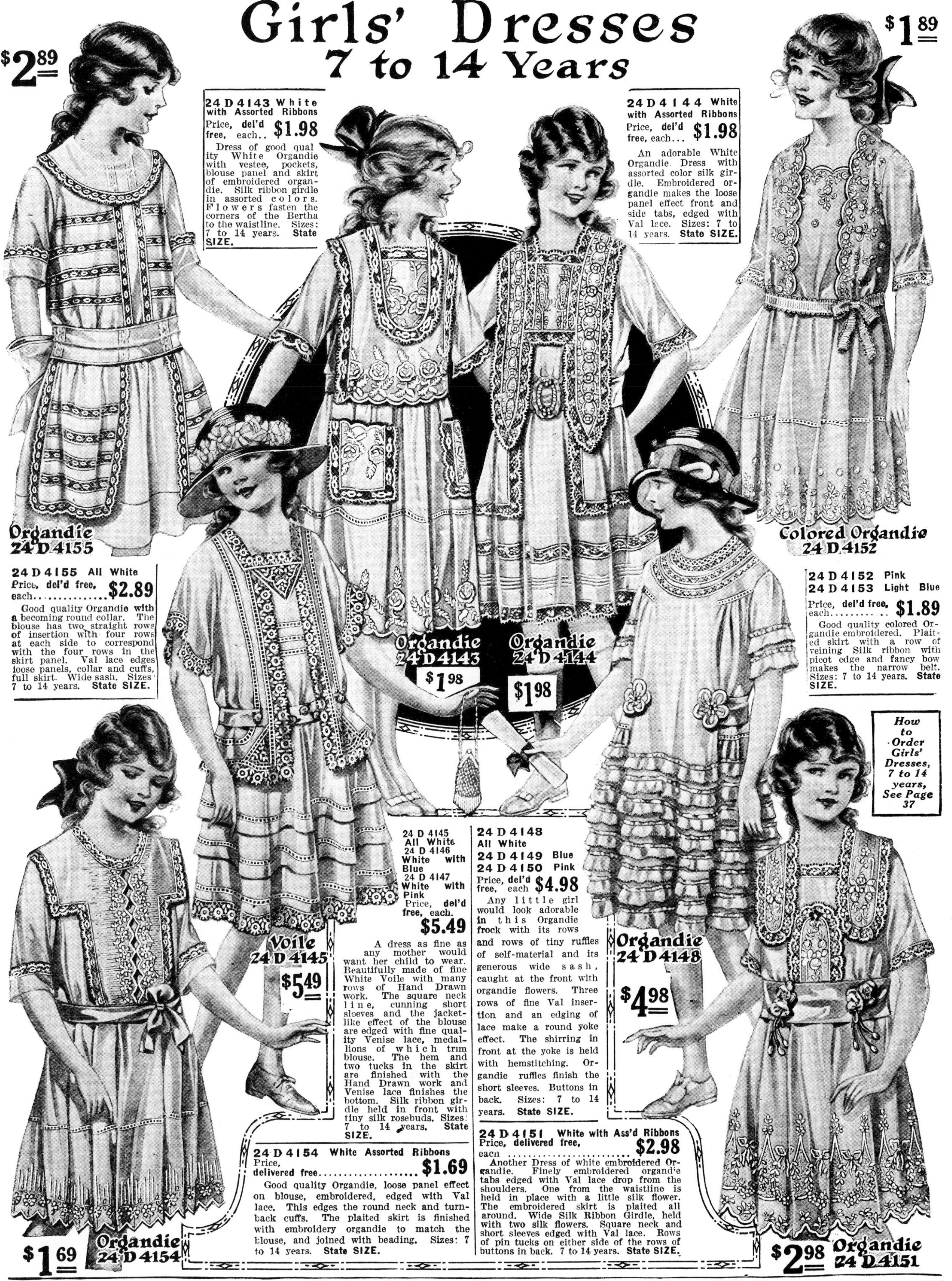


**24 D 4143 White with Assorted Ribbons**
Price, del'd free, each.. **$1.98**
Dress of good quality White Organdie with vestee, pockets, blouse panel and skirt of embroidered organdie. Silk ribbon girdle in assorted colors. Flowers fasten the corners of the Bertha to the waistline. Sizes: 7 to 14 years. State **SIZE.**

**24 D 4144 White with Assorted Ribbons**
Price, del'd free, each... **$1.98**
An adorable White Organdie Dress with assorted color silk girdle. Embroidered organdie makes the loose panel effect front and side tabs, edged with Val lace. Sizes: 7 to 14 years. State **SIZE.**

**24 D 4155 All White**
Price, del'd free, each............. **$2.89**
Good quality Organdie with a becoming round collar. The blouse has two straight rows of insertion with four rows at each side to correspond with the four rows in the skirt panel. Val lace edges loose panels, collar and cuffs, full skirt. Wide sash. Sizes 7 to 14 years. State **SIZE.**

**24 D 4152 Pink**
**24 D 4153 Light Blue**
Price, del'd free, each......... .. **$1.89**
Good quality colored Organdie embroidered. Plaited skirt with a row of veining Silk ribbon with picot edge and fancy bow makes the narrow belt. Sizes: 7 to 14 years. State **SIZE.**

*How to Order Girls' Dresses, 7 to 14 years, See Page 37*

**24 D 4145 All White**
**24 D 4146 White with Blue**
**24 D 4147 White with Pink**
Price, del'd free, each. **$5.49**
A dress as fine as any mother would want her child to wear. Beautifully made of fine White Voile with many rows of Hand Drawn work. The square neck line, cunning short sleeves and the jacket-like effect of the blouse are edged with fine quality Venise lace, medallions of which trim blouse. The hem and two tucks in the skirt are finished with the Hand Drawn work and Venise lace finishes the bottom. Silk ribbon girdle held in front with tiny silk rosebuds. Sizes: 7 to 14 years. State **SIZE.**

**24 D 4148 All White**
**24 D 4149 Blue**
**24 D 4150 Pink**
Price, del'd free, each **$4.98**
Any little girl would look adorable in this Organdie frock with its rows and rows of tiny ruffles of self-material and its generous wide sash, caught at the front with organdie flowers. Three rows of fine Val insertion and an edging of lace make a round yoke effect. The shirring in front at the yoke is held with hemstitching. Organdie ruffles finish the short sleeves. Buttons in back. Sizes: 7 to 14 years. State **SIZE.**

**24 D 4154 White Assorted Ribbons**
Price, delivered free........................ **$1.69**
Good quality Organdie, loose panel effect on blouse, embroidered, edged with Val lace. This edges the round neck and turn-back cuffs. The plaited skirt is finished with embroidery organdie to match the blouse, and joined with beading. Sizes: 7 to 14 years. State **SIZE.**

**24 D 4151 White with Ass'd Ribbons**
Price, delivered free, eacn ........................ **$2.98**
Another Dress of white embroidered Organdie. Finely embroidered organdie tabs edged with Val lace drop from the shoulders. One from the waistline is held in place with a little silk flower. The embroidered skirt is plaited all around. Wide Silk Ribbon Girdle, held with two silk flowers. Square neck and short sleeves edged with Val lace. Rows of pin tucks on either side of the rows of buttons in back. 7 to 14 years. State **SIZE.**

# "The Materials are The Better Sort"

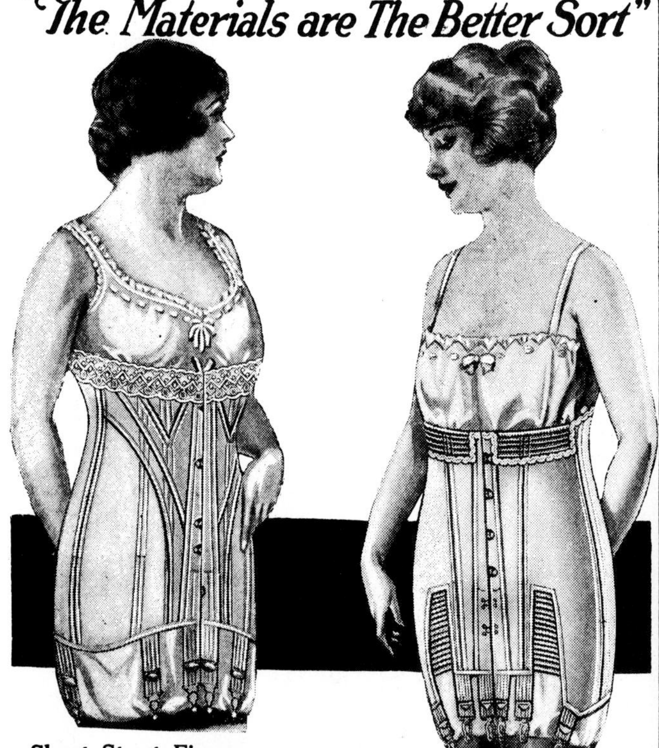

**Short Stout Figures.**

**18K462** White Coutil. **$2.48**

***Medium bust, 3½ in. Skirt, 12½ in. Clasp, 10 in. Sizes, 22 to 30.***

Ample fullness in skirt to care for large hips. Comfortable and roomy bust. Firmly boned. Strong broad end front clasp. **State corset size.**

**18K463**—Same style as 18K462, but in extra sizes, 32, 34 and 36. Price.................. **$2.65**

**Average to Full Figures.**

**18K173** Pink Coutil. **$2.50**

***Low bust, 2 in. Skirt, 15 in. Broad end front clasp, 9 in. Sizes, 21 to 30; also 32.***

A graceful low bust model with higher back to support flesh at shoulders. Elastic insertion on each side at top allows for freedom of diaphragm. Custom inserted wide diagonal elastic gores at bottom of skirt. Fine pink coutil body material, moderately stayed with double strength boning. Six strong supporters. **State corset size.**

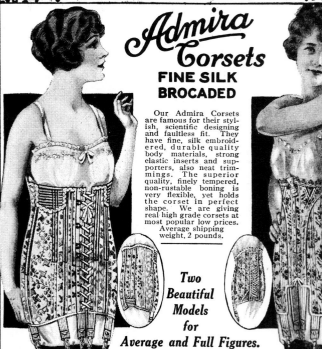

## Admira Corsets

### FINE SILK BROCADED

Our Admira Corsets are famous for their stylish, scientific designing and faultless fit. They have fine, silk embroidered, durable quality body materials, strong elastic inserts and supporters, also neat trimmings. The superior quality, finely tempered, non-rustable boning is very flexible, yet holds the corset in perfect shape. We are giving real high grade corsets at most popular low prices. Average shipping weight, 2 pounds.

***Two Beautiful Models for Average and Full Figures.***

**18K211** Pink Brocade. **$4.45**

***Low bust, 2¾ inches. Skirt, 13½ inches. Clasp, 8½ inches. Sizes, 21 to 30.***

One of this season's newest front lacing corsets. The body material is very rich looking, heavy pink silk brocade, and will give good wear. Has extra firm quality surgical elastic inserts at top, also insert at bottom of back. Well stayed with fine, flexible, double strength boning. Has boned tongue behind lacers and six high grade supporters. **State corset size.**

**18K203** Pink Brocade. **$4.45**

***Very low bust, 1¾ in. Skirt, 14¾ in. Clasp, 8½ in. Hook and lacing below. Sizes, 21 to 30.***

Very fashionable girdle top corset with comfortable low bust and higher back to support flesh at shoulders. High grade fancy silk brocaded pink material. Well stayed with superior quality boning. Elastic section in back at bottom. Splendidly modeled. Six strong supporters. **State corset size.**

***Average Shipping Weight, 2 Lbs.***

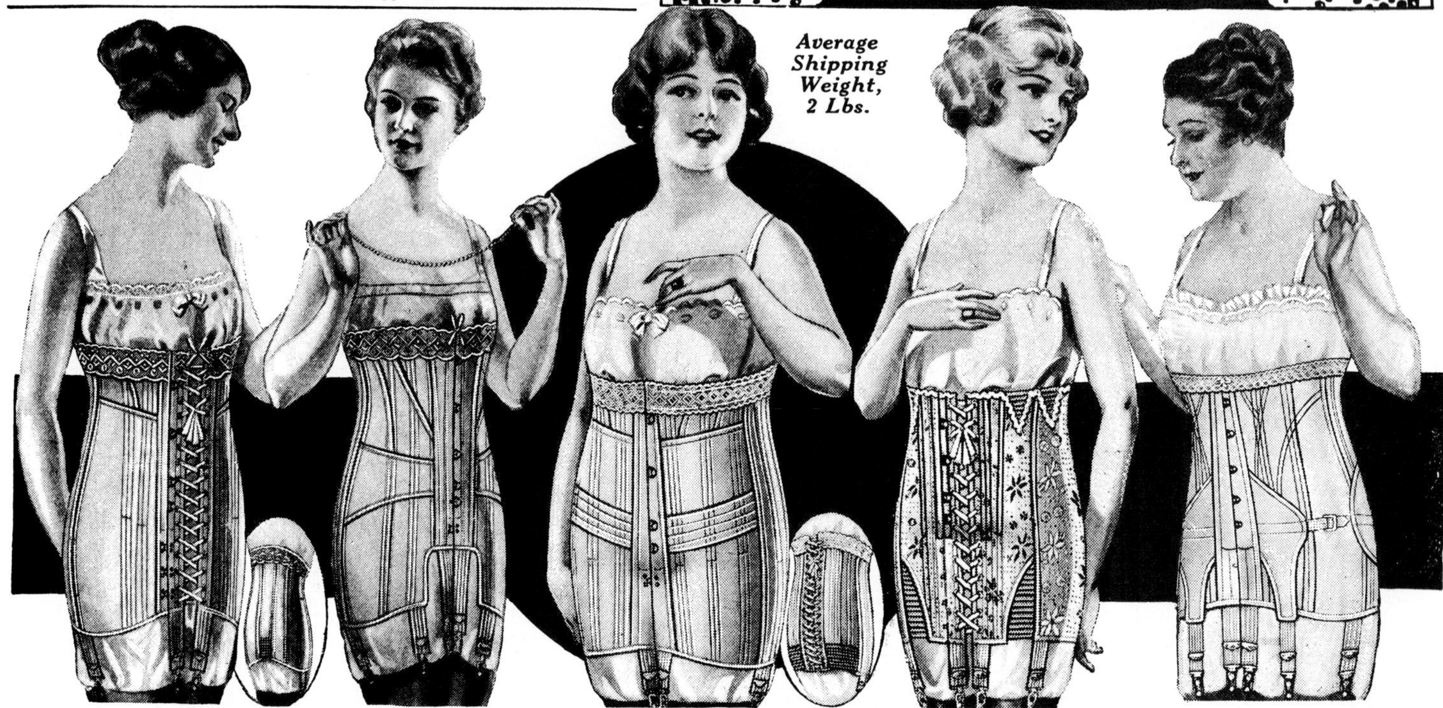

**Average Figures.**

**18K476** White Coutil. **$2.35**

***Medium bust, 3½ in. Skirt, 14 in. Clasp, 9½ in. Sizes, 20 to 30.***

Firmly boned front lacing corset which will give good support and excellent figure lines. Elastic insert in bottom of skirt at back. Stayed tongue behind lacers. Four good hose supporters. **State corset size.**

**Average Figures.**

**18K235** White Coutil. **$2.69**

***High bust, 5 in. Skirt, 15 in. Clasp, 11 in. Sizes, 20 to 30.***

Roomy gored bust cares for well developed figures. Double sections across abdomen to add strength where needed. High, restful back. The cut-out front makes this corset very comfortable. **State corset size.**

**Reducer for Full and Stout Figures.**

**18K404** Pink Coutil. **$2.59**

***Medium bust, 3 in. Skirt, 14 in. Clasp, 10 in. Sizes, 23 to 30.***

A great favorite Reducing Corset, designed to give apparent reduction to the figure without any straps or adjusting devices. Heavy 3-inch width elastic at each side of back; sewed in reinforcing sections across abdomen. Made of firm pink coutil; well boned.

**18K405**—Extra sizes, 32, 34 and 36. Price.......... **$2.89**

**Slender and Average Figures.**

**18K105** Pink only. **$2.39**

***Low bust, 2½ in. Skirt, 14 in. Clasp, 8 in.; 3 hooks below. Sizes, 21 to 30.***

Front Lacing Corset made of medium weight fancy figured pink material. Four elastic gores in bust, two elastic sections in skirt. Boned tongue behind lacers. Moderately boned.

**State corset size.**

**Reducer for Stout Figures.**

**18K245** White Coutil. **$2.35**

***Medium bust, 3 in. Skirt, 13 in. Clasp, 9½ in. Sizes, 22 to 30.***

Stout women appear thinner in this corset. Very firmly boned. Roomy bust. Full skirt to care for large abdomen and hips. Non-elastic straps to tighten reducing sections. Broad end front clasp.

**18K250**—Same style as 18K245, but in extra sizes, 32, 34 and 36. Price.................. **$2.59**

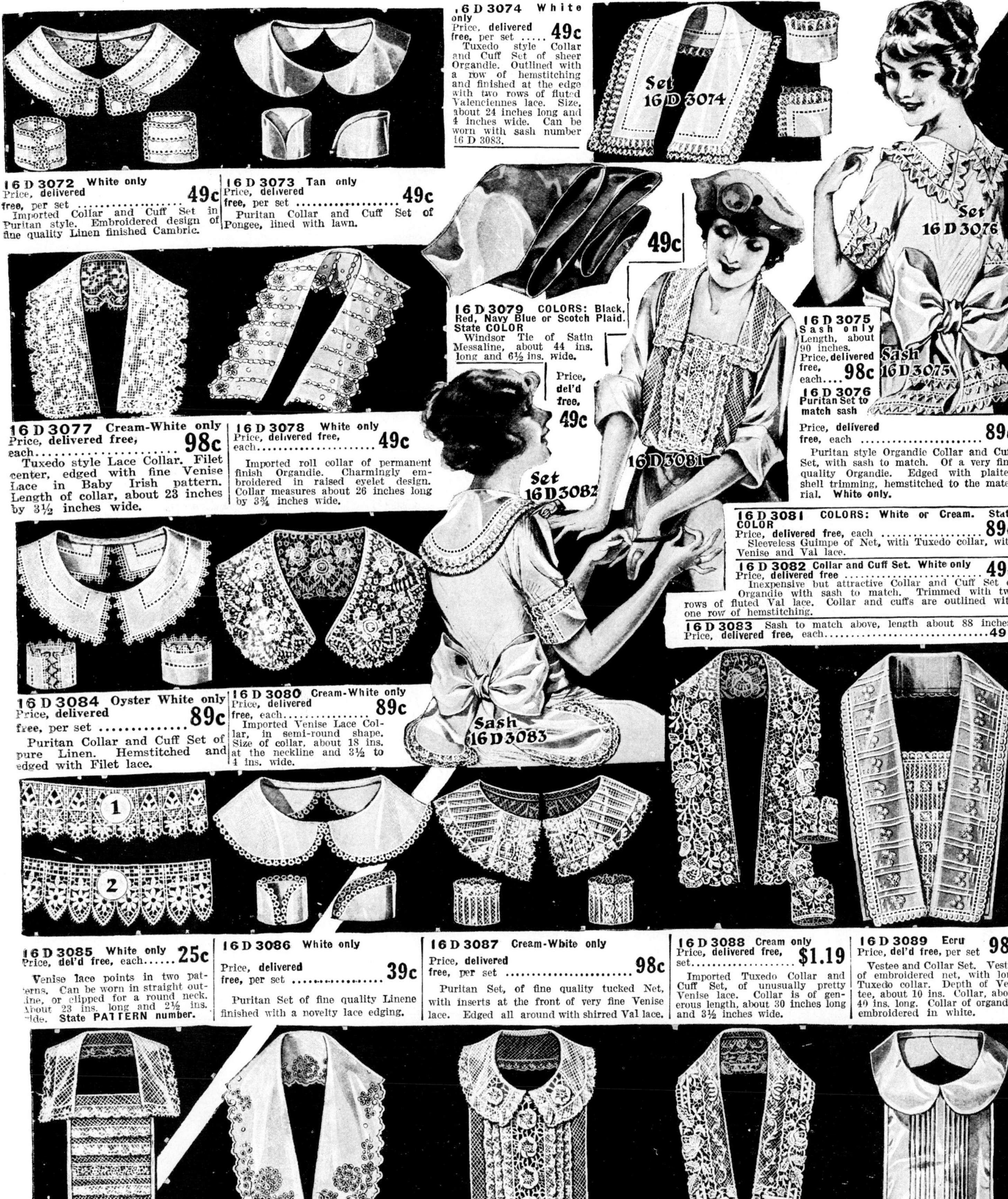


**16 D 3074** White only
Price, delivered free, per set ..... **49c**
Tuxedo style Collar and Cuff Set of sheer Organdie. Outlined with a row of hemstitching and finished at the edge with two rows of fluted Valenciennes lace. Size, about 24 inches long and 4 inches wide. Can be worn with sash number 16 D 3083.

**16 D 3072** White only
Price, delivered free, per set .................. **49c**
Imported Collar and Cuff Set in Puritan style. Embroidered design of fine quality Linen finished Cambric.

**16 D 3073** Tan only
Price, delivered free, per set .................. **49c**
Puritan Collar and Cuff Set of Pongee, lined with lawn.

**16 D 3079** COLORS: Black, Red, Navy Blue or Scotch Plaid. State COLOR
Windsor Tie of Satin Messaline, about 44 ins. long and 6½ ins. wide.
Price, del'd free. **49c**

**16 D 3075** Sash only
Length, about 90 inches.
Price, delivered free, each.... **98c**

**16 D 3076** Puritan Set to match sash
Price, delivered free, each ...................... **89c**
Puritan style Organdie Collar and Cuff Set, with sash to match. Of a very fine quality Organdie. Edged with plaited shell trimming, hemstitched to the material. White only.

**16 D 3077** Cream-White only
Price, delivered free, each **98c**
Tuxedo style Lace Collar. Filet center, edged with fine Venise Lace in Baby Irish pattern. Length of collar, about 23 inches by 3½ inches wide.

**16 D 3078** White only
Price, delivered free, each.................... **49c**
Imported roll collar of permanent finish Organdie. Charmingly embroidered in raised eyelet design. Collar measures about 26 inches long by 3¾ inches wide.

**16 D 3081** COLORS: White or Cream. State COLOR
Price, delivered free, each ................. **89c**
Sleeveless Guimpe of Net, with Tuxedo collar, with Venise and Val lace.

**16 D 3082** Collar and Cuff Set. White only
Price, delivered free ................................. **49c**
Inexpensive but attractive Collar and Cuff Set of Organdie with sash to match. Trimmed with two rows of fluted Val lace. Collar and cuffs are outlined with one row of hemstitching.

**16 D 3083** Sash to match above, length about 88 inches.
Price, delivered free, each................................**49c**

**16 D 3084** Oyster White only
Price, delivered free, per set .............. **89c**
Puritan Collar and Cuff Set of pure Linen. Hemstitched and edged with Filet lace.

**16 D 3080** Cream-White only
Price, delivered free, each.............. **89c**
Imported Venise Lace Collar, in semi-round shape. Size of collar, about 18 ins. at the neckline and 3½ to 4 ins. wide.

**16 D 3085** White only
Price, del'd free, each...... **25c**
Venise lace points in two patterns. Can be worn in straight outline, or clipped for a round neck. About 23 ins. long and 2½ ins. wide. State PATTERN number.

**16 D 3086** White only
Price, delivered free, per set .................. **39c**
Puritan Set of fine quality Linene finished with a novelty lace edging.

**16 D 3087** Cream-White only
Price, delivered free, per set ........................ **98c**
Puritan Set, of fine quality tucked Net, with inserts at the front of very fine Venise lace. Edged all around with shirred Val lace.

**16 D 3088** Cream only
Price, delivered free, set.................... **$1.19**
Imported Tuxedo Collar and Cuff Set, of unusually pretty Venise lace. Collar is of generous length, about 30 inches long and 3½ inches wide.

**16 D 3089** Ecru
Price, del'd free, per set **98c**
Vestee and Collar Set. Vestee of embroidered net, with long Tuxedo collar. Depth of Vestee, about 10 ins. Collar, about 40 ins. long. Collar of organdie embroidered in white.

**; D 3090** Cream-White only
. ice, delivered free, each .............. **49c**
Vestee of Net with Tuxedo Col-lar. Trimmed with Val and Venise lace. Vestee about 15 ins. long; collar about 22 ins.

**16 D 3091** White only
Price, delivered free, per set.............. **49c**
Embroidered Tuxedo Collar, made of fine quality Cambric in a pretty eyelet pattern. Cuffs to match.

**16 D 3092** COLORS: White or Cream. State COLOR.
Price, del'd free, each.......... **98c**
Vestee with Peter Pan Collar. Trimmed with wide Venise lace edged with shirred Val lace. Depth of vestee, about 12 inches.

**16 D 3093** Cream-White only
Price, delivered free, each.......................... **59c**
Tuxedo Collar and Cuff Set of Venise lace, edging an embroidered Net lace. Length of collar, about 23 inches. Width, about 3 inches.

**16 D 3094** White only
Price, delivered free, each.......................... **98c**
High Neck Vestee with Puritan Collar; made of good quality Satin. Trimmed with many rows of pin tucks. Length, about 13 ins.

# Attractive Values in New Hand Bags

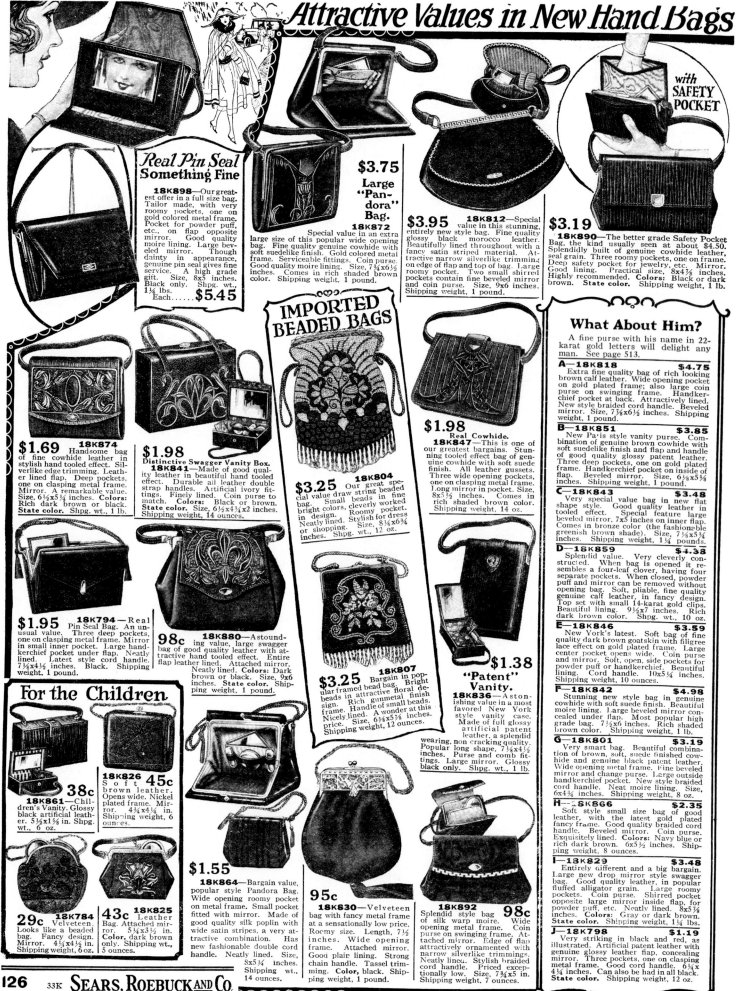

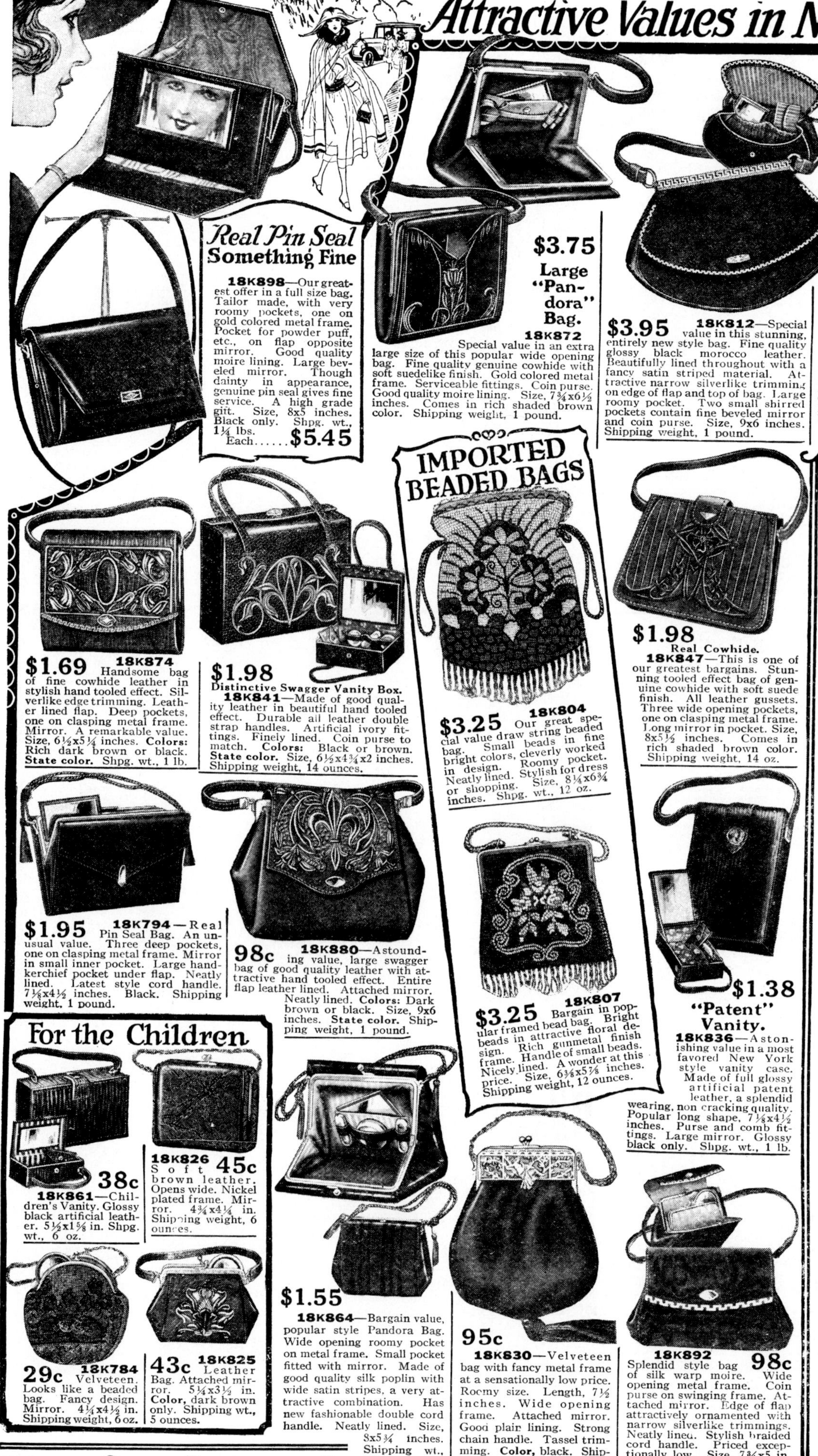

## Real Pin Seal Something Fine

**18K898**—Our greatest offer in a full size bag. Tailor made, with very roomy pockets, one on gold colored metal frame. Pocket for powder puff, etc., on flap opposite mirror. Good quality moire lining. Large beveled mirror. Though dainty in appearance, genuine pin seal gives fine service. A high grade gift. Size, 8x5 inches. Black only. Shpg. wt., 1¼ lbs. Each......**$5.45**

**$3.75** Large "Pandora" Bag.

**18K872** Special value in an extra large size of this popular wide opening bag. Fine quality genuine cowhide with soft suedelike finish. Gold colored metal frame. Serviceable fittings. Coin purse. Good quality moire lining. Size, 7¾x6½ inches. Comes in rich shaded brown color. Shipping weight, 1 pound.

**$3.95** **18K812**—Special value in this stunning, entirely new style bag. Fine quality glossy black morocco leather. Beautifully lined throughout with a fancy satin striped material. Attractive narrow silverlike trimming on edge of flap and top of bag. Large roomy pocket. Two small shirred pockets contain fine beveled mirror and coin purse. Size, 9x6 inches. Shipping weight, 1 pound.

with SAFETY POCKET

**$3.19** **18K890**—The better grade Safety Pocket Bag, the kind usually seen at about $4.50. Splendidly built of genuine cowhide leather, seal grain. Three roomy pockets, one on frame. Deep safety pocket for jewelry, etc. Mirror. Good lining. Practical size, 8x4⅞ inches. Highly recommended. **Colors:** Black or dark brown. **State color.** Shipping weight, 1 lb.

**$1.69** **18K874** Handsome bag of fine cowhide leather in stylish hand tooled effect. Silverlike edge trimming. Leather lined flap. Deep pockets, one on clasping metal frame. Mirror. A remarkable value. Size, 6½x5¼ inches. **Colors:** Rich dark brown or black. **State color.** Shpg. wt., 1 lb.

**$1.98** **Distinctive Swagger Vanity Box.** **18K841**—Made of good quality leather in beautiful hand tooled effect. Durable all leather double strap handles. Artificial ivory fittings. Finely lined. Coin purse to match. **Colors:** Black or brown. **State color.** Size, 6½x4¾x2 inches. Shipping weight, 14 ounces.

## IMPORTED BEADED BAGS

**$3.25** **18K804** Our great special value draw string beaded bag. Small beads in fine bright colors, cleverly worked in design. Roomy pocket. Neatly lined. Stylish for dress or shopping. Size, 8¼x6¾ inches. Shpg. wt., 12 oz.

**$3.25** **18K807** Bargain in popular framed bead bag. Bright beads in attractive floral design. Rich gunmetal finish frame. Handle of small beads. Nicely lined. A wonder at this price. Size, 6¾x5⅞ inches. Shipping weight, 12 ounces.

**$1.98** Real Cowhide. **18K847**—This is one of our greatest bargains. Stunning tooled effect bag of genuine cowhide with soft suede finish. All leather gussets. Three wide opening pockets, one on clasping metal frame. Long mirror in pocket. Size, 8x5½ inches. Comes in rich shaded brown color. Shipping weight, 14 oz.

**$1.95** **18K794**—Real Pin Seal Bag. An unusual value. Three deep pockets, one on clasping metal frame. Mirror in small inner pocket. Large handkerchief pocket under flap. Neatly lined. Latest style cord handle. 7⅛x4½ inches. Black. Shipping weight, 1 pound.

**98c** **18K880**—Astounding value, large swagger bag of good quality leather with attractive hand tooled effect. Entire flap leather lined. Attached mirror. Neatly lined. **Colors:** Dark brown or black. Size, 9x6 inches. **State color.** Shipping weight, 1 pound.

**$1.38** "Patent" Vanity. **18K836**—Astonishing value in a most favored New York style vanity case. Made of full glossy artificial patent leather, a splendid wearing, non cracking quality. Popular long shape, 7⅛x4½ inches. Purse and comb fittings. Large mirror. Glossy black only. Shpg. wt., 1 lb.

## For the Children

**38c** **18K861**—Children's Vanity. Glossy black artificial leather. 5½x1⅝ in. Shpg. wt., 6 oz.

**18K826** **45c** Soft brown leather. Opens wide. Nickel plated frame. Mirror. 4¾x4¼ in. Shipping weight, 6 ounces.

**29c** **18K784** Velveteen. Looks like a beaded bag. Fancy design. Mirror. 4¼x4½ in. Shipping weight, 6 oz.

**43c** **18K825** Leather Bag. Attached mirror. 5¼x3½ in. **Color,** dark brown only. Shipping wt., 5 ounces.

**$1.55** **18K864**—Bargain value, popular style Pandora Bag. Wide opening roomy pocket on metal frame. Small pocket fitted with mirror. Made of good quality silk poplin with wide satin stripes, a very attractive combination. Has new fashionable double cord handle. Neatly lined. Size, 8x5¾ inches. Shipping wt., 14 ounces.

**95c** **18K830**—Velveteen bag with fancy metal frame at a sensationally low price. Roomy size. Length, 7½ inches. Wide opening frame. Attached mirror. Good plain lining. Strong chain handle. Tassel trimming. **Color,** black. Shipping weight, 1 pound.

**18K892** **98c** Splendid style bag of silk warp moire. Wide opening metal frame. Coin purse on swinging frame. Attached mirror. Edge of flap attractively ornamented with narrow silverlike trimmings. Neatly lined. Stylish braided cord handle. Priced exceptionally low. Size, 7¾x5 in. Shipping weight, 7 ounces.

## What About Him?

A fine purse with his name in 22-karat gold letters will delight any man. See page 513.

**A—18K818** **$4.75**
Extra fine quality bag of rich looking brown calf leather. Wide opening pocket on gold plated frame; also large coin purse on swinging frame. Handkerchief pocket at back. Attractively lined. New style braided cord handle. Beveled mirror. Size, 7⅞x6½ inches. Shipping weight, 1 pound.

**B—18K851** **$3.85**
New Paris style vanity purse. Combination of genuine brown cowhide with soft suedelike finish and flap and handle of good quality glossy patent leather. Three deep pockets, one on gold plated frame. Handkerchief pocket on inside of flap. Beveled mirror. Size, 6⅛x5⅝ inches. Shipping weight, 1 pound.

**C—18K843** **$3.48**
Very special value bag in new flat shape style. Good quality leather in tooled effect. Special feature large beveled mirror, 7x5 inches on inner flap. Comes in bronze color (the fashionable greenish brown shade). Size, 7⅛x5¾ inches. Shipping weight, 1¼ pounds.

**D—18K859** **$4.38**
Splendid value. Very cleverly constructed. When bag is opened it resembles a four-leaf clover, having four separate pockets. When closed, powder puff and mirror can be removed without opening bag. Soft, pliable, fine quality genuine calf leather, in fancy design. Top set with small 14-karat gold clips. Beautiful lining. 9½x7 inches. Rich dark brown color. Shpg. wt., 10 oz.

**E—18K846** **$3.59**
New York's latest. Soft bag of fine quality dark brown goatskin with filigree lace effect on gold plated frame. Large center pocket opens wide. Coin purse and mirror. Soft, open, side pockets for powder puff or handkerchief. Beautiful lining. Cord handle. 10x5¼ inches. Shipping weight, 10 ounces.

**F—18K842** **$4.98**
Stunning new style bag in genuine cowhide with soft suede finish. Beautiful moire lining. Large beveled mirror concealed under flap. Most popular high grade bag. 7½x6 inches. Rich shaded brown color. Shipping weight, 1 lb.

**G—18K801** **$3.19**
Very smart bag. Beautiful combination of brown, soft, suede finished cowhide and genuine black patent leather. Wide opening metal frame. Fine beveled mirror and change purse. Large outside handkerchief pocket. New style braided cord handle. Neat moire lining. Size, 6x4¾ inches. Shipping weight, 8 oz.

**H—18K866** **$2.35**
Soft style small size bag of good leather, with the latest gold plated fancy frame. Good quality braided cord handle. Beveled mirror. Coin purse. Exquisitely lined. **Colors:** Navy blue or rich dark brown. 6x5½ inches. Shipping weight, 8 ounces.

**I—18K829** **$3.48**
Entirely different and a big bargain. Large new drop mirror style swagger bag. Good quality leather, in popular fluffed alligator grain. Large roomy pockets. Coin purse. Shirred pocket opposite large mirror inside flap, for powder puff, etc. Neatly lined. 8x5⅞ inches. **Colors:** Gray or dark brown. **State color.** Shipping weight, 1¼ lbs.

**J—18K798** **$1.19**
Very striking in black and red, as illustrated. Artificial patent leather with genuine glossy leather flap, concealing mirror. Three pockets, one on clasping metal frame. Good cord handle. 6¼x4¼ inches. Can also be had in all black. **State color.** Shipping weight, 12 oz.

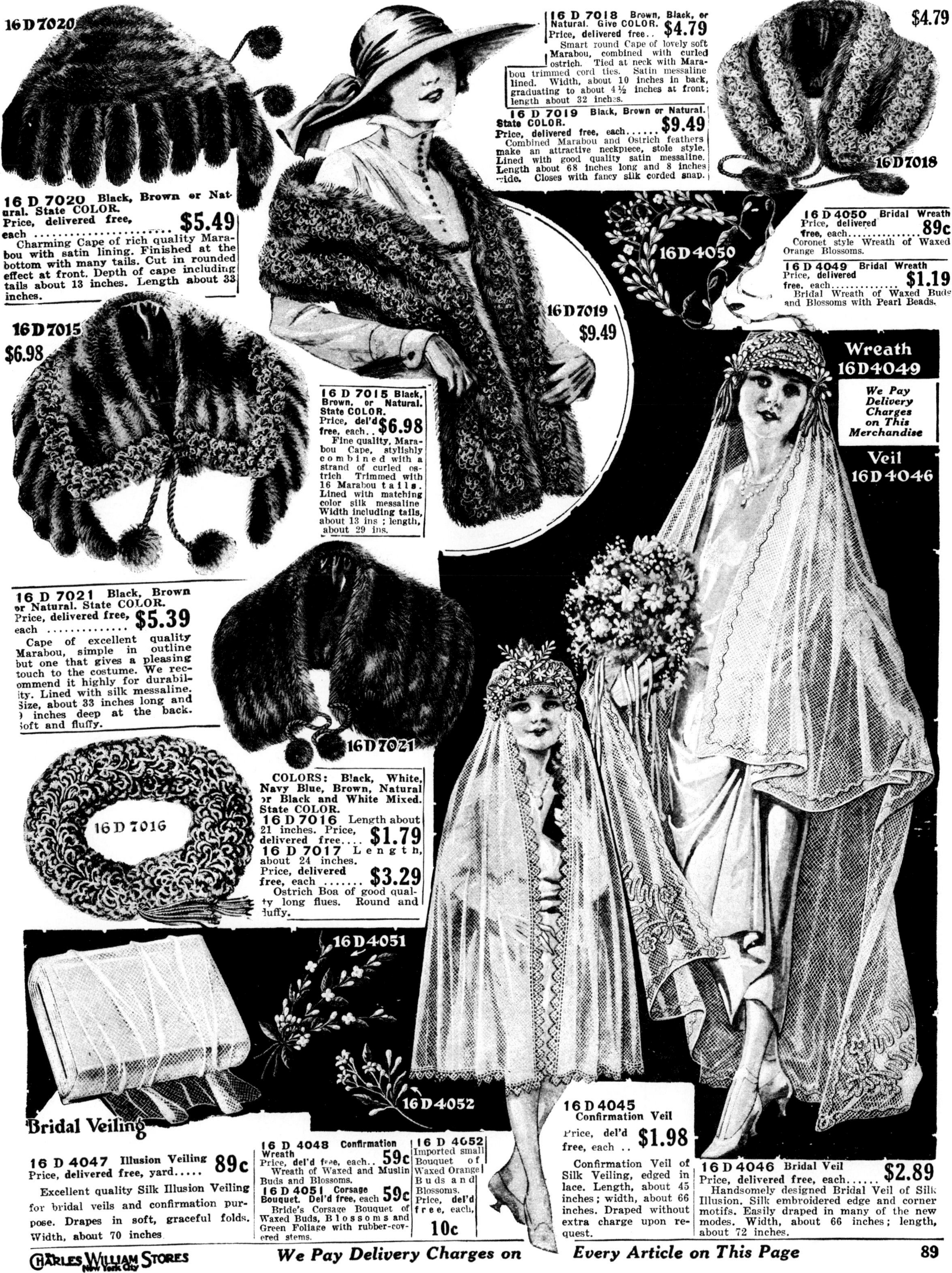
16 D 7020
16 D 7020 Black, Brown or Natural. State COLOR.
Price, delivered free, each .................... $5.49
Charming Cape of rich quality Marabou with satin lining. Finished at the bottom with many tails. Cut in rounded effect at front. Depth of cape including tails about 13 inches. Length about 33 inches.
16 D 7018 Brown, Black, or Natural. Give COLOR. Price, delivered free.. $4.79
Smart round Cape of lovely soft Marabou, combined with curled ostrich. Tied at neck with Marabou trimmed cord ties. Satin messaline lined. Width, about 10 inches in back, graduating to about 4½ inches at front; length about 32 inches.
16 D 7019 Black, Brown or Natural. State COLOR.
Price, delivered free, each...... $9.49
Combined Marabou and Ostrich feathers make an attractive neckpiece, stole style. Lined with good quality satin messaline. Length about 68 inches long and 8 inches wide. Closes with fancy silk corded snap.
$4.79
16 D 7018
16 D 4050
16 D 4050 Bridal Wreath Price, delivered free, each.............. 89c
Coronet style Wreath of Waxed Orange Blossoms.
16 D 4049 Bridal Wreath Price, delivered free, each.............. $1.19
Bridal Wreath of Waxed Buds and Blossoms with Pearl Beads.
16 D 7015
$6.98
16 D 7019
$9.49
Wreath 16 D 4049
We Pay Delivery Charges on This Merchandise
Veil 16 D 4046
16 D 7015 Black, Brown, or Natural. State COLOR.
Price, del'd free, each.. $6.98
Fine quality, Marabou Cape, stylishly combined with a strand of curled ostrich. Trimmed with 16 Marabou tails. Lined with matching color silk messaline Width including tails, about 13 ins; length, about 29 ins.
16 D 7021 Black, Brown or Natural. State COLOR.
Price, delivered free, each ............. $5.39
Cape of excellent quality Marabou, simple in outline but one that gives a pleasing touch to the costume. We recommend it highly for durability. Lined with silk messaline. Size, about 33 inches long and 9 inches deep at the back. Soft and fluffy.
16 D 7021
16 D 7016
COLORS: Black, White, Navy Blue, Brown, Natural or Black and White Mixed. State COLOR.
16 D 7016 Length about 21 inches. Price, delivered free.... $1.79
16 D 7017 Length, about 24 inches. Price, delivered free, each ....... $3.29
Ostrich Boa of good quality long flues. Round and fluffy.
16 D 4051
16 D 4052
Bridal Veiling
16 D 4047 Illusion Veiling Price, delivered free, yard..... 89c
Excellent quality Silk Illusion Veiling for bridal veils and confirmation purpose. Drapes in soft, graceful folds. Width, about 70 inches
16 D 4048 Confirmation Wreath Price, del'd free, each.. 59c
Wreath of Waxed and Muslin Buds and Blossoms.
16 D 4051 Corsage Bouquet. Del'd free, each 59c
Bride's Corsage Bouquet of Waxed Buds, Blossoms and Green Foliage with rubber-covered stems.
16 D 4052 Imported small Bouquet of Waxed Orange Buds and Blossoms. Price, del'd free, each, 10c
16 D 4045 Confirmation Veil
Price, del'd free, each .. $1.98
Confirmation Veil of Silk Veiling, edged in lace. Length, about 45 inches; width, about 66 inches. Draped without extra charge upon request.
16 D 4046 Bridal Veil
Price, delivered free, each...... $2.89
Handsomely designed Bridal Veil of Silk Illusion. Silk embroidered edge and corner motifs. Easily draped in many of the new modes. Width, about 66 inches; length, about 72 inches.

# Women's, Girls' and Children's Arctics, Gaiters, Galoshes

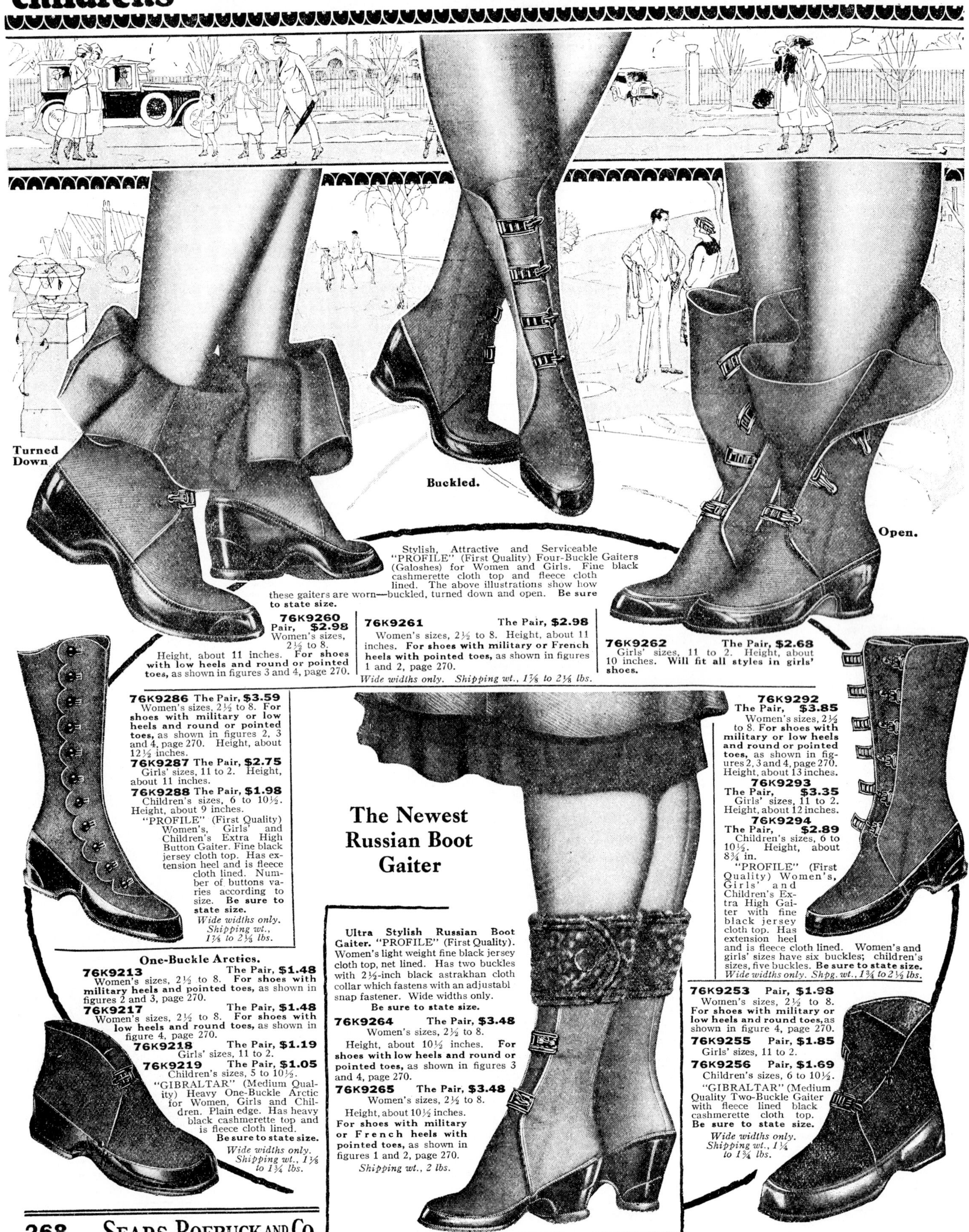

Turned Down
Buckled.
Open.
Stylish, Attractive and Serviceable "PROFILE" (First Quality) Four-Buckle Gaiters (Galoshes) for Women and Girls. Fine black cashmerette cloth top and fleece cloth lined. The above illustrations show how these gaiters are worn—buckled, turned down and open. Be sure to state size.
76K9260 Pair, $2.98 Women's sizes, 2½ to 8. Height, about 11 inches. For shoes with low heels and round or pointed toes, as shown in figures 3 and 4, page 270.
76K9261 The Pair, $2.98 Women's sizes, 2½ to 8. Height, about 11 inches. For shoes with military or French heels with pointed toes, as shown in figures 1 and 2, page 270.
Wide widths only. Shipping wt., 1⅞ to 2⅛ lbs.
76K9262 The Pair, $2.68 Girls' sizes, 11 to 2. Height, about 10 inches. Will fit all styles in girls' shoes.
76K9286 The Pair, $3.59 Women's sizes, 2½ to 8. For shoes with military or low heels and round or pointed toes, as shown in figures 2, 3 and 4, page 270. Height, about 12¼ inches.
76K9287 The Pair, $2.75 Girls' sizes, 11 to 2. Height, about 11 inches.
76K9288 The Pair, $1.98 Children's sizes, 6 to 10½. Height, about 9 inches.
"PROFILE" (First Quality) Women's, Girls' and Children's Extra High Button Gaiter. Fine black jersey cloth top. Has extension heel and is fleece cloth lined. Number of buttons varies according to size. Be sure to state size.
Wide widths only. Shipping wt., 1⅞ to 2⅛ lbs.
The Newest Russian Boot Gaiter
76K9292 The Pair, $3.85 Women's sizes, 2½ to 8. For shoes with military or low heels and round or pointed toes, as shown in figures 2, 3 and 4, page 270. Height, about 13 inches.
76K9293 The Pair, $3.35 Girls' sizes, 11 to 2. Height, about 12 inches.
76K9294 The Pair, $2.89 Children's sizes, 6 to 10½. Height, about 8¾ in.
"PROFILE" (First Quality) Women's, Girls' and Children's Extra High Gaiter with fine black jersey cloth top. Has extension heel and is fleece cloth lined. Women's and girls' sizes have six buckles; children's sizes, five buckles. Be sure to state size.
Wide widths only. Shpg. wt., 1¾ to 2½ lbs.
One-Buckle Arctics.
76K9213 The Pair, $1.48 Women's sizes, 2½ to 8. For shoes with military heels and pointed toes, as shown in figures 2 and 3, page 270.
76K9217 The Pair, $1.48 Women's sizes, 2½ to 8. For shoes with low heels and round toes, as shown in figure 4, page 270.
76K9218 The Pair, $1.19 Girls' sizes, 11 to 2.
76K9219 The Pair, $1.05 Children's sizes, 5 to 10½.
"GIBRALTAR" (Medium Quality) Heavy One-Buckle Arctic for Women, Girls and Children. Plain edge. Has heavy black cashmerette top and is fleece cloth lined. Be sure to state size.
Wide widths only. Shipping wt., 1⅛ to 1¾ lbs.
Ultra Stylish Russian Boot Gaiter. "PROFILE" (First Quality). Women's light weight fine black jersey cloth top, net lined. Has two buckles with 2½-inch black astrakhan cloth collar which fastens with an adjustabl snap fastener. Wide widths only.
Be sure to state size.
76K9264 The Pair, $3.48 Women's sizes, 2½ to 8. Height, about 10½ inches. For shoes with low heels and round or pointed toes, as shown in figures 3 and 4, page 270.
76K9265 The Pair, $3.48 Women's sizes, 2½ to 8. Height, about 10½ inches. For shoes with military or French heels with pointed toes, as shown in figures 1 and 2, page 270.
Shipping wt., 2 lbs.
76K9253 Pair, $1.98 Women's sizes, 2½ to 8. For shoes with military or low heels and round toes, as shown in figure 4, page 270.
76K9255 Pair, $1.85 Girls' sizes, 11 to 2.
76K9256 Pair, $1.69 Children's sizes, 6 to 10½.
"GIBRALTAR" (Medium Quality Two-Buckle Gaiter with fleece lined black cashmerette cloth top. Be sure to state size.
Wide widths only. Shipping wt., 1¼ to 1¾ lbs.

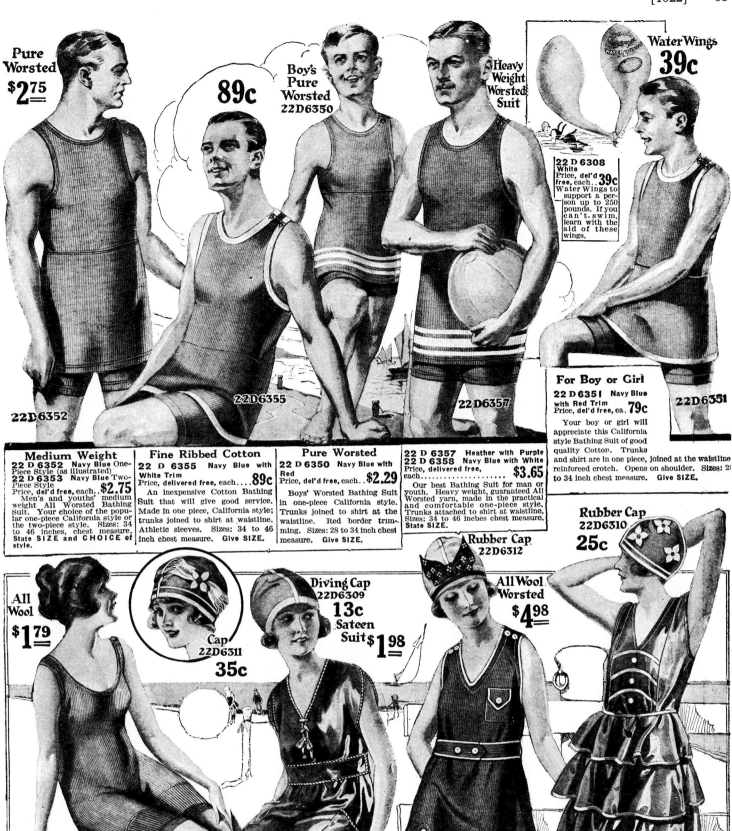

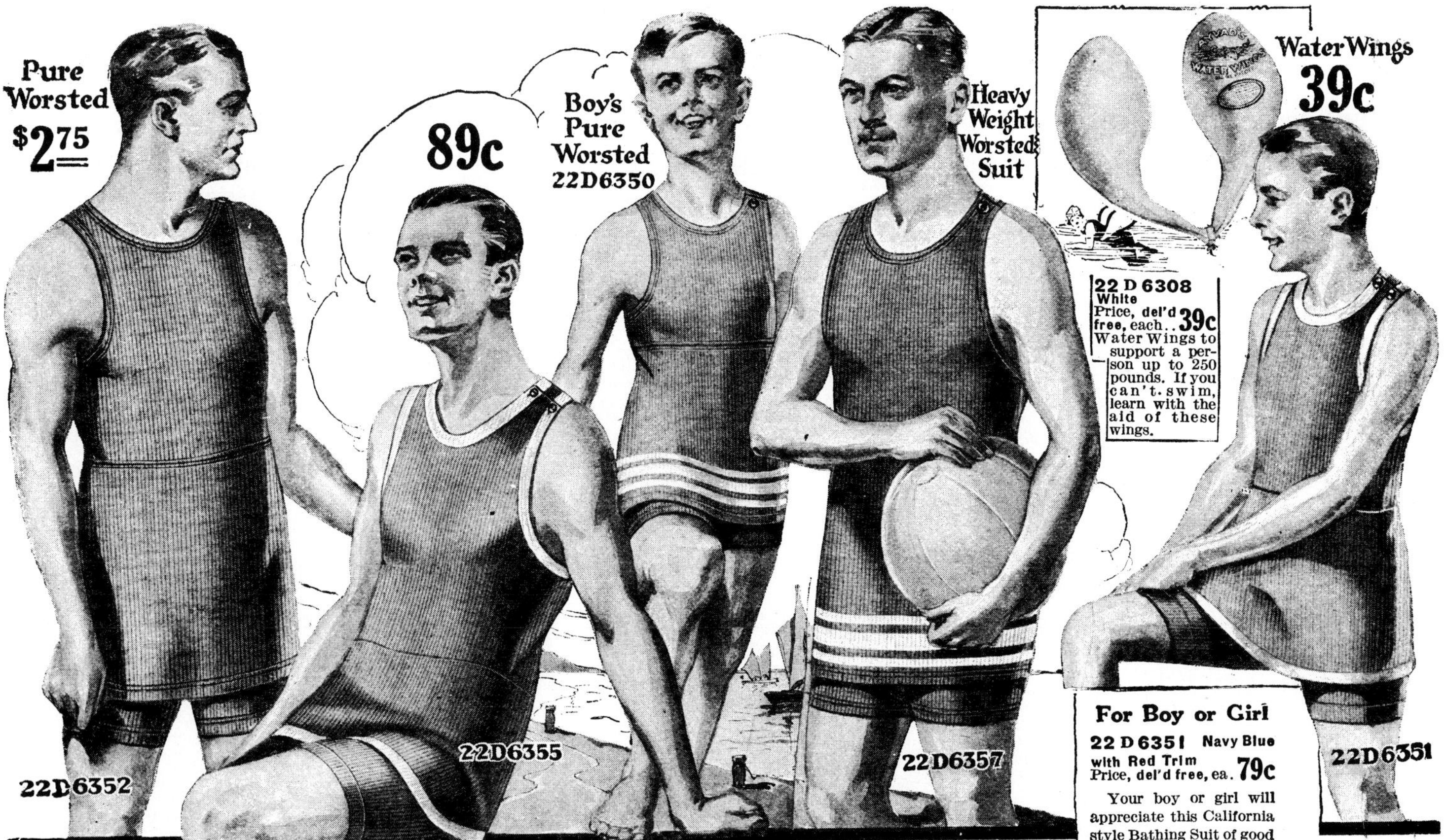

Pure Worsted $2.75

89c

Boy's Pure Worsted 22D6350

Heavy Weight Worsted Suit

Water Wings 39c

22 D 6308 White
Price, del'd free, each.. 39c
Water Wings to support a person up to 250 pounds. If you can't swim, learn with the aid of these wings.

22D6352

22D6355

22D6357

For Boy or Girl
22 D 6351 Navy Blue with Red Trim
Price, del'd free, ea. 79c
Your boy or girl will appreciate this California style Bathing Suit of good quality Cotton. Trunks and shirt are in one piece, joined at the waistline; reinforced crotch. Opens on shoulder. Sizes: 28 to 34 inch chest measure. Give SIZE.

22D6351

**Medium Weight**
22 D 6352 Navy Blue One-Piece Style (as illustrated)
22 D 6353 Navy Blue Two-Piece Style
Price, del'd free, each.. $2.75
Men's and youths' medium weight All Worsted Bathing Suit. Your choice of the popular one-piece California style or the two-piece style. Sizes: 34 to 46 inches, chest measure. State SIZE and CHOICE of style.

**Fine Ribbed Cotton**
22 D 6355 Navy Blue with White Trim
Price, delivered free, each.... 89c
An inexpensive Cotton Bathing Suit that will give good service. Made in one piece, California style; trunks joined to shirt at waistline. Athletic sleeves. Sizes: 34 to 46 inch chest measure. Give SIZE.

**Pure Worsted**
22 D 6350 Navy Blue with Red
Price, del'd free, each.. $2.29
Boys' Worsted Bathing Suit in one-piece California style. Trunks joined to shirt at the waistline. Red border trimming. Sizes: 28 to 34 inch chest measure. Give SIZE.

22 D 6357 Heather with Purple
22 D 6358 Navy Blue with White
Price, delivered free, each.................. $3.65
Our best Bathing Suit for man or youth. Heavy weight, guaranteed All Worsted yarn, made in the practical and comfortable one-piece style. Trunks attached to shirt at waistline. Sizes: 34 to 46 inches chest measure. State SIZE.

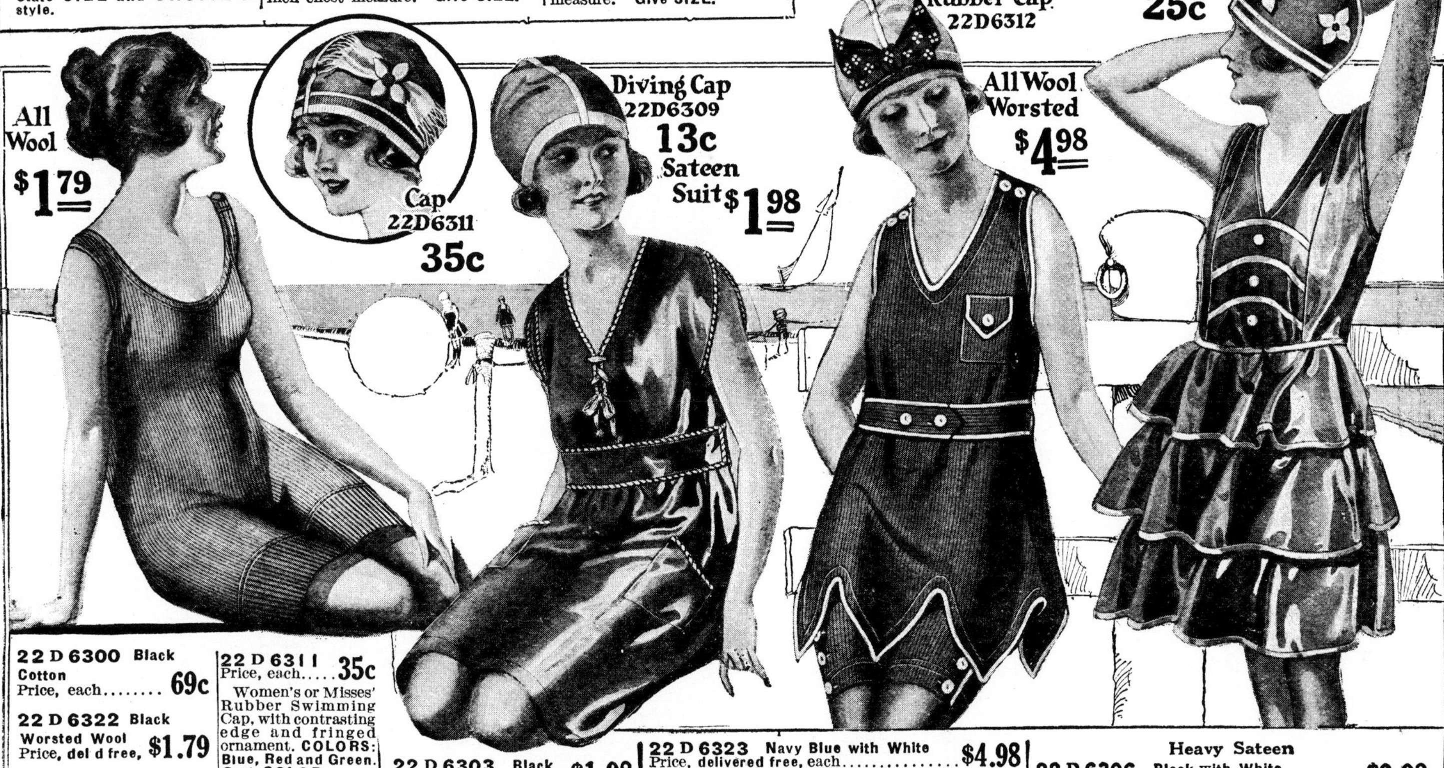


22 D 6300 Black Cotton
Price, each........ 69c
22 D 6322 Black Worsted Wool
Price, del'd free, $1.79
One-piece undergarment for women and girls. Closely knit, in fine elastic stitch. Warm and durable. Elastic ribbed cuffs. Sizes: 28 to 44 inches bust measure. Give SIZE.

22 D 6311 Price, each..... 35c
Women's or Misses' Rubber Swimming Cap, with contrasting edge and fringed ornament. COLORS: Blue, Red and Green. Give COLOR.

22 D 6303 Black
Price, del'd free, each.. $1.98
Black Sateen Bathing Suit for women and girls. Has belt and pockets. For undergarment see 22 D 6300. Sizes: 28 to 44 inches bust. Give SIZE.
22 D 6309 Assorted Colors
Price, each.......................... 13c
Two for 25c
Rubber diving cap for women and misses.

22 D 6323 Navy Blue with White
Price, delivered free, each.......... $4.98
All-Wool Worsted Bathing Suit, in fine Jersey knit, suitable for women and misses. Scalloped skirt edged with white; trunks have three pearl buttons at each side. Has belt and pocket. Sizes: 34 to 44 inches bust measure. State SIZE.
22 D 6312 Rubber Cap
Price, delivered free, each.................. 49c
Good quality Rubber Cap, with "Kiss-Me" bow. COLORS: Blue, Green and Red. State COLOR.

**Heavy Sateen**
22 D 6306 Black with White
Price, delivered free, each.................. $2.98
Lustrous Black Sateen Bathing Suit. Ruffles piped with white Sateen. For undergarment, see 22 D 6300. Sizes: 34 to 44 inches bust measure. State SIZE.
22 D 6310 Rubber Cap
Price, delivered free, each.................. 25c
Good quality Rubber Cap, with flower design. COLORS: Blue, Red and Green. State COLOR.

# Cool Athletic Underwear

**VALUES**

On these pages you will find seasonable underwear for every member of the family. Made in a variety of fabrics, of materials selected for long wearing qualities. Every garment is designed and made for comfort and service. We have many styles in all weights and lengths of underwear.

## Athletic Style

**15 D 1825** Shirt
**15 D 1827** Drawers

Sizes: Shirt, 34 to 46 chest. Drawers, 32 to 44 waist. State SIZE.
Price, delivered free, each........................ **47c**

An especially comfortable style for summer wear. Cool Undergarments of White Crossbar Nainsook in popular sleeveless athletic style. Well finished. Closes with pearl buttons. The knee length drawers have a double waistband; laced in the back.

## Athletic Shirt and Drawers

**15 D 1817** Shirt
Sizes: 34 to 46 chest measure. State SIZE.
**15 D 1819** Drawers
Sizes: 32 to 44 waist measure. State SIZE.
Price, delivered free, each...... **69c**

Summer weight Athletic Undergarments. Shirt is made in a flat knit elastic stitch of white Cotton. Pulls over the head. Deep elastic hem of self-material on the neck and armholes. Drawers are knee length, finished with an elastic hem. Heavy muslin waistband double stitched. Suspender straps and tie tape in back.

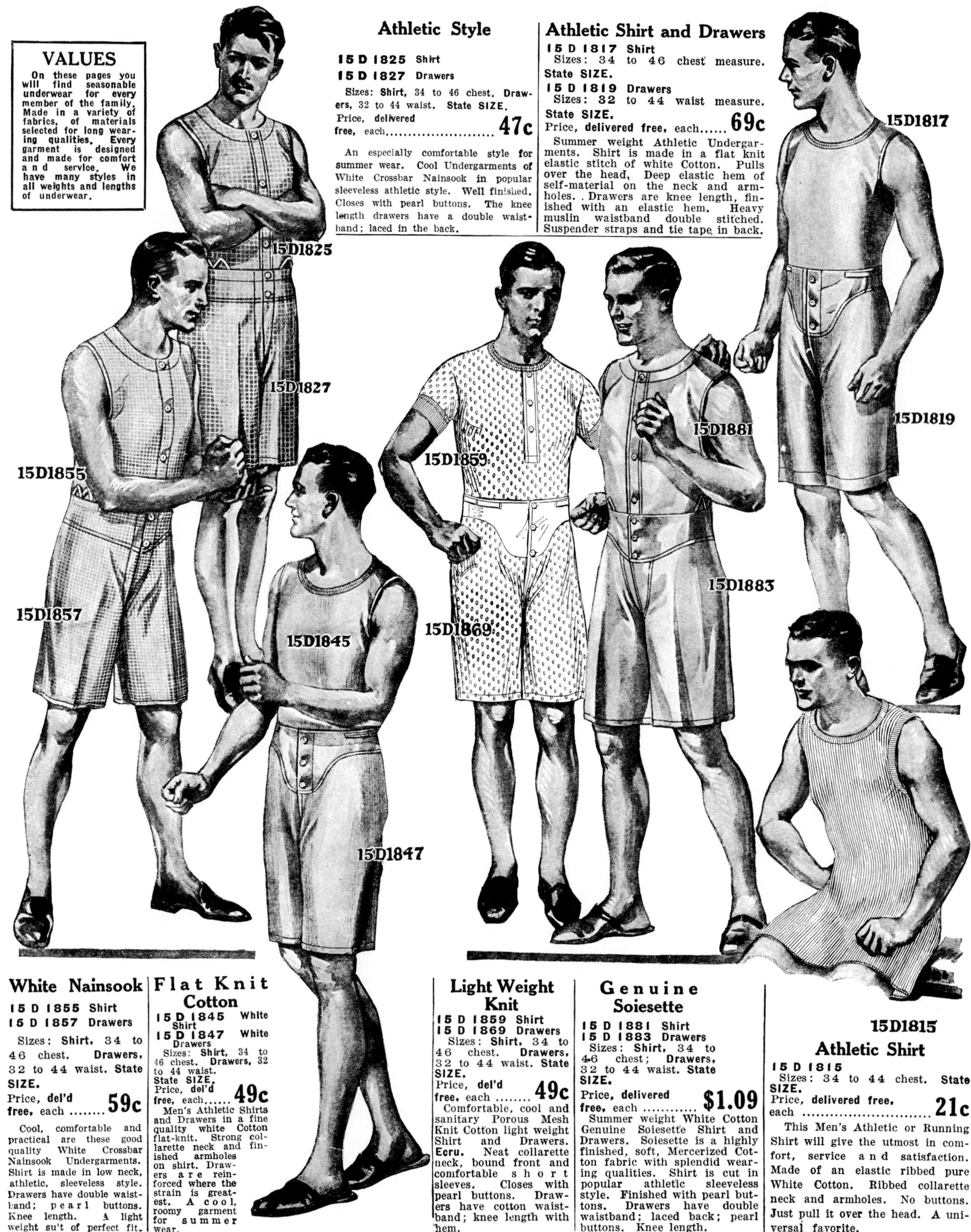


## White Nainsook

**15 D 1855** Shirt
**15 D 1857** Drawers

Sizes: Shirt, 34 to 46 chest. Drawers, 32 to 44 waist. State SIZE.
Price, del'd free, each ........ **59c**

Cool, comfortable and practical are these good quality White Crossbar Nainsook Undergarments. Shirt is made in low neck, athletic, sleeveless style. Drawers have double waistband; pearl buttons. Knee length. A light weight suit of perfect fit.

## Flat Knit Cotton

**15 D 1845** White Shirt
**15 D 1847** White Drawers

Sizes: Shirt, 34 to 46 chest. Drawers, 32 to 44 waist. State SIZE.
Price, del'd free, each...... **49c**

Men's Athletic Shirts and Drawers in a fine quality white Cotton flat-knit. Strong collarette neck and finished armholes on shirt. Drawers are reinforced where the strain is greatest. A cool, roomy garment for summer wear.

## Light Weight Knit

**15 D 1859** Shirt
**15 D 1869** Drawers

Sizes: Shirt, 34 to 46 chest. Drawers, 32 to 44 waist. State SIZE.
Price, del'd free, each ........ **49c**

Comfortable, cool and sanitary Porous Mesh Knit Cotton light weight Shirt and Drawers. Ecru. Neat collarette neck, bound front and comfortable short sleeves. Closes with pearl buttons. Drawers have cotton waistband; knee length with hem.

## Genuine Soiesette

**15 D 1881** Shirt
**15 D 1883** Drawers

Sizes: Shirt, 34 to 46 chest; Drawers, 32 to 44 waist. State SIZE.
Price, delivered free, each ........... **$1.09**

Summer weight White Cotton Genuine Soiesette Shirt and Drawers. Soiesette is a highly finished, soft, Mercerized Cotton fabric with splendid wearing qualities. Shirt is cut in popular athletic sleeveless style. Finished with pearl buttons. Drawers have double waistband; laced back; pearl buttons. Knee length.

15D1815

## Athletic Shirt

**15 D 1815**
Sizes: 34 to 44 chest. State SIZE.
Price, delivered free, each ........................... **21c**

This Men's Athletic or Running Shirt will give the utmost in comfort, service and satisfaction. Made of an elastic ribbed pure White Cotton. Ribbed collarette neck and armholes. No buttons. Just pull it over the head. A universal favorite.

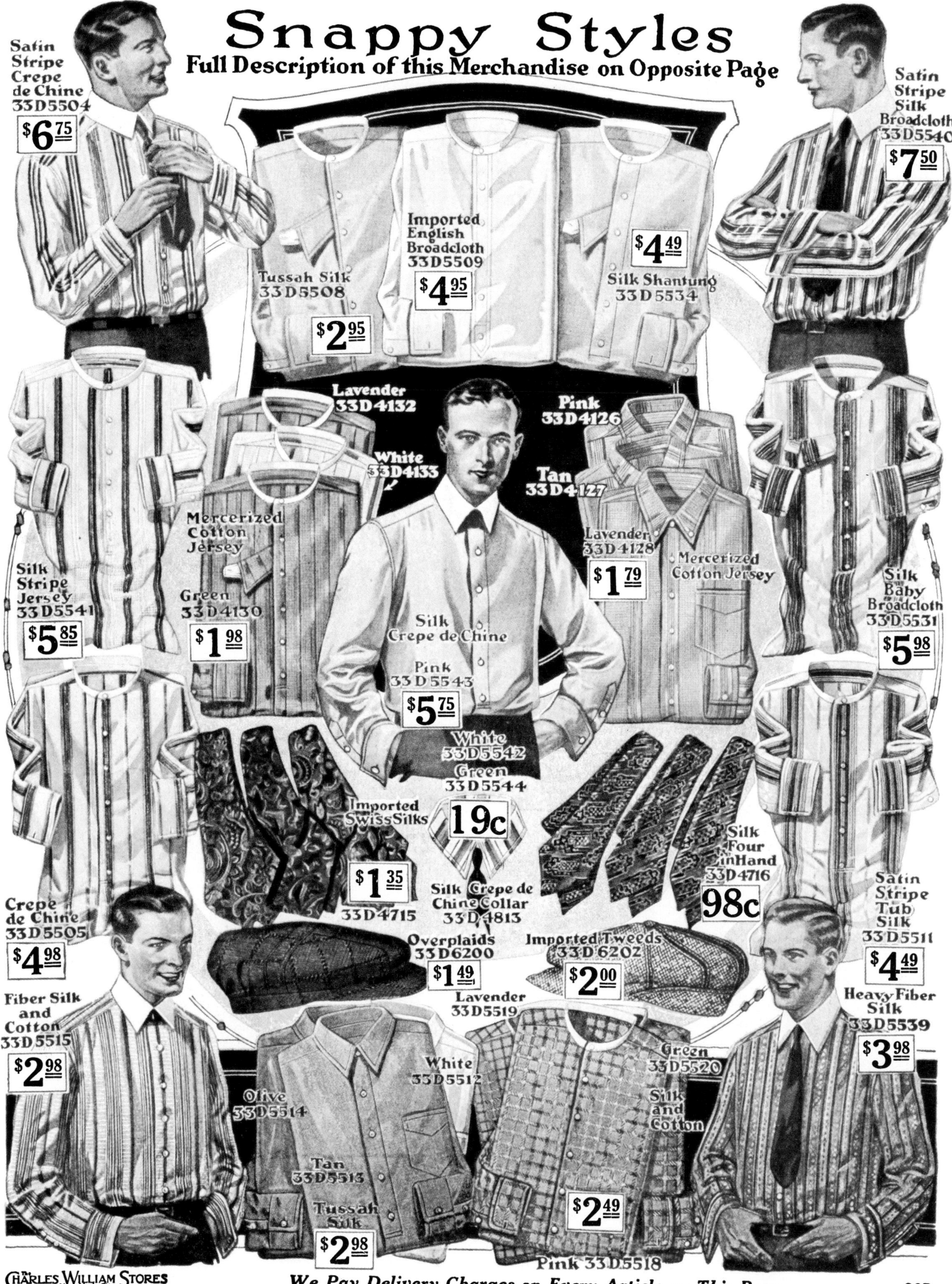
Snappy Styles
Full Description of this Merchandise on Opposite Page
Satin Stripe Crepe de Chine 33D5504 $6.75
Satin Stripe Silk Broadcloth 33D5540 $7.50
Imported English Broadcloth 33D5509 $4.95
Tussah Silk 33D5508 $2.95
$4.49 Silk Shantung 33D5534
Lavender 33D4132
White 33D4133
Pink 33D4126
Tan 33D4127
Mercerized Cotton Jersey
Green 33D4130 $1.98
Lavender 33D4128 $1.79
Mercerized Cotton Jersey
Silk Stripe Jersey 33D5541 $5.85
Silk Baby Broadcloth 33D5531 $5.98
Silk Crepe de Chine Pink 33D5543 $5.75
White 33D5542
Green 33D5544
Imported Swiss Silks $1.35 33D4715
19c
Silk Crepe de Chine Collar 33D4813
Silk Four in Hand 33D4716 98c
Crepe de Chine 33D5505 $4.98
Satin Stripe Tub Silk 33D5511 $4.49
Overplaids 33D6200 $1.49
Imported Tweeds 33D6202 $2.00
Fiber Silk and Cotton 33D5515 $2.98
Heavy Fiber Silk 33D5539 $3.98
Lavender 33D5519
White 33D5512
Olive 33D5514
Tan 33D5513
Tussah Silk $2.98
Green 33D5520
Silk and Cotton
$2.49
Pink 33D5518

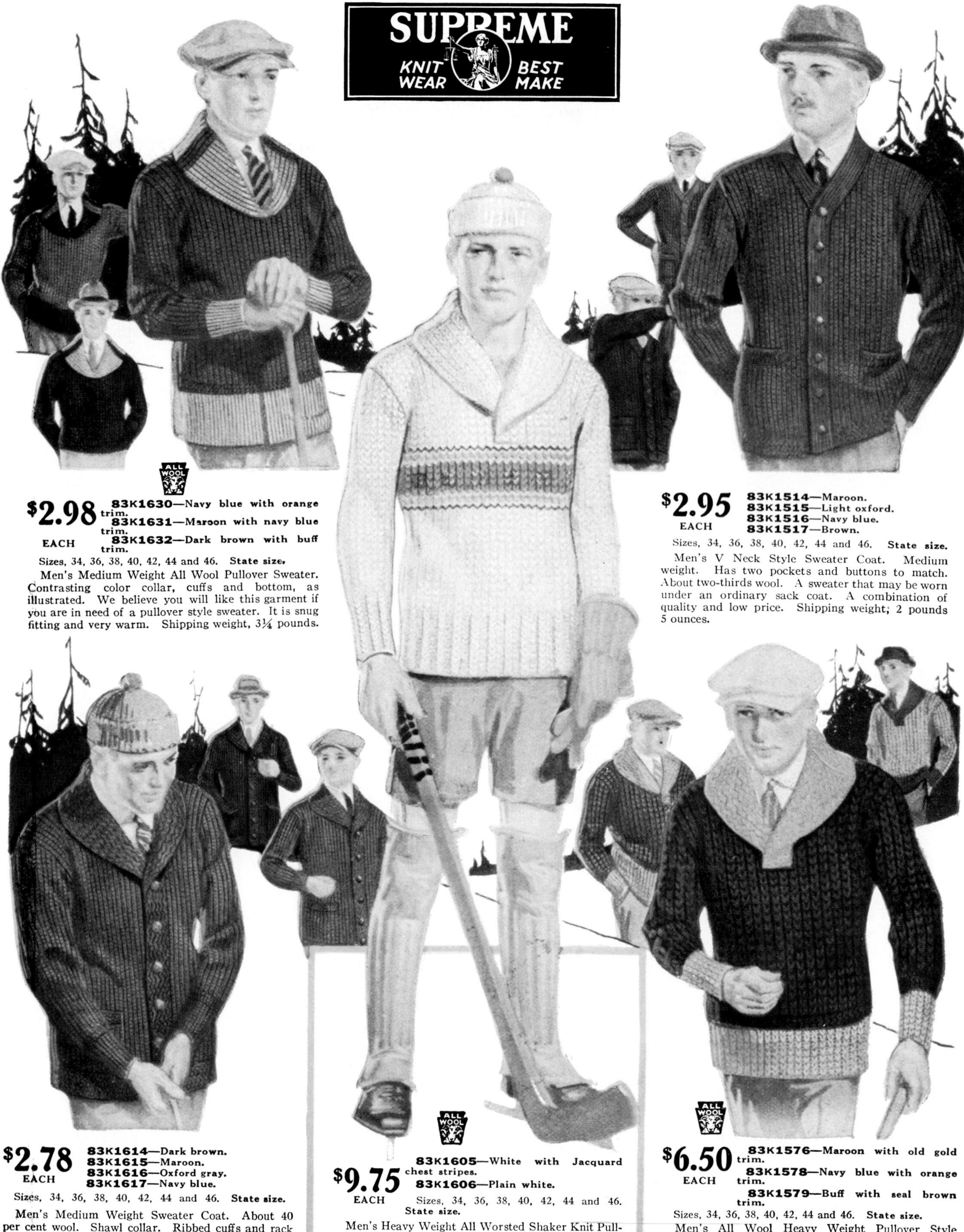


**$2.98** EACH
**83K1630**—Navy blue with orange trim.
**83K1631**—Maroon with navy blue trim.
**83K1632**—Dark brown with buff trim.

Sizes, 34, 36, 38, 40, 42, 44 and 46. **State size.**

Men's Medium Weight All Wool Pullover Sweater. Contrasting color collar, cuffs and bottom, as illustrated. We believe you will like this garment if you are in need of a pullover style sweater. It is snug fitting and very warm. Shipping weight, 3¼ pounds.

**$2.95** EACH
**83K1514**—Maroon.
**83K1515**—Light oxford.
**83K1516**—Navy blue.
**83K1517**—Brown.

Sizes, 34, 36, 38, 40, 42, 44 and 46. **State size.**

Men's V Neck Style Sweater Coat. Medium weight. Has two pockets and buttons to match. About two-thirds wool. A sweater that may be worn under an ordinary sack coat. A combination of quality and low price. Shipping weight, 2 pounds 5 ounces.

**$2.78** EACH
**83K1614**—Dark brown.
**83K1615**—Maroon.
**83K1616**—Oxford gray.
**83K1617**—Navy blue.

Sizes, 34, 36, 38, 40, 42, 44 and 46. **State size.**

Men's Medium Weight Sweater Coat. About 40 per cent wool. Shawl collar. Ribbed cuffs and rack knit front and bottom. Made with two pockets. Trimmed with pearl buttons. Can be buttoned closely about neck in severe weather, if desired. **Extremely low priced.** Will wear well. Truly a wonderful bargain at our low price. Shipping weight, 2¾ pounds.

**$9.75** EACH
**83K1605**—White with Jacquard chest stripes.
**83K1606**—Plain white.

Sizes, 34, 36, 38, 40, 42, 44 and 46. **State size.**

Men's Heavy Weight All Worsted Shaker Knit Pullover Sweater. Made with large shawl collar. Handmade and finished throughout. A very high quality garment. In offering this sweater we are giving our customers a chance to buy a real snappy up to the minute sweater, one that is very popular all over the country. A very attractive garment. Shipping weight, 3½ pounds.

**$6.50** EACH
**83K1576**—Maroon with old gold trim.
**83K1578**—Navy blue with orange trim.
**83K1579**—Buff with seal brown trim.

Sizes, 34, 36, 38, 40, 42, 44 and 46. **State size.**

Men's All Wool Heavy Weight Pullover Style Sweater. Body of this coat is made in heavy rope stitch and the large shawl collar, cuffs and bottom are in rack stitch. Collars, cuffs and bottom trimmed with contrasting colors as illustrated. A fine quality garment. Shipping weight, 3½ pounds.

See How to Measure Scale on Page 351.

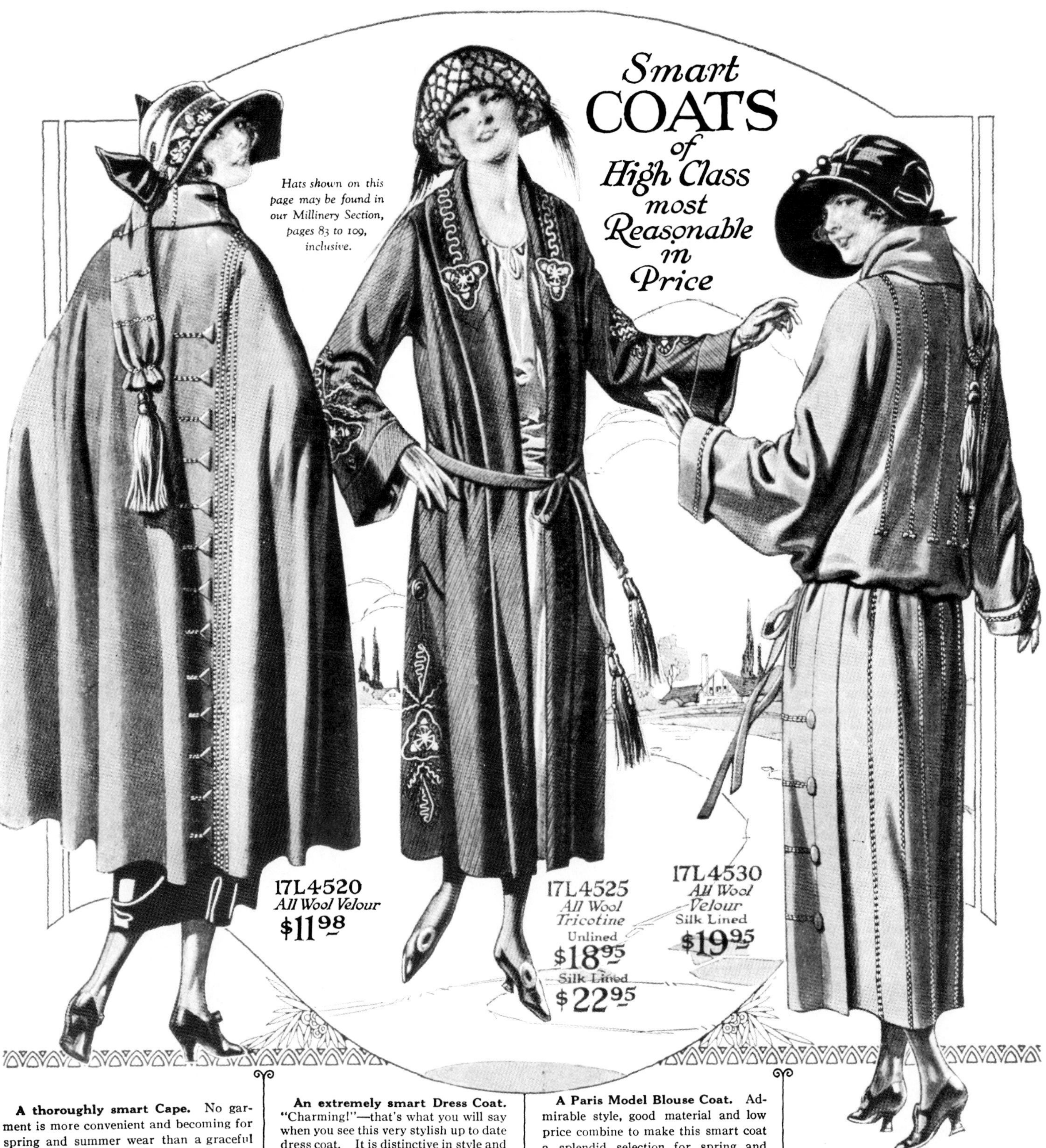


**A thoroughly smart Cape.** No garment is more convenient and becoming for spring and summer wear than a graceful circular cape like the one pictured above. This model is made of good quality **all wool velour** in spring weight. It is cut with ample fullness, falling in graceful rippling folds, and is elaborated on the back with full length rows of heavy embroidery stitching and oddly shaped self covered buttons. Attached to the cape is a stylish throw scarf collar of the same material, finished with embroidery stitching and tasseled ends. Cape is unlined and is 43 inches long. **A highly satisfactory garment very reasonably priced.**

WOMEN'S AND MISSES' SIZES—34 to 46 inches bust measure. **State size.** Shipping weight, 3½ pounds.

**17L4520**—Tan.
**17L4521**—Liberty blue. **$11.98**

**An extremely smart Dress Coat.** "Charming!"—that's what you will say when you see this very stylish up to date dress coat. It is distinctive in style and ideal for dress occasions during the spring and summer. The coat is made of high grade spring weight **all wool tricotine.** It is a loose fitting model held at waist by a tasseled tie sash. The collar, bell sleeves and the panels on the sides of coat are richly adorned with a tasteful design of heavy embroidery in contrasting colors. Note also the graceful turned back revers extending down the front of the model. Coat is 43 inches long and may be had unlined or lined with fancy silk. **A splendid value.**

WOMEN'S AND MISSES' SIZES—34 to 46 inches bust measure. **State size.** Shpg. wt., 3¾ lbs.

**Unlined.**
**17L4525**—Navy blue.
**17L4526**—Black. **$18.95**

**Full Fancy Silk Lined.**
**17L4527**—Navy blue.
**17L4528** Black. **$22.95**

**A Paris Model Blouse Coat.** Admirable style, good material and low price combine to make this smart coat a splendid selection for spring and summer. It is made of durable quality spring weight **all wool velour,** and is designed with a stylish blouse back as pictured. Back of coat is trimmed with embroidery stitching in self color, and the cuffs on the loose mandarin sleeves, also front of model, are adorned with embroidery stitching to match back. Another smart style feature is the graceful throw scarf collar which is trimmed with long tassels. Tie sash is of self material. Two pockets. This coat is 46 inches long and is richly lined throughout with fancy silk. **A wonderful value.**

WOMEN'S AND MISSES' SIZES—34 to 46 inches bust measure. **State size.** Shipping weight, 3½ pounds.

**17L4530**—Taupe.
**17L4531** Reindeer tan. **$19.95**

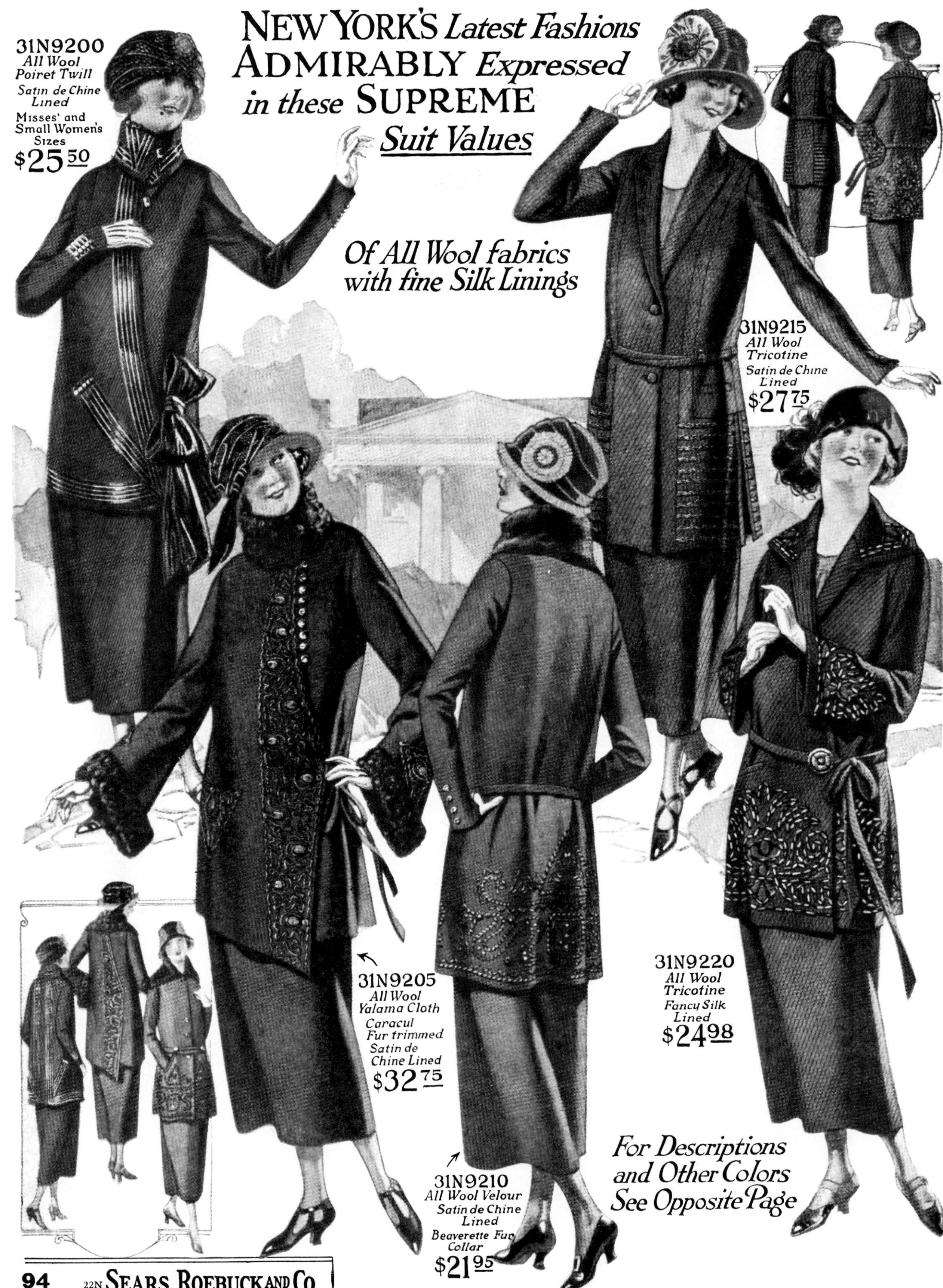
NEW YORK'S Latest Fashions
ADMIRABLY Expressed
in these SUPREME
Suit Values
Of All Wool fabrics
with fine Silk Linings
31N9200
All Wool
Poiret Twill
Satin de Chine
Lined
Misses' and
Small Women's
Sizes
$25.50
31N9215
All Wool
Tricotine
Satin de Chine
Lined
$27.75
31N9205
All Wool
Yalama Cloth
Caracul
Fur trimmed
Satin de
Chine Lined
$32.75
31N9220
All Wool
Tricotine
Fancy Silk
Lined
$24.98
31N9210
All Wool Velour
Satin de Chine
Lined
Beaverette Fur
Collar
$21.95
For Descriptions
and Other Colors
See Opposite Page

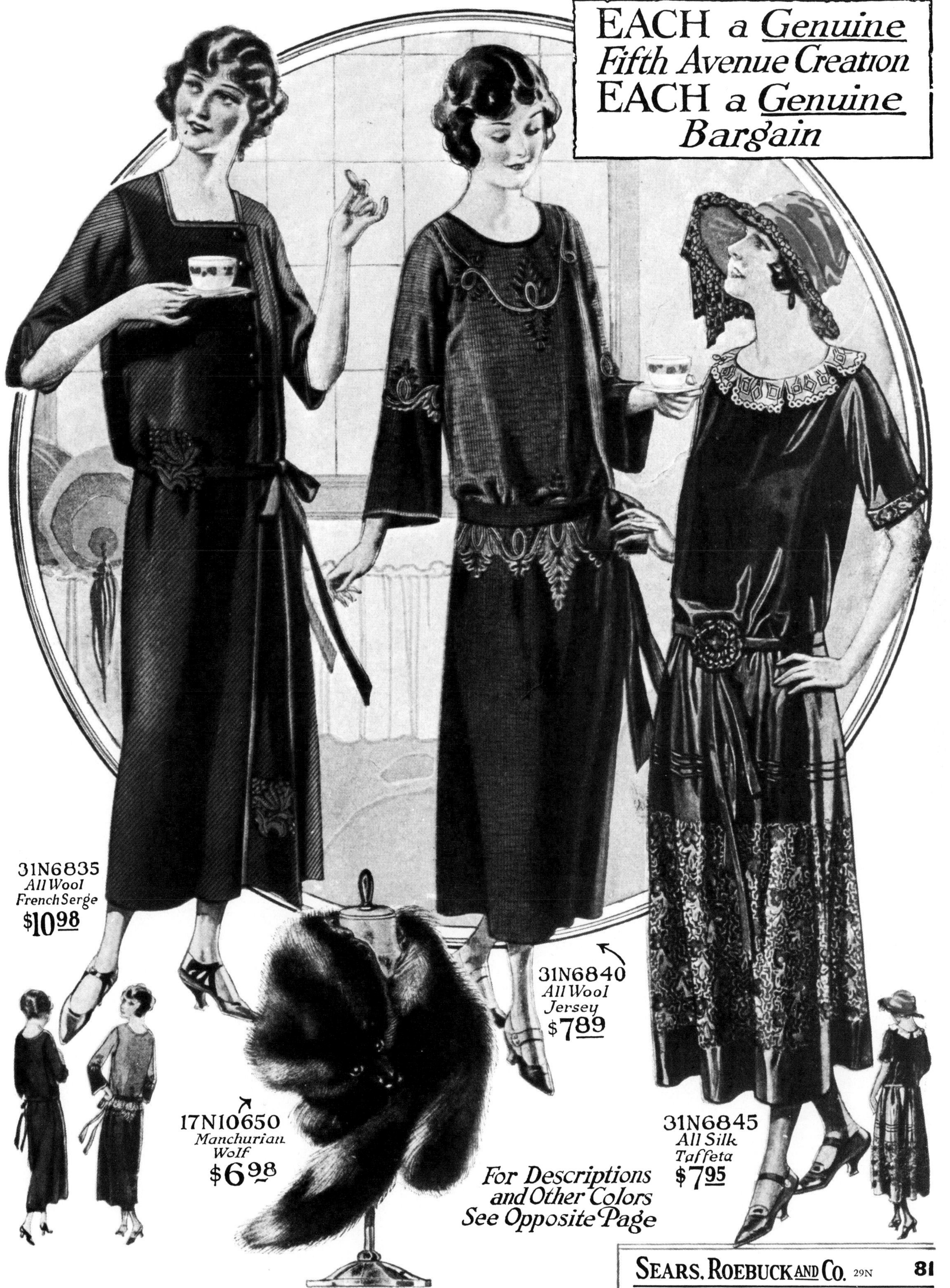
EACH a Genuine
Fifth Avenue Creation
EACH a Genuine
Bargain
31N6835
All Wool
French Serge
$10.98
31N6840
All Wool
Jersey
$7.89
17N10650
Manchurian
Wolf
$6.98
31N6845
All Silk
Taffeta
$7.95
For Descriptions
and Other Colors
See Opposite Page
SEARS, ROEBUCK AND CO. 29N 81

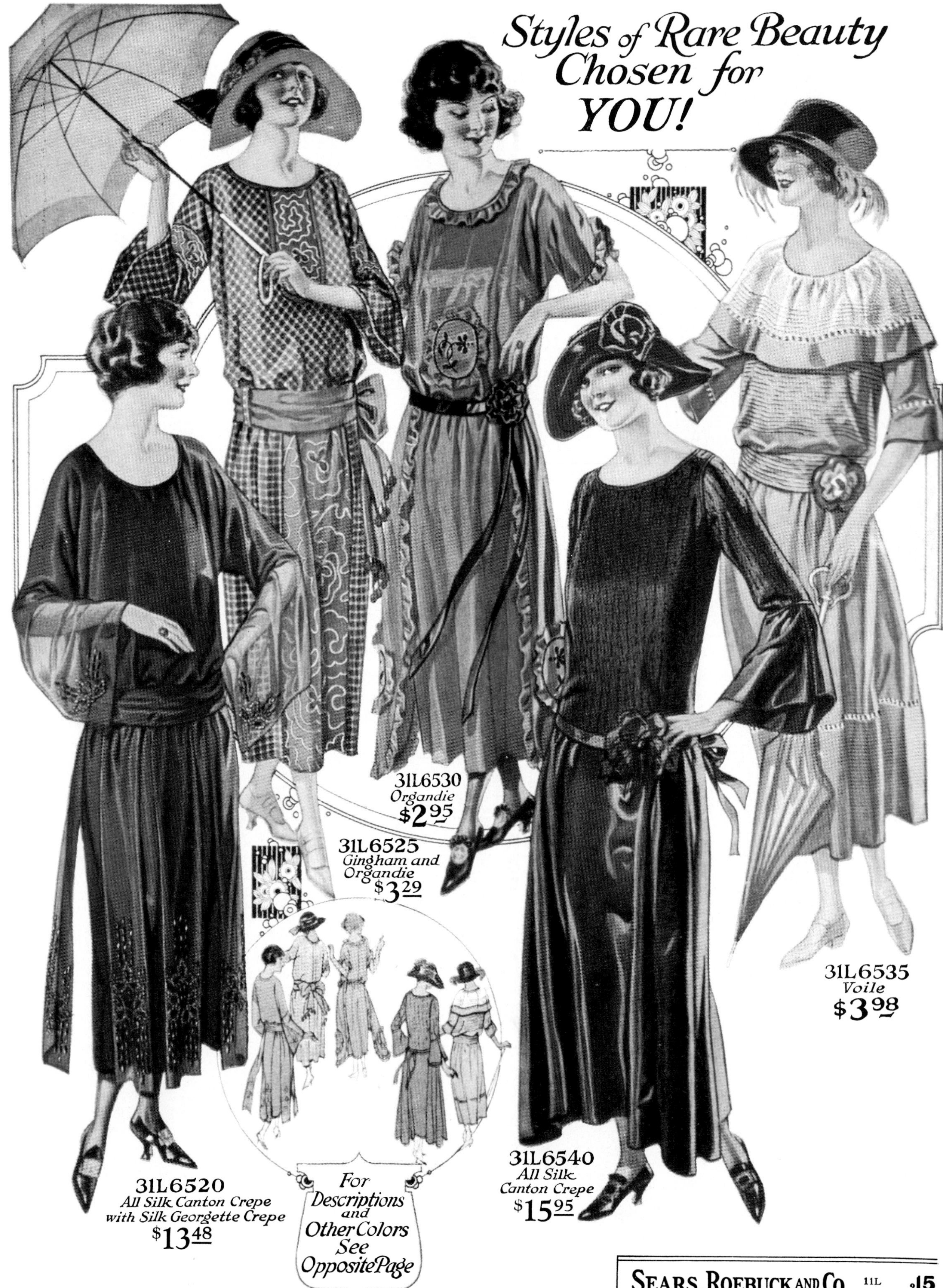
Styles of Rare Beauty Chosen for YOU!
31L6530
Organdie
$2.95
31L6525
Gingham and Organdie
$3.29
31L6535
Voile
$3.98
31L6520
All Silk Canton Crepe with Silk Georgette Crepe
$13.48
For Descriptions and Other Colors See Opposite Page
31L6540
All Silk Canton Crepe
$15.95

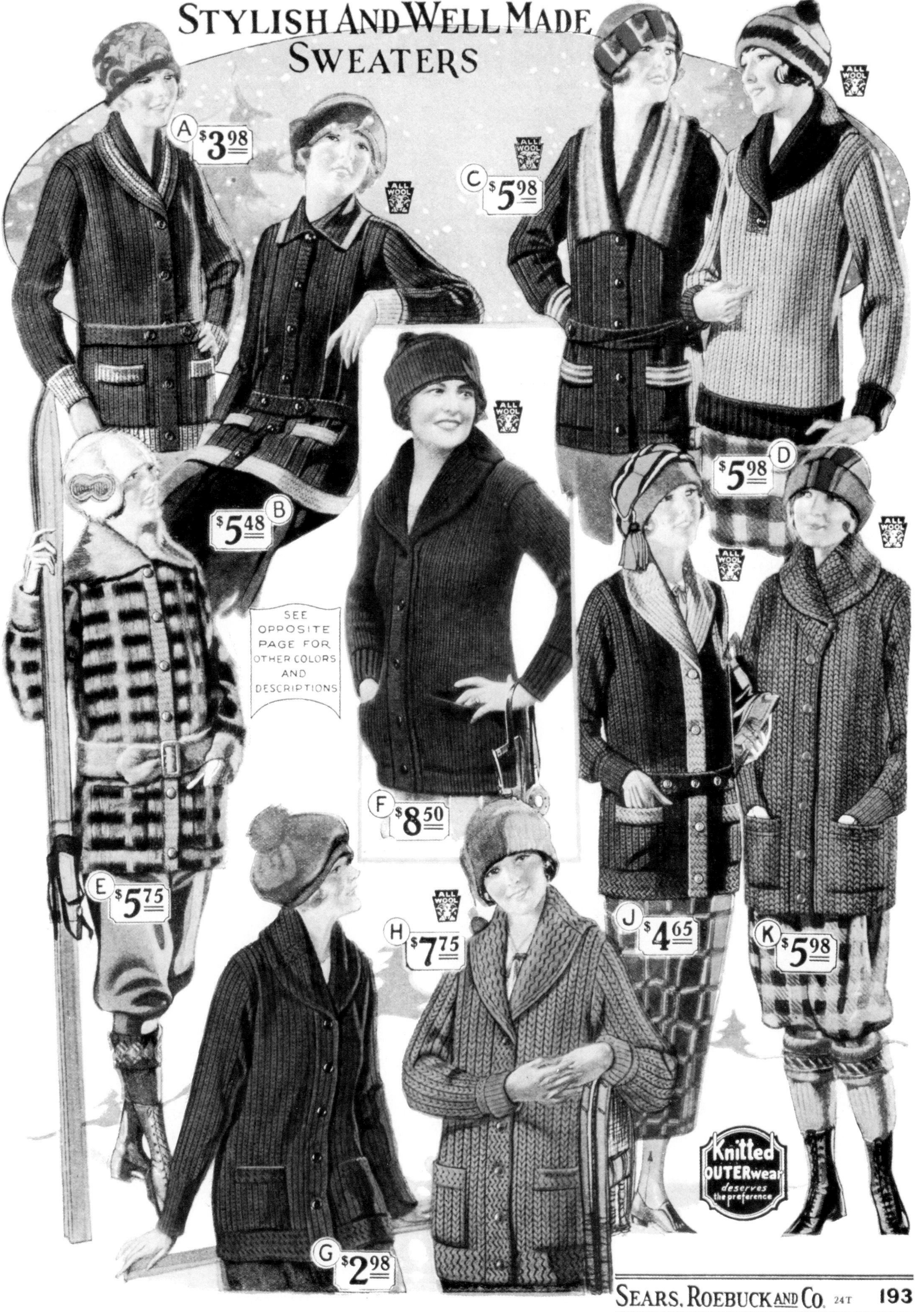
STYLISH AND WELL MADE SWEATERS
A $3.98
B $5.48
C $5.98
D $5.98
E $5.75
F $8.50
G $2.98
H $7.75
J $4.65
K $5.98
ALL WOOL
SEE OPPOSITE PAGE FOR OTHER COLORS AND DESCRIPTIONS
Knitted OUTERwear deserves the preference

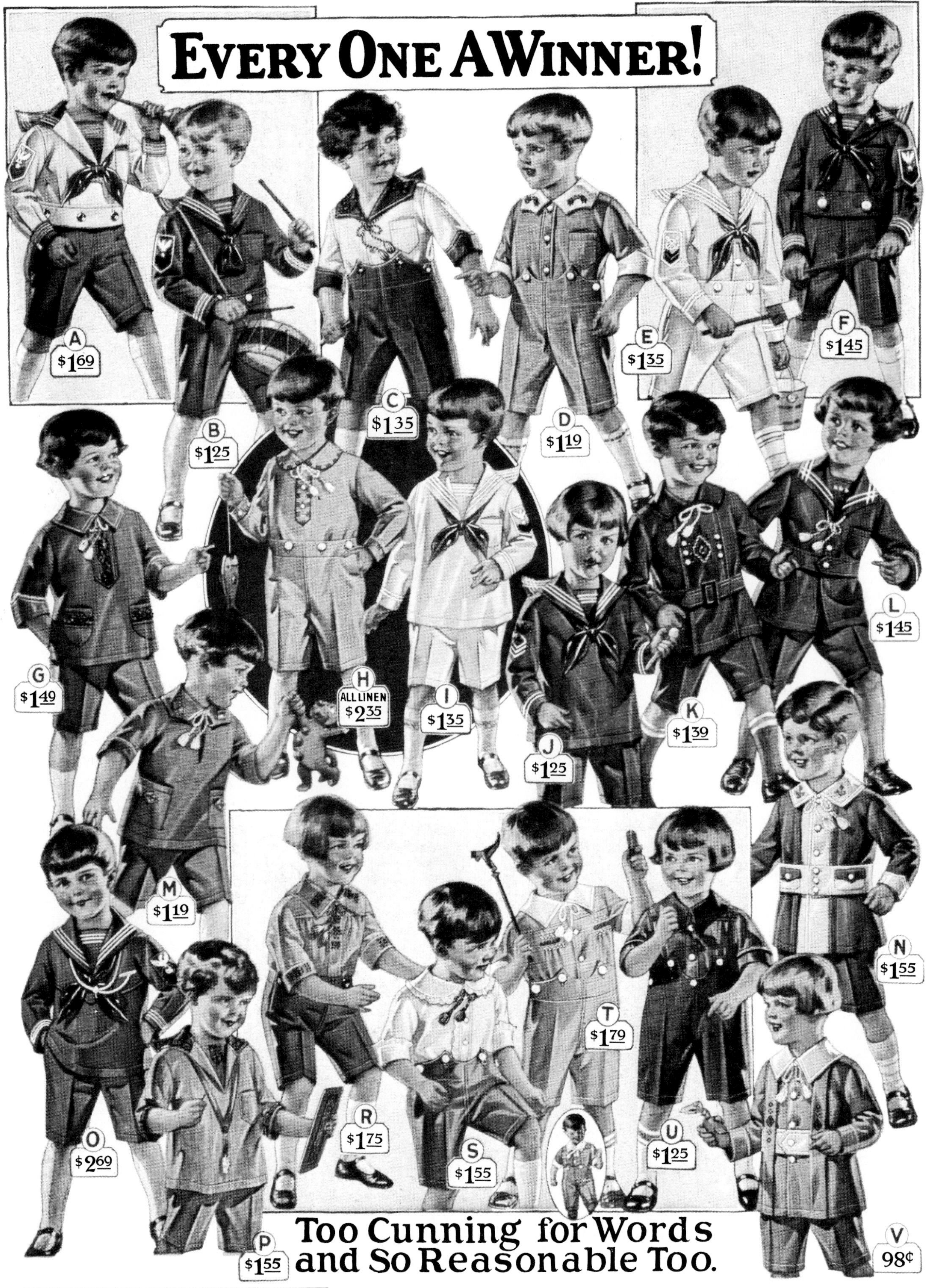




*See Opposite Page for Descriptions*

# Part Two: 1925-1931

Beginning in 1925, the standards and range of women's fashions offered in mail-order catalogs started to decline. The available selection diminished. The most expensive coats and dresses offered were nearly half the price of those offered in 1919. The same was true of men's dress clothes. One of the reasons for this, although by no means the only one, was the lure of the automobile.

In the mid-1920s, through technological advances and because of an unprecedented growth of prosperity, the automobile came within the reach of the average middle-class American. Quite naturally it was a class symbol to own a car. What was more important was the freedom of movement it provided. Within a short time America was in the grip of a full-blown love affair with the car. No sacrifice seemed too great for this new infatuation. Installment buying had become an accepted practice and now millions of Americans were buying automobiles on time. The impact of this development was enormous and touched every facet of life in America, including fashions and the way they were marketed.

Since many of their rural customers could now drive into town to shop, mail-order houses found themselves in competition with city stores. The larger organizations tried to meet this challenge by opening up their own retail stores. The catalogs of the latter part of the 1920s reveal, however, that in the area of wearing apparel, this move met with limited success. Articles such as denim coveralls, long woolen underwear, corsets for older women who from habit found them indispensable, remained fairly constant throughout the decade. But for the fashion-minded, there was less variety, generally duller-looking offerings with a strong accent on economy. Profitable sales in mail orders now lay primarily in their appeal to the isolated, the thrifty or the poor. Those with money, the more discriminating customers, preferred buying in department stores or in specialty shops which had mushroomed all over the country. Not only did they find a richer selection there, but they could also try on and examine the clothes and, having paid for them or charged them, walk out of the store with their purchases. For a great many Americans this was an attractive new experience.

As the price level dropped, mail-order fashions began to fall behind those of Paris and by 1930 the lag increased to about two years. Late and somewhat diluted, the style of the period nevertheless touched even the cheapest wearing apparel. The art movements in Paris and the Exposition Internationale des Arts Décoratifs of 1925 managed eventually to make their influence felt on the farms of Iowa, Nebraska and Kansas, and in the ghettos of the large cities.

## 1925-26

(pages 87-98)

In the fashions of the second half of the 1920s, in the silhouette, the hair styles, hats, shoes, gloves and the jewelry, as in the paintings of Picasso, Braque, Léger and Matisse, the accent was on the hard edge of geometric forms and the clean beauty of pure line. In clothing design, to relieve the monotony of the spacial forms of rectangles, squares and circles and simple linear outlines, inner planes were broken up with abstract rhythmic patterns of appliqués, piecings, tucks and formalized embroidered patterns.

The focus now was on "the slender mode of youth." The boyish look, totally flat, rectangular, mid-calf in length had arrived. Advertisements for foundations claiming "new freedom in corsetry" actually implied freedom primarily for the waistline. Women endowed with what were formerly considered feminine charms—a full bosom and wide hips—could now correct these "faults" with bust and hip constrictors.

As clothes became more casual, there was less restriction on what was to be worn at different times of the day or for special occasions. Many pieces of apparel once considered purely men's wear and some that were looked on as work clothes were absorbed into women's fashions. Sears, Roebuck copy said, "Being exceedingly smart and practical from every standpoint, the 'Collegiate' slicker or 'Fisherman's Oilskin' has become one of the most popular models in raincoats. It comes in the attractive natural yellow shade and is absolutely waterproof."

Primarily through the influence of the movies, cosmetics were now offering a wide range of powders, rouges, lipsticks, black and brown mascaras and eyelash curlers. Although liquid nail polish "for highly tinted brilliance" was for sale, the average American woman did not sport scarlet nails until the next decade.

## 1927-28

(pages 99-120)

There were no dramatic changes this year. Coats remained the same as before. The belts on dresses tightened at the hips to produce a blousing above. Skirt portions, diminished in size, were designed for the swinging motion of easy movement through pleats, gathers, shirrings and insets.

The quest to look like an underdeveloped youth continued—so much so that, except for the fact that they were scaled for smaller figures, fashions for schoolgirls were much the same as those designed for their mothers.

Rayon had become an accepted substitute for silk in hosiery, women's dresses and underwear. Now artificial effects such as alligator patterned rubber and synthetic materials such as leatherette were also used. "New automatic fasteners" (zippers) appeared on overshoes. Footwear in general became more imaginative. Even some sneakers were decorated. Women who wished to elongate their legs and to look taller and more slender could buy shoes with spike heels. Gloves and other accessories grew in variety and embellishment, and were an important part of a total ensemble.

In men's wear, suits, although reflecting the new slimness and straighter lines, retained traditional styles. Informal and work clothes, however, showed a new burst of creativity and design.

## 1928-29

(pages 121-134)

In Paris, hemlines had begun to dip downwards and waistlines started to climb up to the natural level. This step toward a new cycle in fashion was not yet in evidence in mail-order catalogs where the cresting of the hem at the top of the knee that was seen in the haute couture of 1927 finally occurred. Except for further detailed treatment of flat planes and the addition of asymmetry, the styles differed little from the year before.

This year, however, more adventuresome young men could buy "Broadway's favorite" or "Collegiate" style suits. Made of boldly striped wool, some had contrasting waistcoats. Others had double-breasted vests that were either collared or collarless. "Black bottom" cuffs on trousers could also be ordered.

## 1930-31

(pages 135-152)

"The trend is toward femininity." The adult female figure returned to fashion. Hemlines dropped below the knee and the waistline became defined at its normal position. In France, Madeleine Vionnet, by using material cut on the bias, was creating beautiful figure-molding gowns. However, because bias construction, or using fabric on the cross, was expensive and called for great skill in handling, its interpretation was limited and relegated mainly to skirts and minor details.

For this new silhouette, foundation garments and underclothes were shaped to conform to the body. Reflecting the stress on natural form, men's suits also began to curve in at the waist.

The inclusion of slacks or "gob outfits," as they were called, anticipated the oncoming popularity of long pants for women. Shorts were listed, but only for little girls. Pumps became fashionable again and were available with different heels, including four-inch spike heels. The men's section added tuxedos to the selection of suits. Trimmings and surface decorations in most clothes began to fall away as the lure of a totally different look came on the horizon.

With the end of the 1920s came the end of the reign of the preadolescent ideal. The Depression and changing times were forging new fashions.

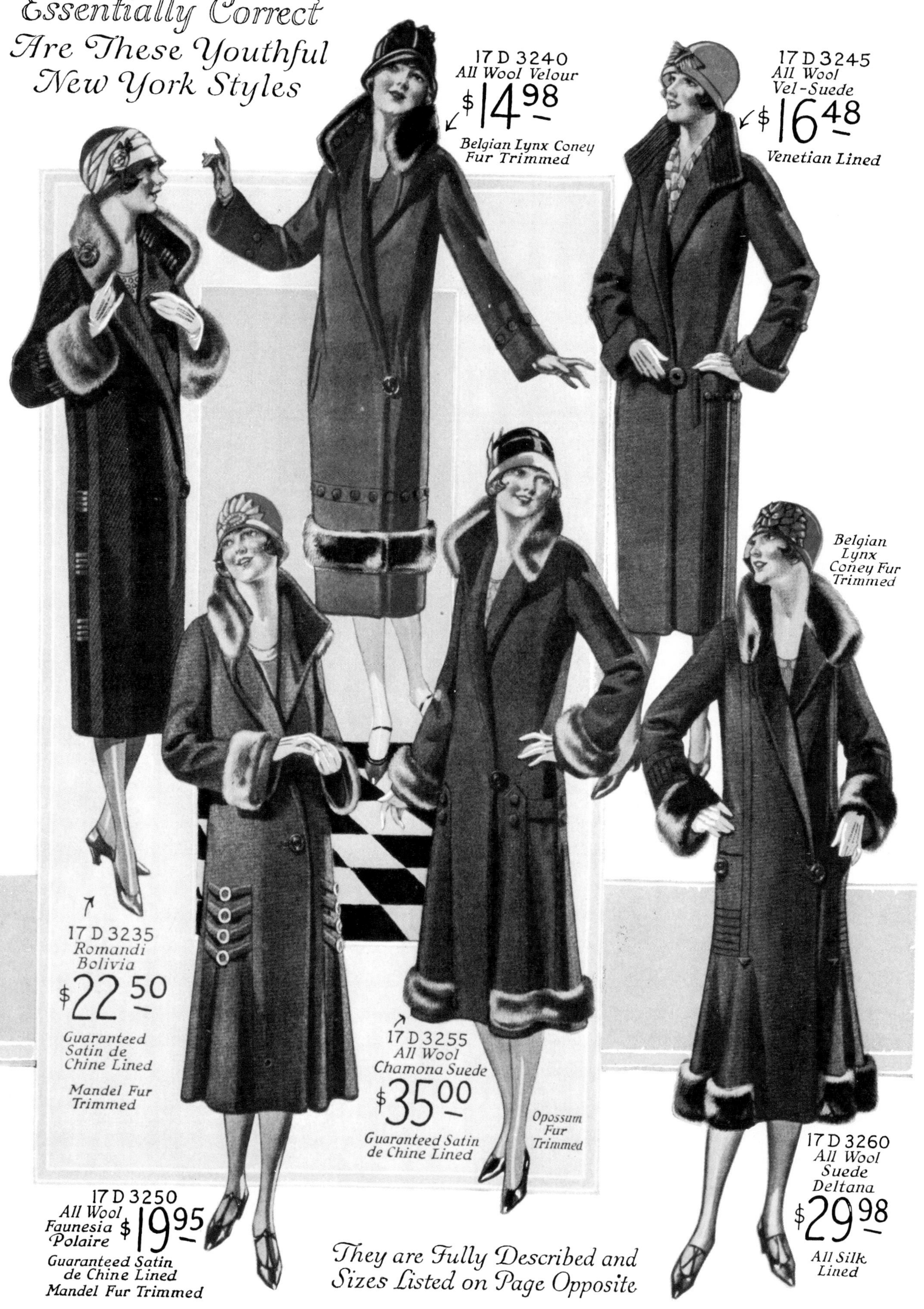
Essentially Correct
Are These Youthful
New York Styles
17 D 3240
All Wool Velour
$14.98
Belgian Lynx Coney
Fur Trimmed
17 D 3245
All Wool
Vel-Suede
$16.48
Venetian Lined
Belgian
Lynx
Coney Fur
Trimmed
17 D 3235
Romandi
Bolivia
$22.50
Guaranteed
Satin de
Chine Lined
Mandel Fur
Trimmed
17 D 3255
All Wool
Chamona Suede
$35.00
Guaranteed Satin
de Chine Lined
Opossum
Fur
Trimmed
17 D 3260
All Wool
Suede
Deltana
$29.98
All Silk
Lined
17 D 3250
All Wool
Faunesia
Polaire
$19.95
Guaranteed Satin
de Chine Lined
Mandel Fur Trimmed
They are Fully Described and
Sizes Listed on Page Opposite

# Fashion Favors the Ensemble Effect

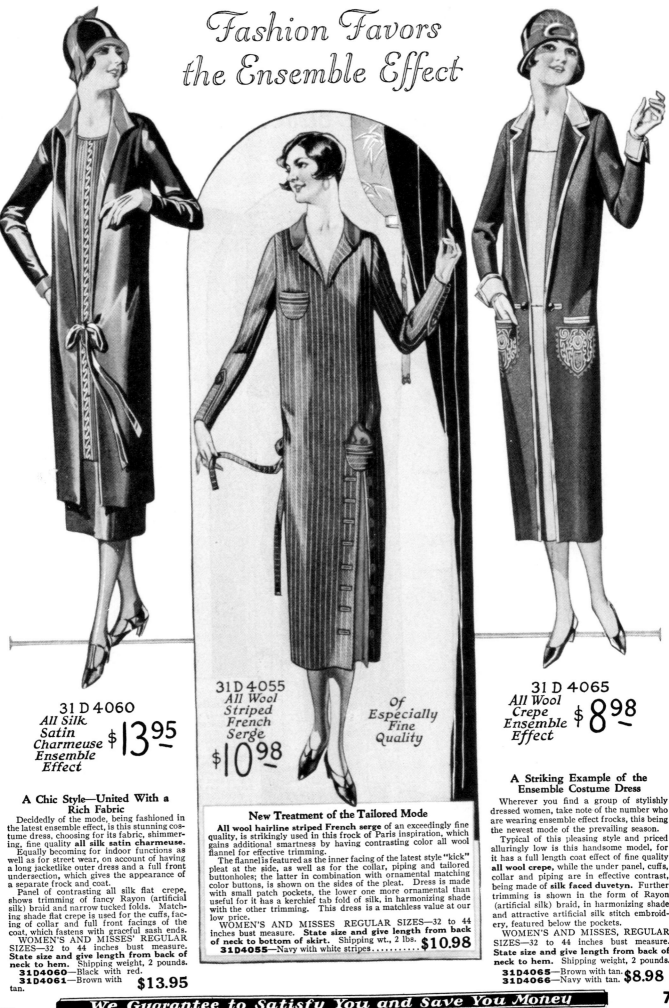

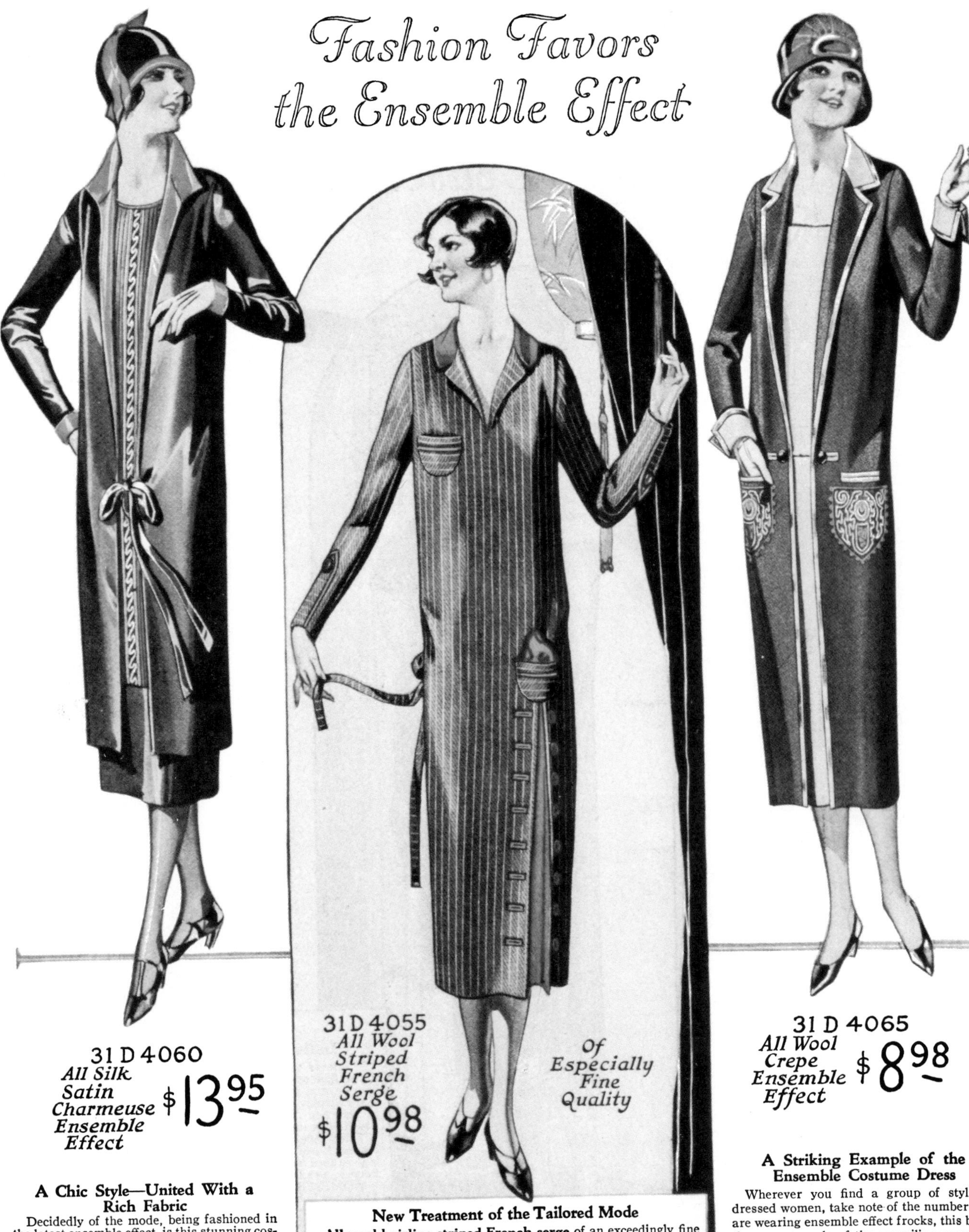


**A Chic Style—United With a Rich Fabric**

Decidedly of the mode, being fashioned in the latest ensemble effect, is this stunning costume dress, choosing for its fabric, shimmering, fine quality **all silk satin charmeuse.**

Equally becoming for indoor functions as well as for street wear, on account of having a long jacketlike outer dress and a full front undersection, which gives the appearance of a separate frock and coat.

Panel of contrasting all silk flat crepe, shows trimming of fancy Rayon (artificial silk) braid and narrow tucked folds. Matching shade flat crepe is used for the cuffs, facing of collar and full front facings of the coat, which fastens with graceful sash ends.

WOMEN'S AND MISSES' REGULAR SIZES—32 to 44 inches bust measure. **State size and give length from back of neck to hem.** Shipping weight, 2 pounds.

**31D4060**—Black with red.
**31D4061**—Brown with tan. **$13.95**

**New Treatment of the Tailored Mode**

**All wool hairline striped French serge** of an exceedingly fine quality, is strikingly used in this frock of Paris inspiration, which gains additional smartness by having contrasting color all wool flannel for effective trimming.

The flannel is featured as the inner facing of the latest style "kick" pleat at the side, as well as for the collar, piping and tailored buttonholes; the latter in combination with ornamental matching color buttons, is shown on the sides of the pleat. Dress is made with small patch pockets, the lower one more ornamental than useful for it has a kerchief tab fold of silk, in harmonizing shade with the other trimming. This dress is a matchless value at our low price.

WOMEN'S AND MISSES REGULAR SIZES—32 to 44 inches bust measure. **State size and give length from back of neck to bottom of skirt.** Shipping wt., 2 lbs.

**31D4055**—Navy with white stripes........... **$10.98**

**A Striking Example of the Ensemble Costume Dress**

Wherever you find a group of stylishly dressed women, take note of the number who are wearing ensemble effect frocks, this being the newest mode of the prevailing season.

Typical of this pleasing style and priced alluringly low is this handsome model, for it has a full length coat effect of fine quality **all wool crepe,** while the under panel, cuffs, collar and piping are in effective contrast, being made of **silk faced duvetyn.** Further trimming is shown in the form of Rayon (artificial silk) braid, in harmonizing shade and attractive artificial silk stitch embroidery, featured below the pockets.

WOMEN'S AND MISSES, REGULAR SIZES—32 to 44 inches bust measure. **State size and give length from back of neck to hem.** Shipping weight, 2 pounds.

**31D4065**—Brown with tan.
**31D4066**—Navy with tan. **$8.98**

**We Guarantee to Satisfy You and Save You Money**

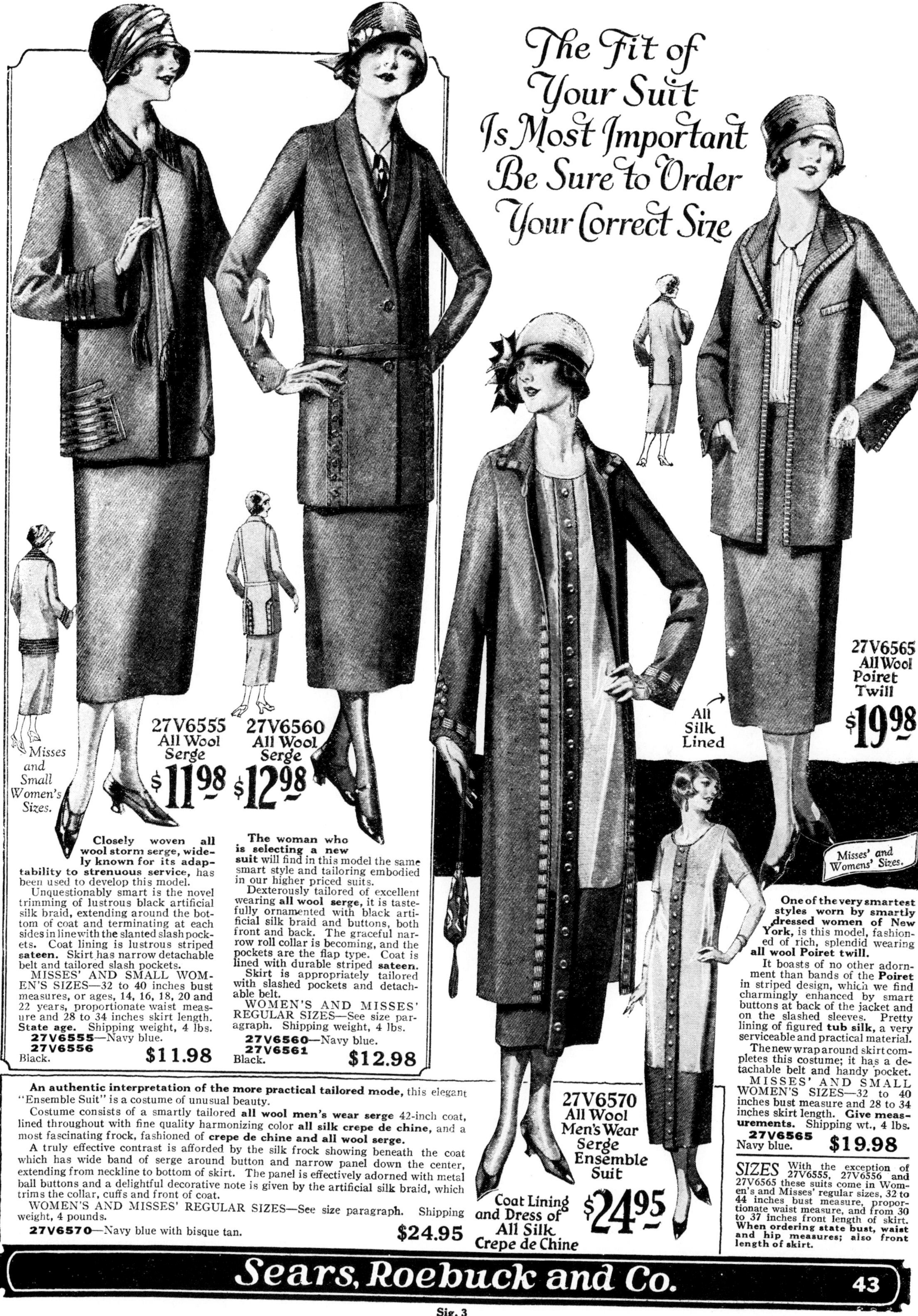

# The Fit of Your Suit Is Most Important Be Sure to Order Your Correct Size

**27V6555** All Wool Serge **$11.98**

Misses and Small Women's Sizes.

**Closely woven all wool storm serge, widely known for its adaptability to strenuous service,** has been used to develop this model.

Unquestionably smart is the novel trimming of lustrous black artificial silk braid, extending around the bottom of coat and terminating at each sides in line with the slanted slash pockets. Coat lining is lustrous striped **sateen.** Skirt has narrow detachable belt and tailored slash pockets.

MISSES' AND SMALL WOMEN'S SIZES—32 to 40 inches bust measures, or ages, 14, 16, 18, 20 and 22 years, proportionate waist measure and 28 to 34 inches skirt length. **State age.** Shipping weight, 4 lbs.

**27V6555**—Navy blue.
**27V6556** Black. **$11.98**

**27V6560** All Wool Serge **$12.98**

**The woman who is selecting a new suit** will find in this model the same smart style and tailoring embodied in our higher priced suits.

Dexterously tailored of excellent wearing **all wool serge,** it is tastefully ornamented with black artificial silk braid and buttons, both front and back. The graceful narrow roll collar is becoming, and the pockets are the flap type. Coat is lined with durable striped **sateen.** Skirt is appropriately tailored with slashed pockets and detachable belt.

WOMEN'S AND MISSES' REGULAR SIZES—See size paragraph. Shipping weight, 4 lbs.

**27V6560**—Navy blue.
**27V6561** Black. **$12.98**

**27V6565** All Wool Poiret Twill **$19.98**

All Silk Lined

Misses' and Womens' Sizes.

**One of the very smartest styles worn by smartly dressed women of New York,** is this model, fashioned of rich, splendid wearing **all wool Poiret twill.**

It boasts of no other adornment than bands of the **Poiret** in striped design, which we find charmingly enhanced by smart buttons at back of the jacket and on the slashed sleeves. Pretty lining of figured **tub silk,** a very serviceable and practical material.

The new wraparound skirt completes this costume; it has a detachable belt and handy pocket.

MISSES' AND SMALL WOMEN'S SIZES—32 to 40 inches bust measure and 28 to 34 inches skirt length. **Give measurements.** Shipping wt., 4 lbs.

**27V6565** Navy blue. **$19.98**

**27V6570** All Wool Men's Wear Serge Ensemble Suit **$24.95**

Coat Lining and Dress of All Silk Crepe de Chine

**An authentic interpretation of the more practical tailored mode,** this elegant "Ensemble Suit" is a costume of unusual beauty.

Costume consists of a smartly tailored **all wool men's wear serge** 42-inch coat, lined throughout with fine quality harmonizing color **all silk crepe de chine,** and a most fascinating frock, fashioned of **crepe de chine and all wool serge.**

A truly effective contrast is afforded by the silk frock showing beneath the coat which has wide band of serge around button and narrow panel down the center, extending from neckline to bottom of skirt. The panel is effectively adorned with metal ball buttons and a delightful decorative note is given by the artificial silk braid, which trims the collar, cuffs and front of coat.

WOMEN'S AND MISSES' REGULAR SIZES—See size paragraph. Shipping weight, 4 pounds.

**27V6570**—Navy blue with bisque tan. **$24.95**

SIZES With the exception of 27V6555, 27V6556 and 27V6565 these suits come in Women's and Misses' regular sizes, 32 to 44 inches bust measure, proportionate waist measure, and from 30 to 37 inches front length of skirt. **When ordering state bust, waist and hip measures; also front length of skirt.**

# Exclusive Creations for Young Women

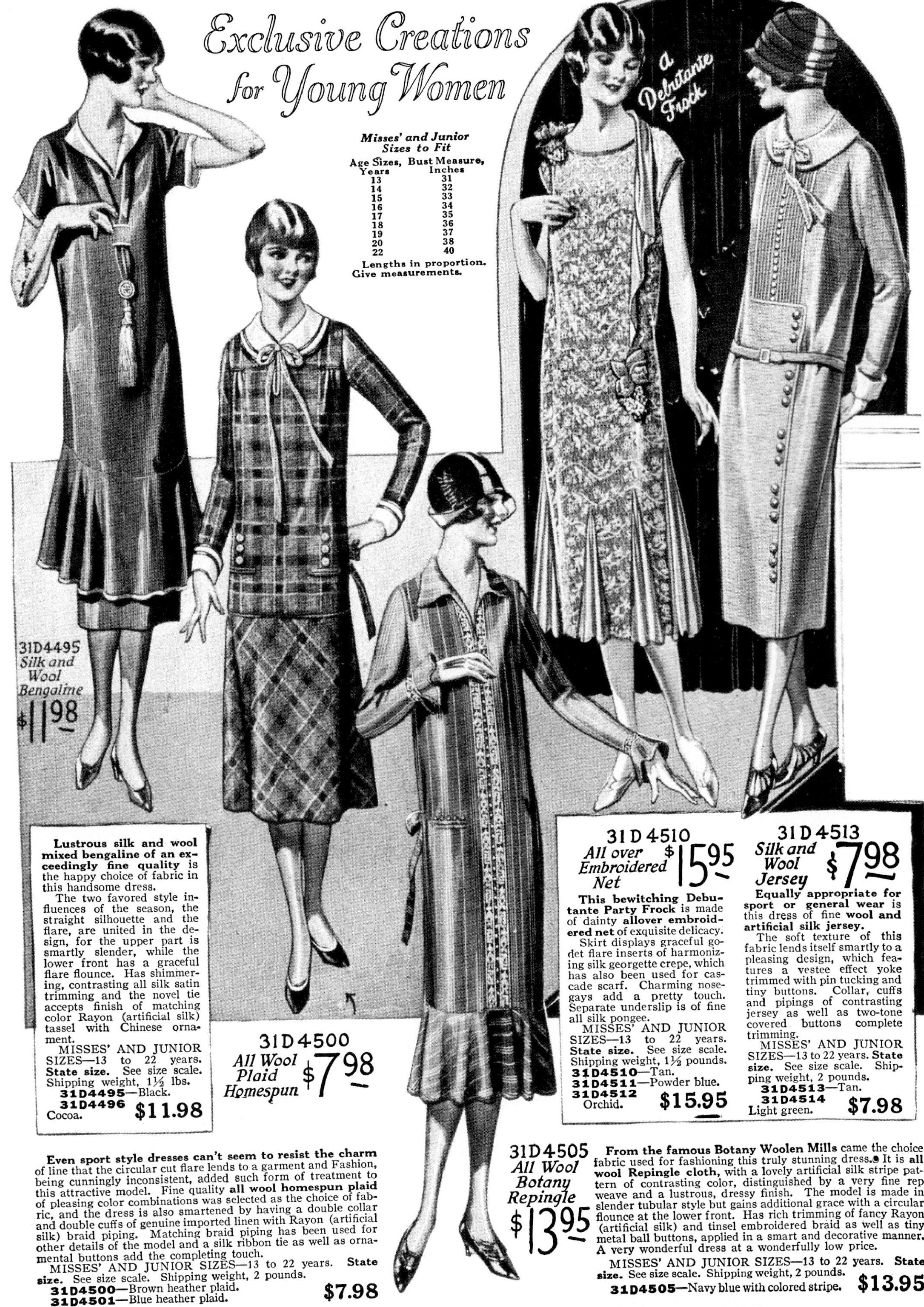


**Misses' and Junior Sizes to Fit**

| Age Sizes, Years | Bust Measure, Inches |
|---|---|
| 13 | 31 |
| 14 | 32 |
| 15 | 33 |
| 16 | 34 |
| 17 | 35 |
| 18 | 36 |
| 19 | 37 |
| 20 | 38 |
| 22 | 40 |

Lengths in proportion. Give measurements.

31D4495
Silk and Wool Bengaline
$11.98

**Lustrous silk and wool mixed bengaline of an exceedingly fine quality** is the happy choice of fabric in this handsome dress.

The two favored style influences of the season, the straight silhouette and the flare, are united in the design, for the upper part is smartly slender, while the lower front has a graceful flare flounce. Has shimmering, contrasting all silk satin trimming and the novel tie accepts finish of matching color Rayon (artificial silk) tassel with Chinese ornament.

MISSES' AND JUNIOR SIZES—13 to 22 years. **State size.** See size scale. Shipping weight, 1½ lbs.
**31D4495**—Black.
**31D4496** Cocoa. **$11.98**

31D4500
All Wool Plaid Homespun
$7.98

**Even sport style dresses can't seem to resist the charm** of line that the circular cut flare lends to a garment and Fashion, being cunningly inconsistent, added such form of treatment to this attractive model. Fine quality **all wool homespun plaid** of pleasing color combinations was selected as the choice of fabric, and the dress is also smartened by having a double collar and double cuffs of genuine imported linen with Rayon (artificial silk) braid piping. Matching braid piping has been used for other details of the model and a silk ribbon tie as well as ornamental buttons add the completing touch.

MISSES' AND JUNIOR SIZES—13 to 22 years. **State size.** See size scale. Shipping weight, 2 pounds.
**31D4500**—Brown heather plaid.
**31D4501**—Blue heather plaid. **$7.98**

31D4510
All over Embroidered Net
$15.95

**This bewitching Debutante Party Frock** is made of dainty **allover embroidered net** of exquisite delicacy.

Skirt displays graceful godet flare inserts of harmonizing silk georgette crepe, which has also been used for cascade scarf. Charming nosegays add a pretty touch. Separate underslip is of fine all silk pongee.

MISSES' AND JUNIOR SIZES—13 to 22 years. **State size.** See size scale. Shipping weight, 1½ pounds.
**31D4510**—Tan.
**31D4511**—Powder blue.
**31D4512** Orchid. **$15.95**

31D4513
Silk and Wool Jersey
$7.98

**Equally appropriate for sport or general wear** is this dress of fine **wool and artificial silk jersey.**

The soft texture of this fabric lends itself smartly to a pleasing design, which features a vestee effect yoke trimmed with pin tucking and tiny buttons. Collar, cuffs and pipings of contrasting jersey as well as two-tone covered buttons complete trimming.

MISSES' AND JUNIOR SIZES—13 to 22 years. **State size.** See size scale. Shipping weight, 2 pounds.
**31D4513**—Tan.
**31D4514** Light green. **$7.98**

31D4505
All Wool Botany Repingle
$13.95

**From the famous Botany Woolen Mills** came the choice fabric used for fashioning this truly stunning dress. It is **all wool Repingle cloth,** with a lovely artificial silk stripe pattern of contrasting color, distinguished by a very fine rep weave and a lustrous, dressy finish. The model is made in slender tubular style but gains additional grace with a circular flounce at the lower front. Has rich trimming of fancy Rayon (artificial silk) and tinsel embroidered braid as well as tiny metal ball buttons, applied in a smart and decorative manner. A very wonderful dress at a wonderfully low price.

MISSES' AND JUNIOR SIZES—13 to 22 years. **State size.** See size scale. Shipping weight, 2 pounds.
**31D4505**—Navy blue with colored stripe. **$13.95**

# GREATEST STORE
Style Leadership

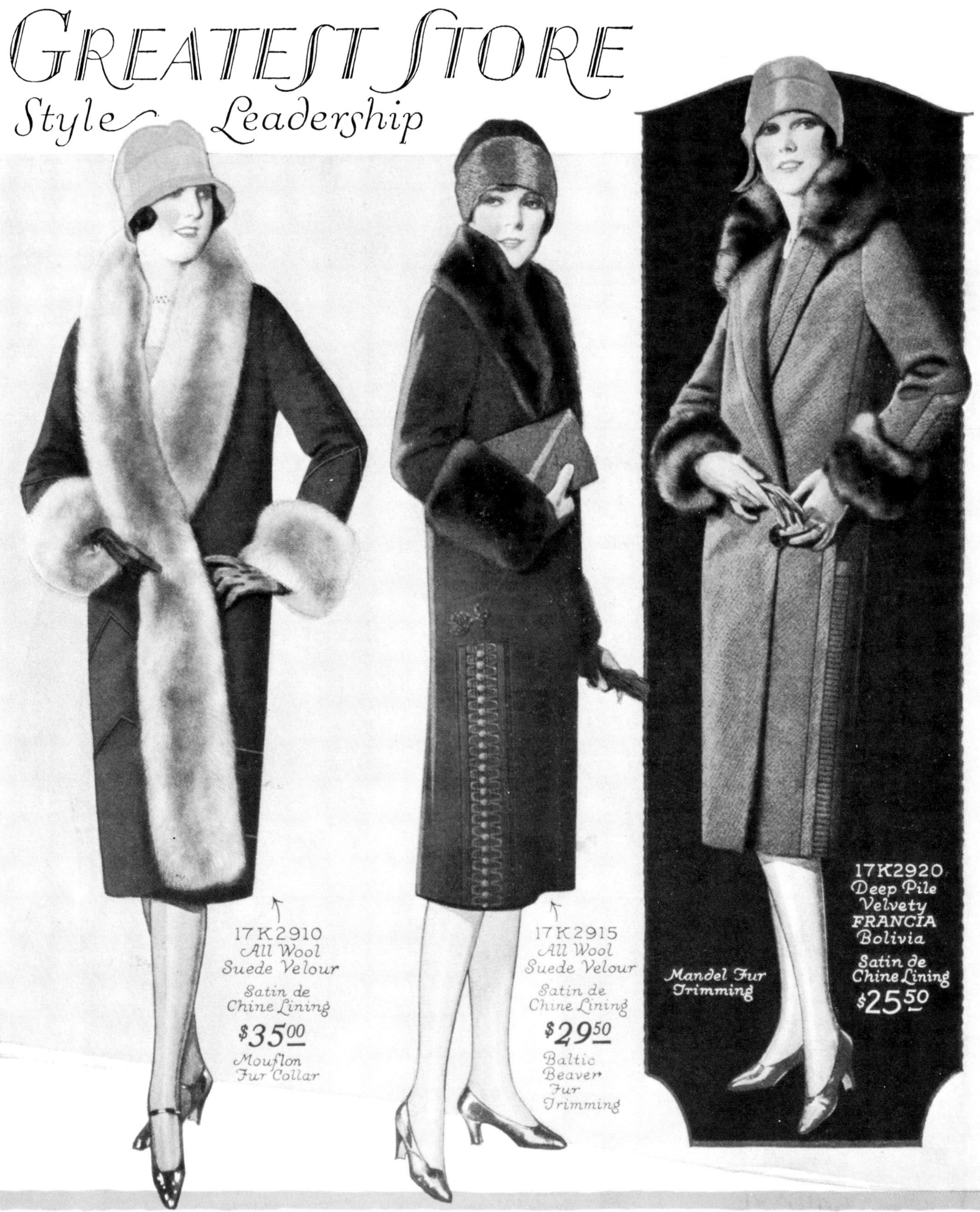


## Paris Inspired Stunning Coat

This beautiful coat is made as Paris makes them this season—elaborately fur trimmed and boasting smart tailored tucking.

Adapted in fine quality warm winterweight *All Wool Suede Velour*, on swagger straight lines, showing a full length shawl collar and deep cuffs of rich silky haired, selected grade gray *Mouflon Fur.*

It is expertly tailored, heavily interlined and lined throughout with guaranteed *Satin de Chine.* Typical of the best New York models. Average length, 44 inches.

*Women's and Misses' Sizes*—34, 36, 38, 40 and 42 inches bust measure. **State size.** See "Measuring Instructions" on page 15. Shipping wt., 6 lbs.

**17K2910**—Grackle Blue. **$35.00**

## Typical Fifth Avenue Style

You will delight in the beauty and luxurious effect of this stunning New York model, with its deep gauntlet cuffs and novel shape collar of rich *Brown Baltic Beaver Fur* (clipped and dyed coney).

Smartly fashioned of fine quality winterweight *All Wool Suede Velour.* The sides of the model show interesting panel treatments, with tailored tucks, novelty *Rayon* embroidery and ornaments of self material.

Heavy interlining; guaranteed *Satin de Chine* lining. Average length, about 44 inches.

*Women's and Misses' Sizes*—34, 36, 38, 40 and 42 inches bust measure. **State size.** See "Measuring Instructions" on page 15. Shipping weight, 6 pounds.

**17K2915**—Cranberry.
**17K2916**—Brown. **$29.50**

## Luxuriously Warm Handsome Model

Presenting a rich, smart appearance, this model will make its appeal to women of conservative taste.

Fashioned of the celebrated *"Francia" Bolivia*—an extra warm winterweight fabric of lovely soft velvety texture; has neat adornment of tailored strap inserts and rows of *Rayon* stitching. Large collar and deep cuffs of selected grade *Mandel Fur.*

Made with heavy interlining and lined with guaranteed *Satin de Chine.* Average length, about 46 inches.

*Women's and Misses' Sizes*—36, 38, 40, 42, 44 and 46 inches bust measure. **State size.** See "Measuring Instructions" on page 15. Shpg. wt., 6 lbs.

**17K2920**—Reindeer Tan.
**17K2921**—Sailor Blue. **$25.50**

**Order Blanks Are in Back of This Catalog**

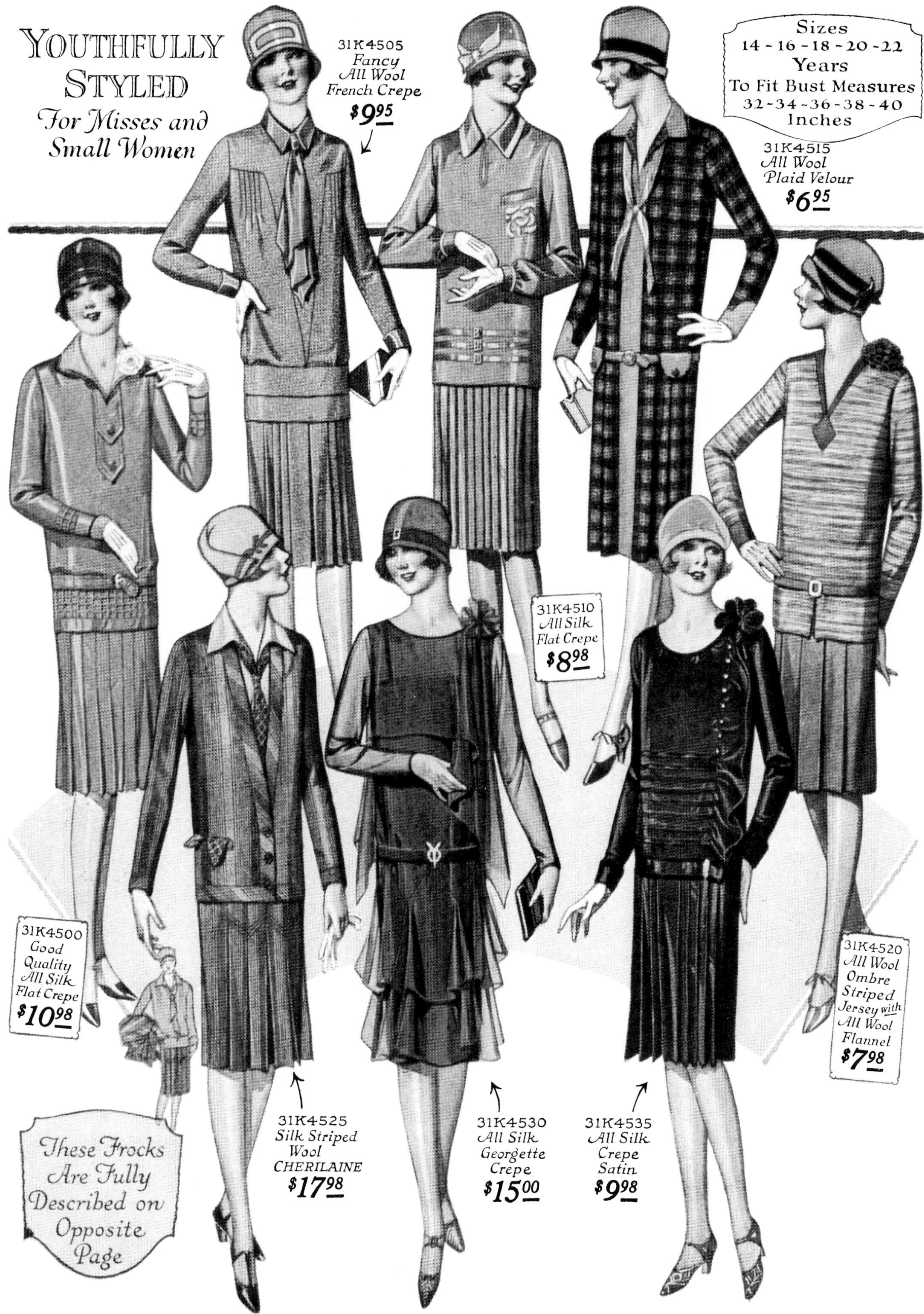
YOUTHFULLY STYLED
For Misses and Small Women
31K4505
Fancy All Wool French Crepe
$9.95
Sizes
14-16-18-20-22
Years
To Fit Bust Measures
32-34-36-38-40
Inches
31K4515
All Wool Plaid Velour
$6.95
31K4510
All Silk Flat Crepe
$8.98
31K4500
Good Quality All Silk Flat Crepe
$10.98
31K4520
All Wool Ombre Striped Jersey with All Wool Flannel
$7.98
31K4525
Silk Striped Wool CHERILAINE
$17.98
31K4530
All Silk Georgette Crepe
$15.00
31K4535
All Silk Crepe Satin
$9.98
These Frocks Are Fully Described on Opposite Page

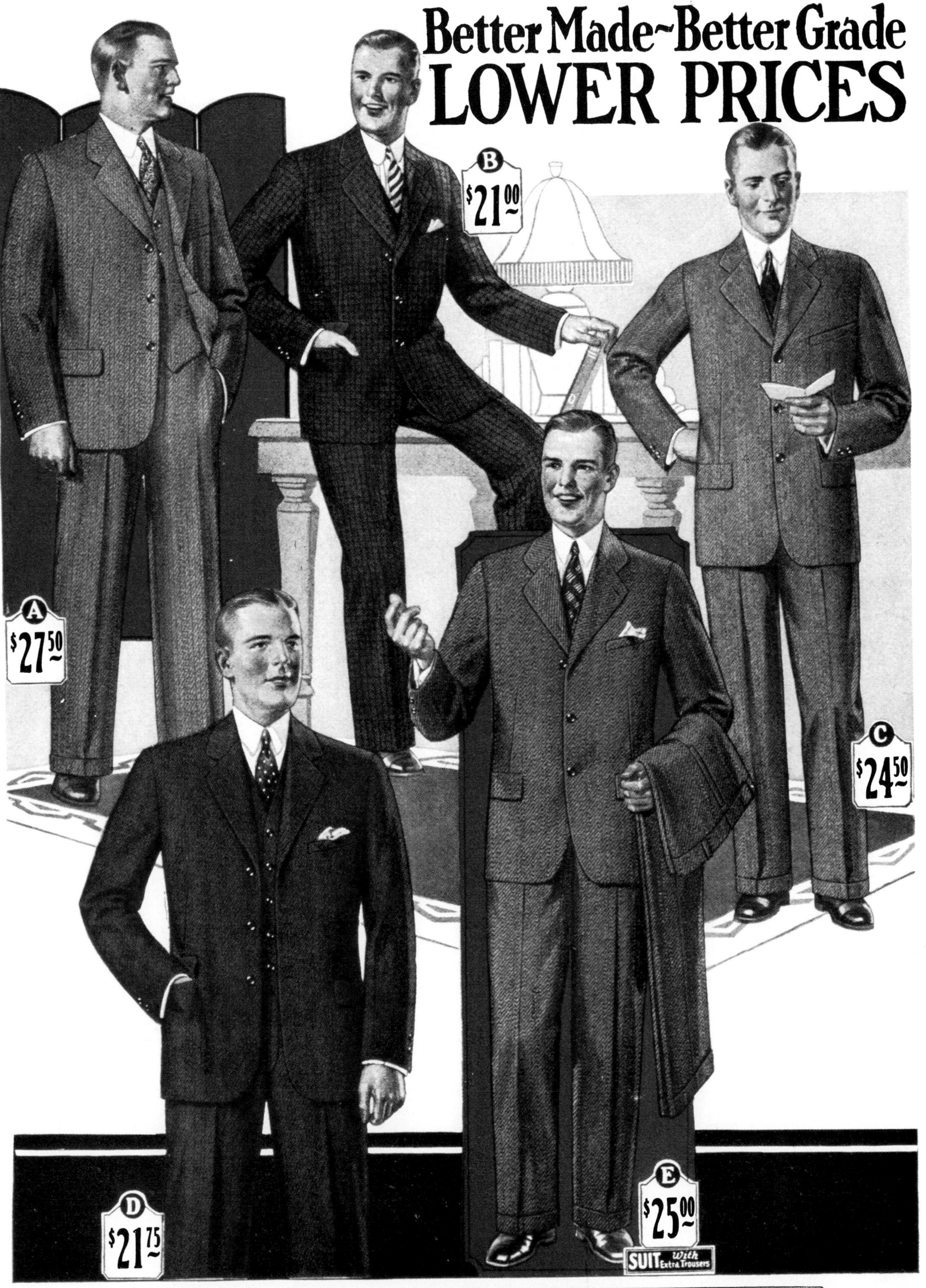


Your Orders Shipped Within 24 Hours!

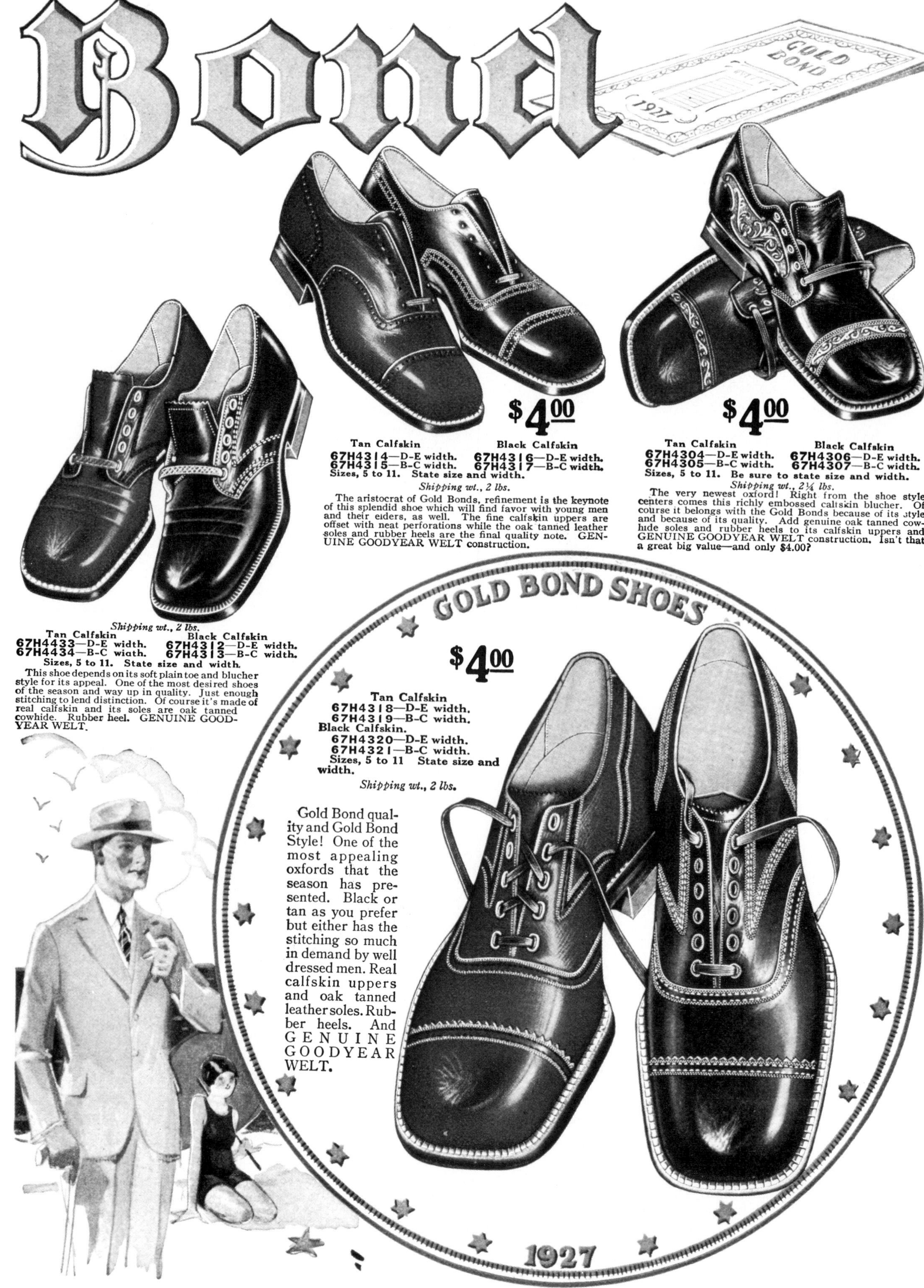
Gold Bond
GOLD BOND
1927
$4.00
Tan Calfskin
67H4314—D-E width.
67H4315—B-C width.
Black Calfskin
67H4316—D-E width.
67H4317—B-C width.
Sizes, 5 to 11. State size and width.
Shipping wt., 2 lbs.
The aristocrat of Gold Bonds, refinement is the keynote of this splendid shoe which will find favor with young men and their elders, as well. The fine calfskin uppers are offset with neat perforations while the oak tanned leather soles and rubber heels are the final quality note. GENUINE GOODYEAR WELT construction.
$4.00
Tan Calfskin
67H4304—D-E width.
67H4305—B-C width.
Black Calfskin
67H4306—D-E width.
67H4307—B-C width.
Sizes, 5 to 11. Be sure to state size and width.
Shipping wt., 2¼ lbs.
The very newest oxford! Right from the shoe style centers comes this richly embossed calfskin blucher. Of course it belongs with the Gold Bonds because of its style and because of its quality. Add genuine oak tanned cowhide soles and rubber heels to its calfskin uppers and GENUINE GOODYEAR WELT construction. Isn't that a great big value—and only $4.00?
Shipping wt., 2 lbs.
Tan Calfskin
67H4433—D-E width.
67H4434—B-C width.
Black Calfskin
67H4312—D-E width.
67H4313—B-C width.
Sizes, 5 to 11. State size and width.
This shoe depends on its soft plain toe and blucher style for its appeal. One of the most desired shoes of the season and way up in quality. Just enough stitching to lend distinction. Of course it's made of real calfskin and its soles are oak tanned cowhide. Rubber heel. GENUINE GOODYEAR WELT.
GOLD BOND SHOES
$4.00
Tan Calfskin
67H4318—D-E width.
67H4319—B-C width.
Black Calfskin.
67H4320—D-E width.
67H4321—B-C width.
Sizes, 5 to 11 State size and width.
Shipping wt., 2 lbs.
Gold Bond quality and Gold Bond Style! One of the most appealing oxfords that the season has presented. Black or tan as you prefer but either has the stitching so much in demand by well dressed men. Real calfskin uppers and oak tanned leather soles. Rubber heels. And GENUINE GOODYEAR WELT.
1927

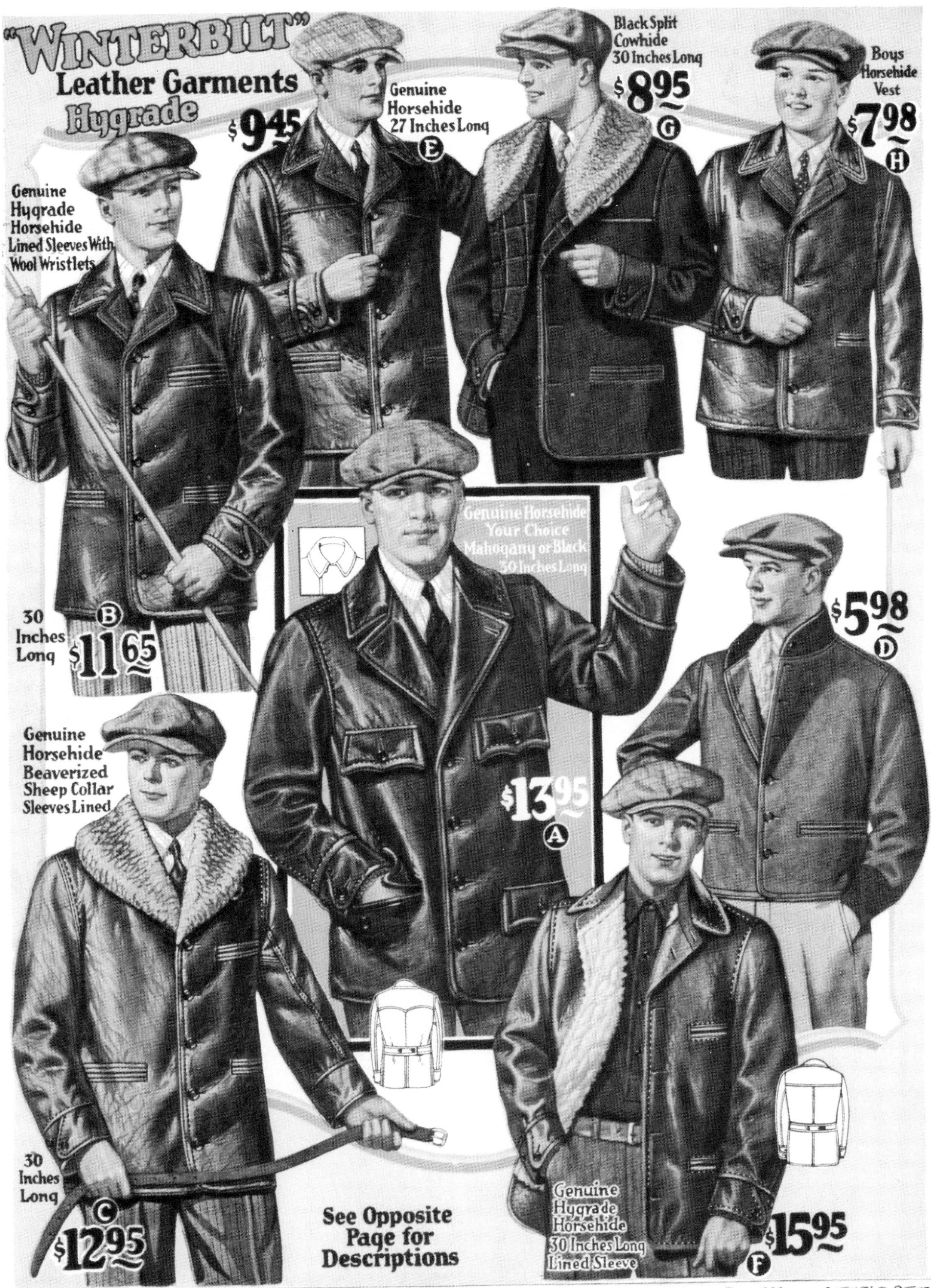


 Satisfaction Guaranteed or Money Refunded    There's a Lot of Money Made in Trapping Furs. Traps and Necessities on Page 386    IT'S EASY TO ORDER

# Pressure Process Cured Super Quality Rubber Footwear

## 4 & 5 Buckle Red Rubber Arctics

### Supreme in Quality Low in Price

### Red Rubber Hip and Short Boot

Any who have worn these Savage super-quality pressure cured red rubber boots will tell you—they are the best there is. Heavy pressure cured gray soles and heels. Reinforced throughout, against cracking. Fully guaranteed to you. Wide widths only. Men's sizes 6 to 12. No half sizes. State size. Ship. wt., 8 lbs.

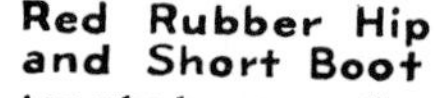

20B872 Knee Boot..$3.98
20B876 Hip Boot.. 5.95

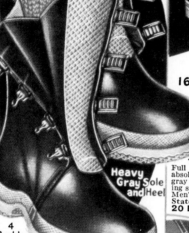

5 Buckles $3.98

4 Buckles $3.49

Heavy Gray Sole and Heel

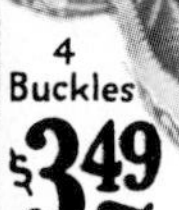

Super-Quality Red Arctics known throughout the world for their long wearing qualities. Special pressure-cured heavy grey rubber soles and heels. Heavy warm lining. Full bellows snow excluding tongue. Heavy chafing strip. Five buckle top affords extra protection, being about 13 inches high. Fully guaranteed. Fresh stock. To be worn over shoes. Men's sizes 6 to 12. No half sizes. State size. Ship. wt., 4¼ lbs.

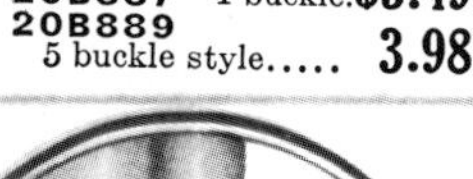

20B887 4 buckle..$3.49
20B889 5 buckle style..... 3.98

### Red Rubber 16 Inch Lace Hi-Cut

$4.95

Rancher Hi-cut Lace Boot adapted to sport and winter wear. Super quality fresh red rubber fully guaranteed. Specially cured under heavy steam pressure giving greatest resilience, life and strength to rubber. To be worn over heavy socks. Full bellows gusset making boot absolutely water-proof. Heavy gray rubber soles, heels and chafing strip. About 16 inches high. Men's sizes 6 to 12. No half sizes. State size. Ship. wt. 5½ lbs.

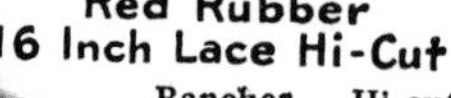

20 B 884..........$4.95

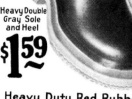

Heavy Double Gray Sole and Heel

$1.59

### Heavy Duty Red Rubber Extra High Cut Vamp

Red Rubber service rubber made by special pressure cured process. Super-quality and fully guaranteed. Heavy double grey rubber soles and heels. Red friction lining. Hi-Cut vamp fits snugly about shoe keeping out dirt, water, snow, etc. Ideal to be worn over either leather or felt shoes. Men's sizes 6 to 12. Wide widths only. Ship. wt., 2½ lbs.

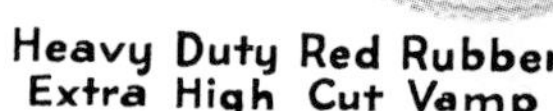

20B863 Red.........$1.59

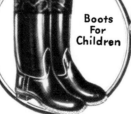

### Boots For Children

Black all rubber boots with pretty red cuff. Wide widths. Ship. wt., 2 lbs.

20B880 Boys and Girls, 5 to 10½.......$1.85
20B879 11 to 2....... 1.98

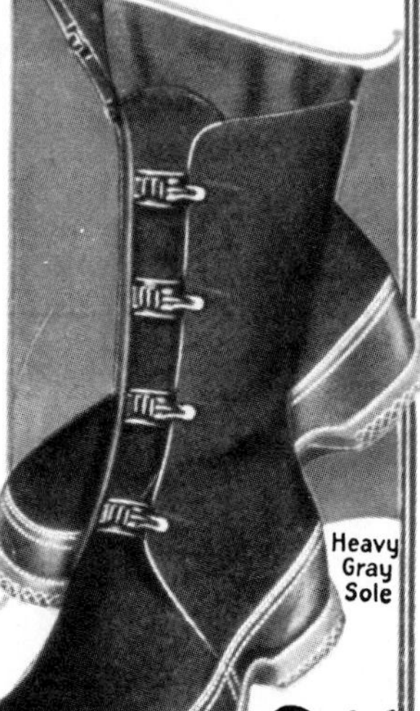

Heavy Gray Sole

$3.45

### Heavy Duty Cloth Top 4 Buckle Arctic

Our best heavy duty men's cloth top arctic. Equipped with the heavy super-quality gray rubber soles and heels. Heavy cashmerette tops with fleece lining. Four buckles reinforced. Men's sizes 6 to 12. No half sizes. State size. Ship. wt., 3 lbs.

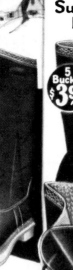

20B946.........$3.45

## Tan Automatic Gaiters Protection with Style

$2.98

Light Color Lining

*Read Description for Information as to Style of Heel to Purchase*

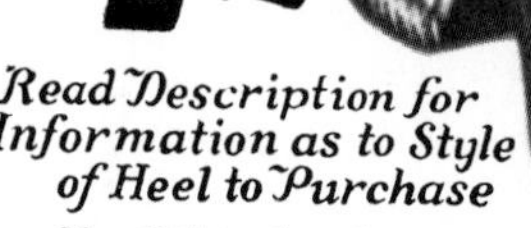

**New light colored overshoes for women are the prevailing style and here is the neatest and most trim of them all.** Made in the high four buckle height, giving ankles and legs protection. Light tan uppers as pictured with tan rubber soles and heels to match. Light colored linings that will not stain the hose. Guaranteed automatic fastener makes it quick to slip on and off. Shipping weight, 2¼ lbs. Tan only. Women's sizes 2½ to 9. Wide widths.

20B919 For medium and high heels as shown in figures 1 and 2 Page 76. Price..............$2.98
20B915 For low heels as shown in figure 3 Page 76. Price........................ 2.98

### Overettes

*The Fashionable Tan Gaiter*
*The Neatest-Smartest Style Ever*

**New tan 7-inch gaiter is a big favorite with the young women of today.** Neatly made with collar which can be turned up in stormy weather. Sizes 2½ to 9. Adjustable collar flap insures neat, trim fit about the ankle. Ship. wt., 2 lbs.

20B907 Low heel shoes shown in figure 3 Page 76.
20B908 Medium and high heel shoes shown in figures 1 and 2 Page 76.

$1.88

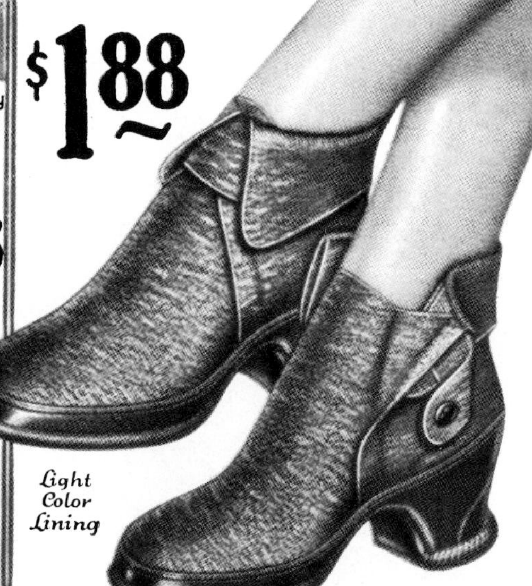

Light Color Lining

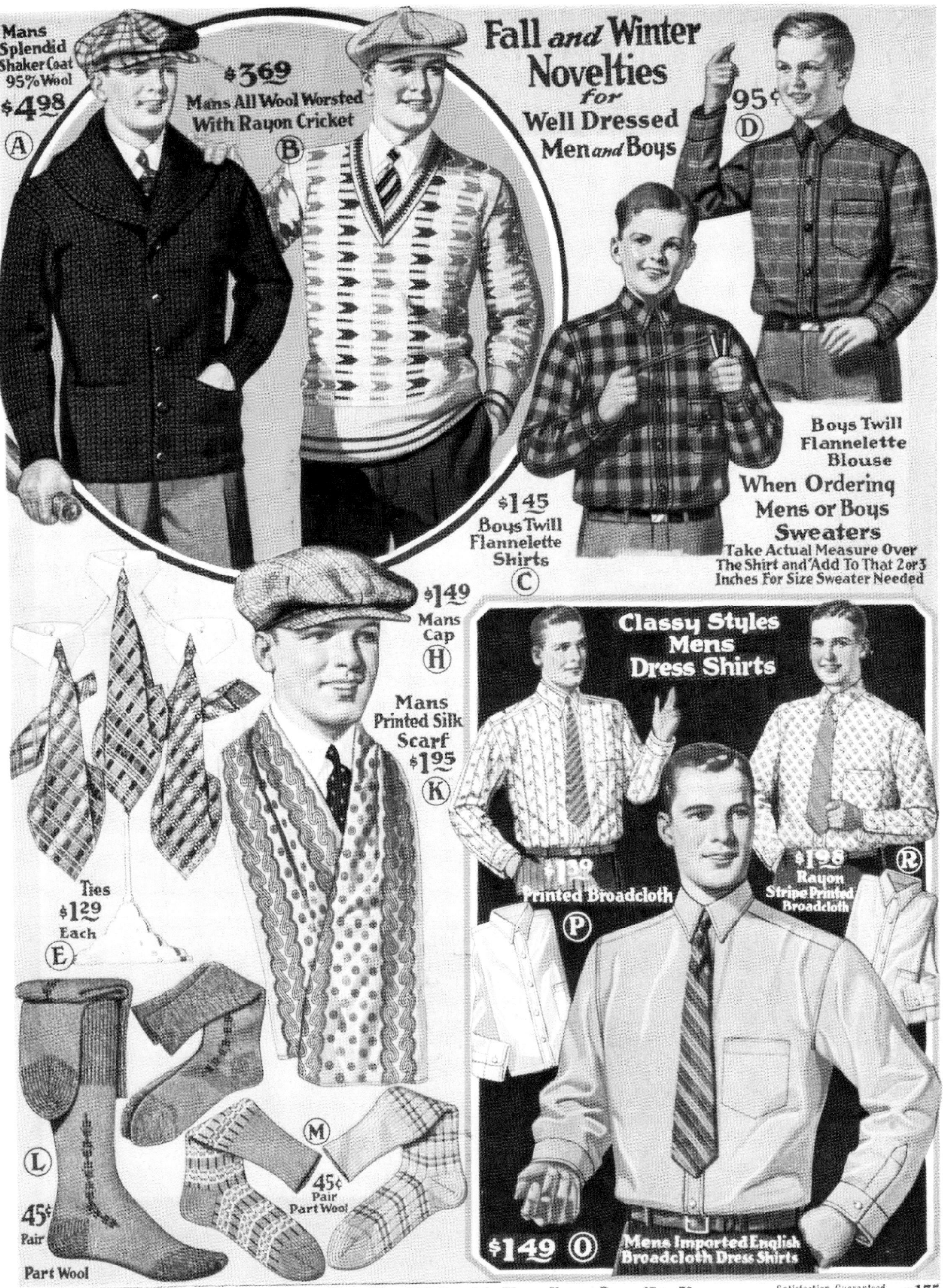
Fall and Winter Novelties for Well Dressed Men and Boys
Mans Splendid Shaker Coat 95% Wool
$4.98
A
$3.69
Mans All Wool Worsted With Rayon Cricket
B
95¢
D
Boys Twill Flannelette Blouse
When Ordering Mens or Boys Sweaters
Take Actual Measure Over The Shirt and Add To That 2 or 3 Inches For Size Sweater Needed
$1.45
Boys Twill Flannelette Shirts
C
$1.49
Mans Cap
H
Mans Printed Silk Scarf
$1.95
K
Ties $1.29 Each
E
Classy Styles Mens Dress Shirts
Printed Broadcloth
P
$1.98
Rayon Stripe Printed Broadcloth
R
L
45¢ Pair
Part Wool
M
45¢ Pair Part Wool
$1.49
O
Mens Imported English Broadcloth Dress Shirts

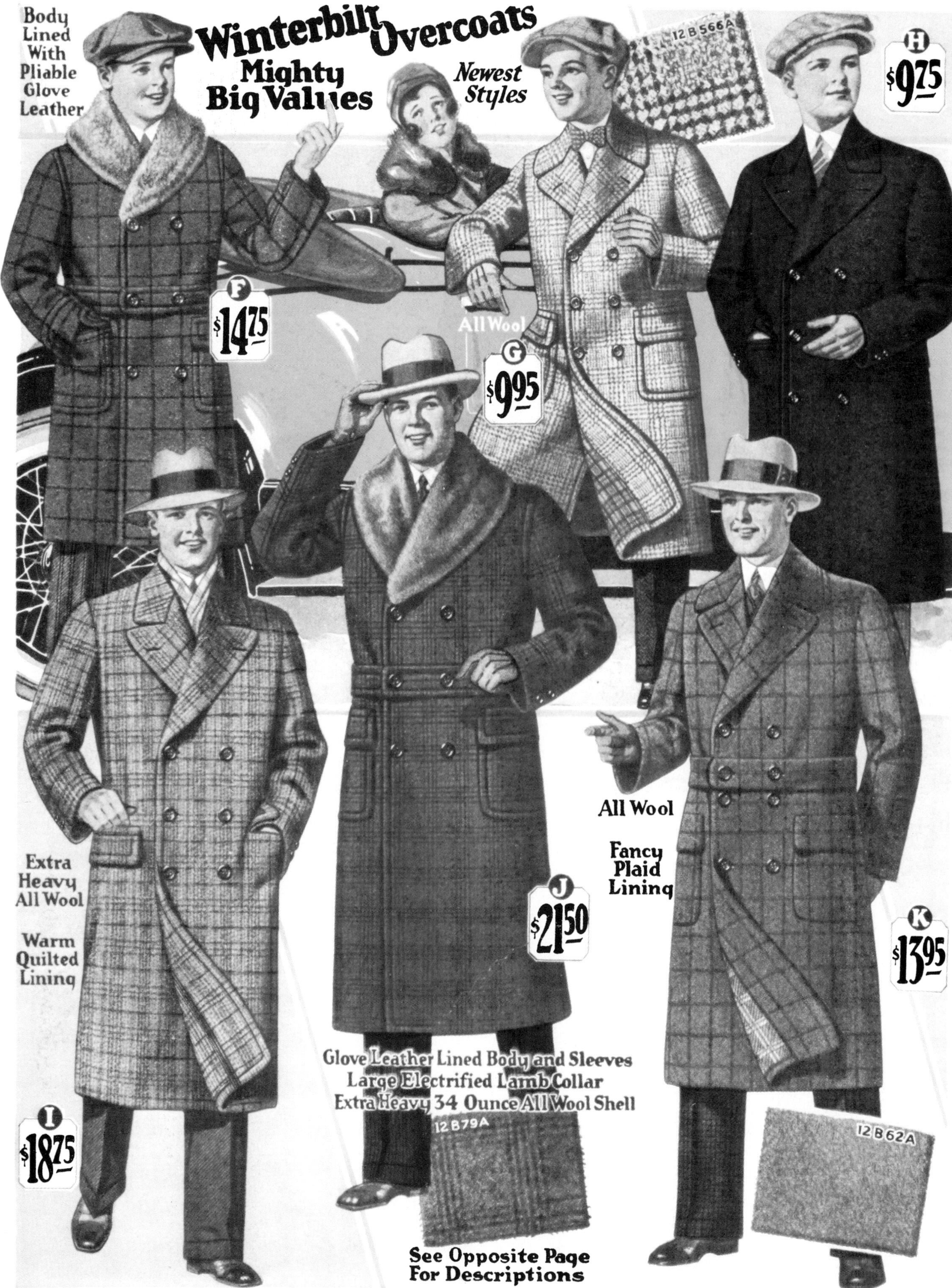
Winterbilt Overcoats
Mighty Big Values
Newest Styles
Body Lined With Pliable Glove Leather
F $14.75
All Wool
G $9.95
H $9.75
12 B 566A
Extra Heavy All Wool
Warm Quilted Lining
I $18.75
J $21.50
Glove Leather Lined Body and Sleeves
Large Electrified Lamb Collar
Extra Heavy 34 Ounce All Wool Shell
12 B 79A
All Wool
Fancy Plaid Lining
K $13.95
12 B 62A
See Opposite Page For Descriptions

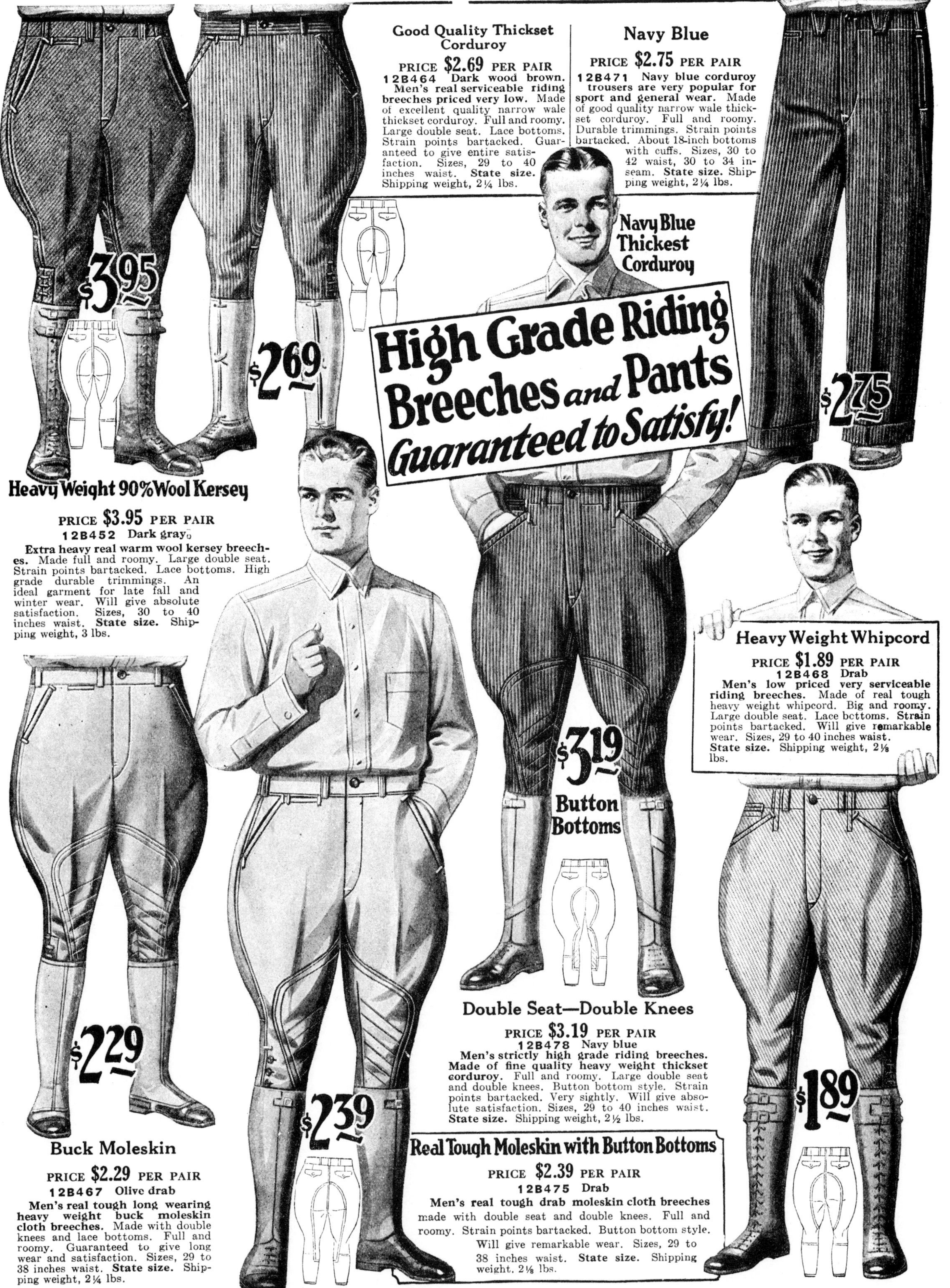


**Good Quality Thickset Corduroy**

PRICE **$2.69** PER PAIR
**12B464** **Dark wood brown. Men's real serviceable riding breeches priced very low.** Made of excellent quality narrow wale thickset corduroy. Full and roomy. Large double seat. Lace bottoms. Strain points bartacked. Guaranteed to give entire satisfaction. Sizes, 29 to 40 inches waist. **State size.** Shipping weight, 2¼ lbs.

**Navy Blue**

PRICE **$2.75** PER PAIR
**12B471** **Navy blue corduroy trousers are very popular for sport and general wear.** Made of good quality narrow wale thickset corduroy. Full and roomy. Durable trimmings. Strain points bartacked. About 18-inch bottoms with cuffs. Sizes, 30 to 42 waist, 30 to 34 inseam. **State size.** Shipping weight, 2¼ lbs.

**Heavy Weight 90% Wool Kersey**

PRICE **$3.95** PER PAIR
**12B452** Dark gray
**Extra heavy real warm wool kersey breeches.** Made full and roomy. Large double seat. Strain points bartacked. Lace bottoms. High grade durable trimmings. An ideal garment for late fall and winter wear. Will give absolute satisfaction. Sizes, 30 to 40 inches waist. **State size.** Shipping weight, 3 lbs.

**Heavy Weight Whipcord**

PRICE **$1.89** PER PAIR
**12B468** Drab
**Men's low priced very serviceable riding breeches.** Made of real tough heavy weight whipcord. Big and roomy. Large double seat. Lace bottoms. Strain points bartacked. Will give remarkable wear. Sizes, 29 to 40 inches waist. **State size.** Shipping weight, 2⅛ lbs.

**Double Seat—Double Knees**

PRICE **$3.19** PER PAIR
**12B478** Navy blue
**Men's strictly high grade riding breeches. Made of fine quality heavy weight thickset corduroy.** Full and roomy. Large double seat and double knees. Button bottom style. Strain points bartacked. Very sightly. Will give absolute satisfaction. Sizes, 29 to 40 inches waist. **State size.** Shipping weight, 2½ lbs.

**Buck Moleskin**

PRICE **$2.29** PER PAIR
**12B467** Olive drab
**Men's real tough long wearing heavy weight buck moleskin cloth breeches.** Made with double knees and lace bottoms. Full and roomy. Guaranteed to give long wear and satisfaction. Sizes, 29 to 38 inches waist. **State size.** Shipping weight, 2¼ lbs.

**Real Tough Moleskin with Button Bottoms**

PRICE **$2.39** PER PAIR
**12B475** Drab
**Men's real tough drab moleskin cloth breeches** made with double seat and double knees. Full and roomy. Strain points bartacked. Button bottom style. Will give remarkable wear. Sizes, 29 to 38 inches waist. **State size.** Shipping weight, 2⅛ lbs.

# Suits *for* Play *and* Everyday

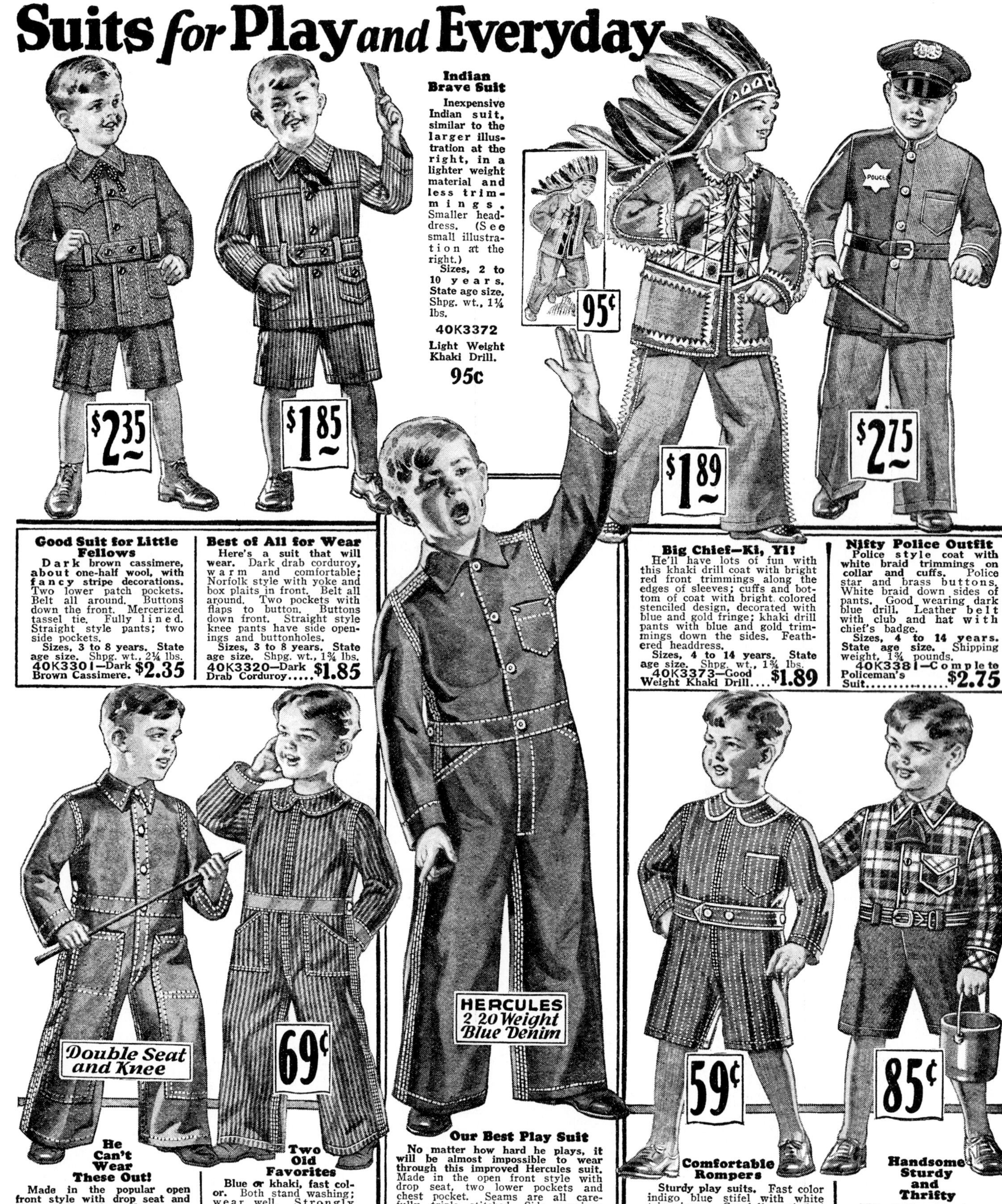


**Indian Brave Suit**

Inexpensive Indian suit, similar to the larger illustration at the right, in a lighter weight material and less trimmings. Smaller headdress. (See small illustration at the right.) Sizes, 2 to 10 years. State age size. Shpg. wt., 1¼ lbs.

40K3372 Light Weight Khaki Drill. **95c**

**Good Suit for Little Fellows**

Dark brown cassimere, about one-half wool, with fancy stripe decorations. Two lower patch pockets. Belt all around. Buttons down the front. Mercerized tassel tie. Fully lined. Straight style pants; two side pockets.

Sizes, 3 to 8 years. State age size. Shpg. wt., 2¼ lbs.

40K3301—Dark Brown Cassimere. **$2.35**

**Best of All for Wear**

Here's a suit that will wear. Dark drab corduroy, warm and comfortable; Norfolk style with yoke and box plaits in front. Belt all around. Two pockets with flaps to button. Buttons down front. Straight style knee pants have side openings and buttonholes.

Sizes, 3 to 8 years. State age size. Shpg. wt., 1¾ lbs.

40K3320—Dark Drab Corduroy..... **$1.85**

**Big Chief—Ki, Yi!**

He'll have lots of fun with this khaki drill coat with bright red front trimmings along the edges of sleeves; cuffs and bottom of coat with bright colored stenciled design, decorated with blue and gold fringe; khaki drill pants with blue and gold trimmings down the sides. Feathered headdress.

Sizes, 4 to 14 years. State age size. Shpg. wt., 1¾ lbs.

40K3373—Good Weight Khaki Drill.... **$1.89**

**Nifty Police Outfit**

Police style coat with white braid trimmings on collar and cuffs. Police star and brass buttons. White braid down sides of pants. Good wearing dark blue drill. Leather belt with club and hat with chief's badge.

Sizes, 4 to 14 years. State age size. Shipping weight, 1¾ pounds.

40K3381—Complete Policeman's Suit.............. **$2.75**

**He Can't Wear These Out!**

Made in the popular open front style with drop seat and shirt style collar. Seams are strongly stitched and buttonholes carefully made. Bar tacked at all points of strain. Double seat and knees for double wear. Riveted brass buttons will not come off or rust. Medium heavy weight, fast color, double and twist indigo blue denim or fast color fine weave khaki twill. Wash, wear well.

Sizes, 3 to 8 years. State size. Shipping weight, 1 pound.

40K3631—Fast Color Indigo Blue Denim....... **85c**

40K3633—Fast Color Khaki Twill............. **85c**

**Two Old Favorites**

Blue or khaki, fast color. Both stand washing; wear well. Strongly stitched seams. Bar tacked at all points of strain. Open back, drop seat. Blue trimmed. Riveted brass buttons, don't come off or rust. Full and roomy.

Sizes, 2 to 8 years. State age size. Shipping weight, ¾ pound.

40K3604—Fast Color Medium Heavy Weight Indigo Blue Stifel Drill......... **69c**

40K3606—Fast Color Khaki Twill............. **69c**

**Our Best Play Suit**

No matter how hard he plays, it will be almost impossible to wear through this improved Hercules suit. Made in the open front style with drop seat, two lower pockets and chest pocket. Seams are all carefully triple stitched. Side openings have continuous facings and cannot rip. Buttonholes securely stitched. Bar tacked at all points of strain. Covered fly front. Riveted brass buttons will not come off or rust. Made of the well known extra heavy 2.20 white back denim which is so popular in our men's high grade overalls. Cut full and roomy. Shaped sleeves and shoulders.

Sizes, 3 to 8 years. State age size. Shipping weight 1¼ pounds.

40K3620—2.20 Weight White Back Indigo Blue Denim **$1.00**

**Comfortable Rompers**

Sturdy play suits. Fast color indigo blue stifel with white trimmings. Carefully stitched seams. Button back, with drop seat.

Sizes, 2 to 7 years. State age size. Shpg. wt., ¾ lb.

40K3614—Fast Color Indigo Blue Stifel......... **59c**

Practical flannel romper, similar to above, but without the trimmings. Good wearing washable flannel, about one-third wool, in plain brown shade. Seams carefully stitched. Button back, with drop seat.

Sizes, 2 to 7 years. State age size. Shpg. wt., 1 lb.

40K3615—Brown Flannel One-Third Wool.. **98c**

**Handsome Sturdy and Thrifty**

This little suit is very attractive and can be worn for dress or play, as it can be very easily washed. Waist is made of good weight, washable cotton material in a fancy brown and tan plaid with blue and green decorations. Brown twill tie. Plain, medium dark brown, washable twill flannel pants which button to waist. Collegiate style bright colored belt.

Sizes, 2 to 8 years. State age size. Shpg. wt., 1 lb.

40K3300 Blazer Suit....... **85c**

*Send Sufficient Money for Postage on Parcel Post Shipments. Any Surplus Will Be Returned*

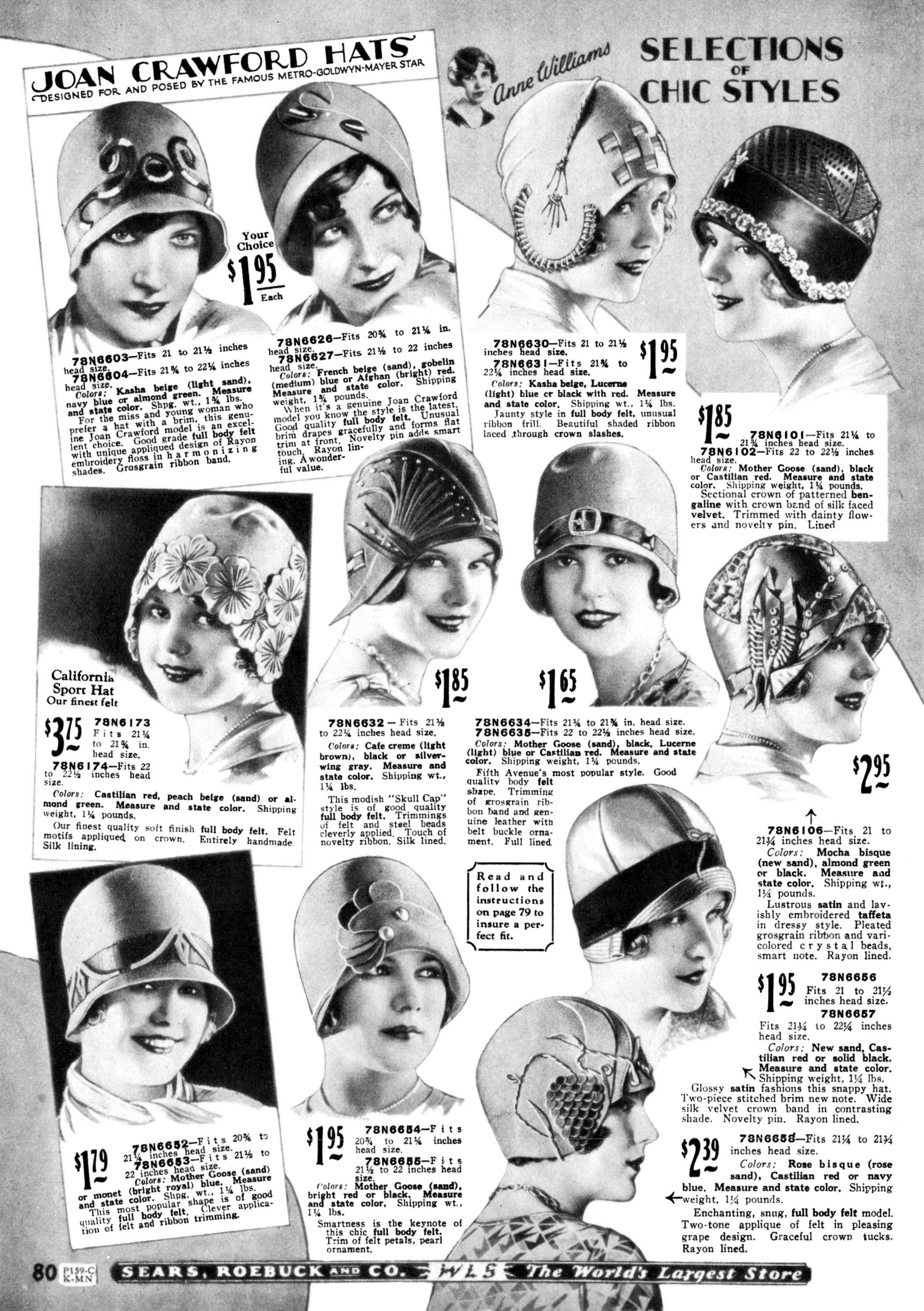

JOAN CRAWFORD HATS
DESIGNED FOR AND POSED BY THE FAMOUS METRO-GOLDWYN-MAYER STAR

Your Choice $1.95 Each

78N6603—Fits 21 to 21½ inches head size.
78N6604—Fits 21¾ to 22¼ inches head size.
*Colors:* Kasha beige (light sand), navy blue or almond green. Measure and state color. Shpg. wt., 1¾ lbs.
For the miss and young woman who prefer a hat with a brim, this genuine Joan Crawford model is an excellent choice. Good grade full body felt with unique appliqued design of Rayon embroidery floss in harmonizing shades. Grosgrain ribbon band.

78N6626—Fits 20¾ to 21¼ in. head size.
78N6627—Fits 21½ to 22 inches head size.
*Colors:* French beige (sand), gobelin (medium) blue or Afghan (bright) red. Measure and state color. Shipping weight, 1¾ pounds.
When it's a genuine Joan Crawford model you know the style is the latest. Good quality full body felt. Unusual brim drapes gracefully and forms flat trim at front. Novelty pin adds smart touch. Rayon lining. A wonderful value.

Anne Williams SELECTIONS OF CHIC STYLES

$1.95
78N6630—Fits 21 to 21½ inches head size.
78N6631—Fits 21¾ to 22¼ inches head size.
*Colors:* Kasha beige, Lucerne (light) blue or black with red. Measure and state color. Shipping wt., 1¼ lbs.
Jaunty style in full body felt, unusual ribbon frill. Beautiful shaded ribbon laced through crown slashes.

$1.85
78N6101—Fits 21¼ to 21¾ inches head size.
78N6102—Fits 22 to 22½ inches head size.
*Colors:* Mother Goose (sand), black or Castilian red. Measure and state color. Shipping weight, 1¼ pounds.
Sectional crown of patterned bengaline with crown band of silk faced velvet. Trimmed with dainty flowers and novelty pin. Lined

California Sport Hat
Our finest felt
$3.75
78N6173 Fits 21¼ to 21¾ in. head size.
78N6174—Fits 22 to 22½ inches head size.
*Colors:* Castilian red, peach beige (sand) or almond green. Measure and state color. Shipping weight, 1¼ pounds.
Our finest quality soft finish full body felt. Felt motifs appliqued on crown. Entirely handmade. Silk lining.

$1.85
78N6632—Fits 21½ to 22¼ inches head size.
*Colors:* Cafe creme (light brown), black or silver-wing gray. Measure and state color. Shipping wt., 1¼ lbs.
This modish "Skull Cap" style is of good quality full body felt. Trimmings of felt and steel beads cleverly applied. Touch of novelty ribbon. Silk lined.

$1.65
78N6634—Fits 21¼ to 21¾ in. head size.
78N6635—Fits 22 to 22½ inches head size.
*Colors:* Mother Goose (sand), black, Lucerne (light) blue or Castilian red. Measure and state color. Shipping weight, 1¼ pounds.
Fifth Avenue's most popular style. Good quality body felt shape. Trimming of grosgrain ribbon band and genuine leather with belt buckle ornament. Full lined.

$2.95
78N6106—Fits 21 to 21¾ inches head size.
*Colors:* Mocha bisque (new sand), almond green or black. Measure and state color. Shipping wt., 1¼ pounds.
Lustrous satin and lavishly embroidered taffeta in dressy style. Pleated grosgrain ribbon and varicolored crystal beads, smart note. Rayon lined.

Read and follow the instructions on page 79 to insure a perfect fit.

$1.95
78N6656 Fits 21 to 21½ inches head size.
78N6657 Fits 21¾ to 22¼ inches head size.
*Colors:* New sand, Castilian red or solid black. Measure and state color. Shipping weight, 1¼ lbs.
Glossy satin fashions this snappy hat. Two-piece stitched brim new note. Wide silk velvet crown band in contrasting shade. Novelty pin. Rayon lined.

$1.79
78N6652—Fits 20¾ to 21¼ inches head size.
78N6653—Fits 21½ to 22 inches head size.
*Colors:* Mother Goose (sand) or monet (bright royal) blue. Measure and state color. Shpg. wt., 1¼ lbs.
This most popular shape is of good quality full body felt. Clever application of felt and ribbon trimming.

$1.95
78N6654—Fits 20¾ to 21¼ inches head size.
78N6655—Fits 21½ to 22 inches head size.
*Colors:* Mother Goose (sand), bright red or black. Measure and state color. Shipping wt., 1¼ lbs.
Smartness is the keynote of this chic full body felt. Trim of felt petals, pearl ornament.

$2.39
78N6658—Fits 21¼ to 21¾ inches head size.
*Colors:* Rose bisque (rose sand), Castilian red or navy blue. Measure and state color. Shipping weight, 1¼ pounds.
Enchanting, snug, full body felt model. Two-tone applique of felt in pleasing grape design. Graceful crown tucks. Rayon lined.

80 P159-C K-MN SEARS, ROEBUCK AND CO. WLS The World's Largest Store

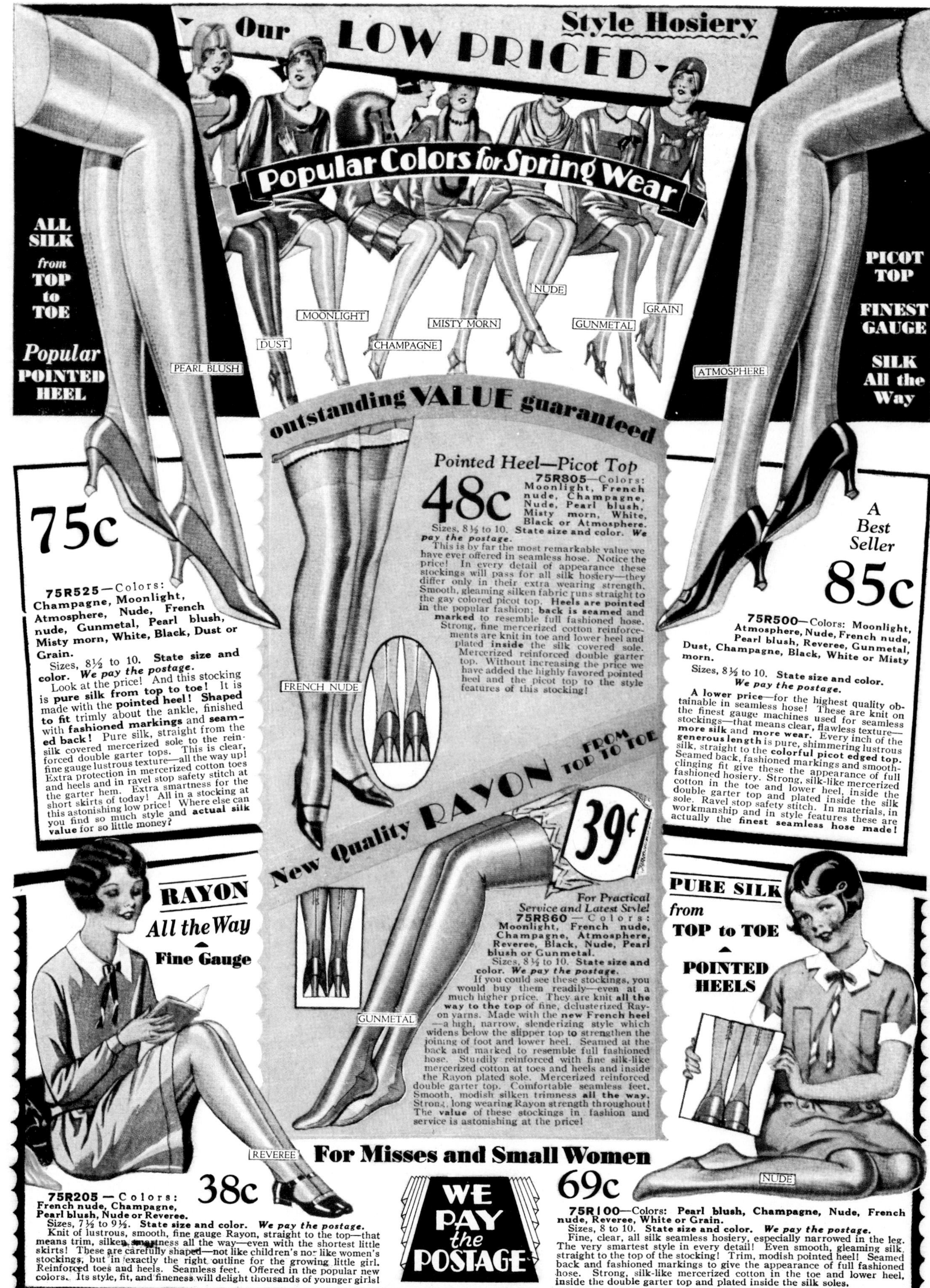
Our LOW PRICED Style Hosiery
Popular Colors for Spring Wear
PEARL BLUSH
DUST
MOONLIGHT
CHAMPAGNE
MISTY MORN
NUDE
GUNMETAL
GRAIN
ATMOSPHERE
ALL SILK from TOP to TOE
Popular POINTED HEEL
PICOT TOP
FINEST GAUGE
SILK All the Way
outstanding VALUE guaranteed
Pointed Heel—Picot Top
48c
75R805—Colors: Moonlight, French nude, Champagne, Nude, Pearl blush, Misty morn, White, Black or Atmosphere.
Sizes, 8½ to 10. State size and color. We pay the postage.
This is by far the most remarkable value we have ever offered in seamless hose. Notice the price! In every detail of appearance these stockings will pass for all silk hosiery—they differ only in their extra wearing strength. Smooth, gleaming silken fabric runs straight to the gay colored picot top. Heels are pointed in the popular fashion; back is seamed and marked to resemble full fashioned hose. Strong, fine mercerized cotton reinforcements are knit in toe and lower heel and plated inside the silk covered sole. Mercerized reinforced double garter top. Without increasing the price we have added the highly favored pointed heel and the picot top to the style features of this stocking!
75c
75R525—Colors: Champagne, Moonlight, Atmosphere, Nude, French nude, Gunmetal, Pearl blush, Misty morn, White, Black, Dust or Grain.
Sizes, 8½ to 10. State size and color. We pay the postage.
Look at the price! And this stocking is pure silk from top to toe! It is made with the pointed heel! Shaped to fit trimly about the ankle, finished with fashioned markings and seamed back! Pure silk, straight from the silk covered mercerized sole to the reinforced double garter tops. This is clear, fine gauge lustrous texture—all the way up! Extra protection in mercerized cotton toes and heels and in ravel stop safety stitch at the garter hem. Extra smartness for the short skirts of today! All in a stocking at this astonishing low price! Where else can you find so much style and actual silk value for so little money?
A Best Seller
85c
75R500—Colors: Moonlight, Atmosphere, Nude, French nude, Pearl blush, Reveree, Gunmetal, Dust, Champagne, Black, White or Misty morn.
Sizes, 8½ to 10. State size and color. We pay the postage.
A lower price—for the highest quality obtainable in seamless hose! These are knit on the finest gauge machines used for seamless stockings—that means clear, flawless texture—more silk and more wear. Every inch of the generous length is pure, shimmering lustrous silk, straight to the colorful picot edged top. Seamed back, fashioned markings and smooth-clinging fit give these the appearance of full fashioned hosiery. Strong, silk-like mercerized cotton in the toe and lower heel, inside the double garter top and plated inside the silk sole. Ravel stop safety stitch. In materials, in workmanship and in style features these are actually the finest seamless hose made!
FRENCH NUDE
New Quality RAYON FROM TOP TO TOE
39¢
For Practical Service and Latest Style!
75R860—Colors: Moonlight, French nude, Champagne, Atmosphere, Reveree, Black, Nude, Pearl blush or Gunmetal.
Sizes, 8½ to 10. State size and color. We pay the postage.
If you could see these stockings, you would buy them readily—even at a much higher price. They are knit all the way to the top of fine, delusterized Rayon yarns. Made with the new French heel—a high, narrow, slenderizing style which widens below the slipper top to strengthen the joining of foot and lower heel. Seamed at the back and marked to resemble full fashioned hose. Sturdily reinforced with fine silk-like mercerized cotton at toes and heels and inside the Rayon plated sole. Mercerized reinforced double garter top. Comfortable seamless feet. Smooth, modish silken trimness all the way. Strong, long wearing Rayon strength throughout! The value of these stockings in fashion and service is astonishing at the price!
GUNMETAL
RAYON All the Way Fine Gauge
PURE SILK from TOP to TOE
POINTED HEELS
For Misses and Small Women
REVEREE
38c
75R205—Colors: French nude, Champagne, Pearl blush, Nude or Reveree.
Sizes, 7½ to 9½. State size and color. We pay the postage.
Knit of lustrous, smooth, fine gauge Rayon, straight to the top—that means trim, silken smartness all the way—even with the shortest little skirts! These are carefully shaped—not like children's nor like women's stockings, but in exactly the right outline for the growing little girl. Reinforced toes and heels. Seamless feet. Offered in the popular new colors. Its style, fit, and fineness will delight thousands of younger girls!
WE PAY the POSTAGE
69c
NUDE
75R100—Colors: Pearl blush, Champagne, Nude, French nude, Reveree, White or Grain.
Sizes, 8 to 10. State size and color. We pay the postage.
Fine, clear, all silk seamless hosiery, especially narrowed in the leg. The very smartest style in every detail! Even smooth, gleaming silk, straight to the top of the stocking! Trim, modish pointed heel! Seamed back and fashioned markings to give the appearance of full fashioned hose. Strong, silk-like mercerized cotton in the toe and lower heel, inside the double garter top and plated inside the silk soles.

# Shoes

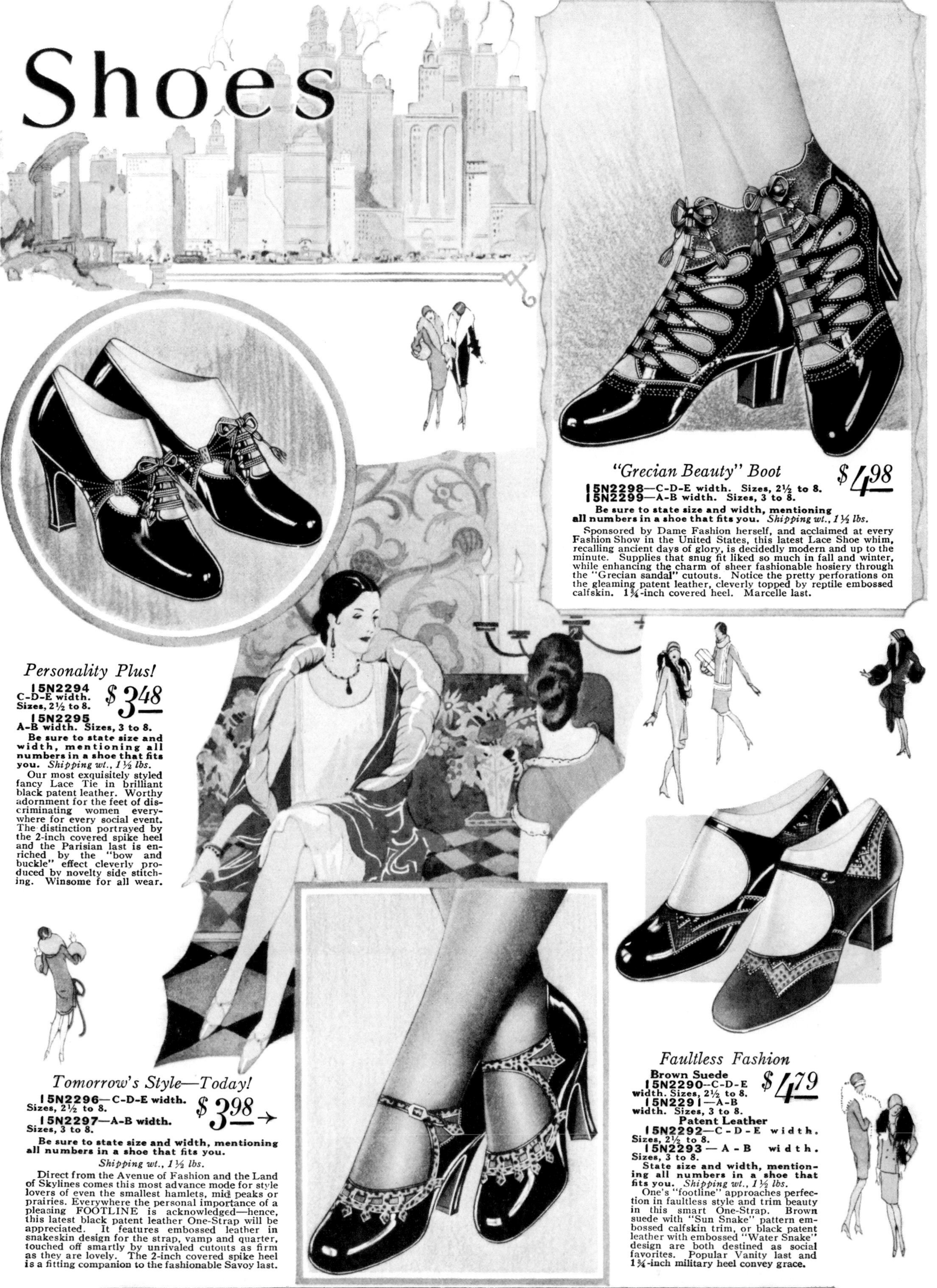

*"Grecian Beauty" Boot* **$4.98**

**15N2298**—C-D-E width. Sizes, 2½ to 8.
**15N2299**—A-B width. Sizes, 3 to 8.

**Be sure to state size and width, mentioning all numbers in a shoe that fits you.** *Shipping wt., 1¼ lbs.*

Sponsored by Dame Fashion herself, and acclaimed at every Fashion Show in the United States, this latest Lace Shoe whim, recalling ancient days of glory, is decidedly modern and up to the minute. Supplies that snug fit liked so much in fall and winter, while enhancing the charm of sheer fashionable hosiery through the "Grecian sandal" cutouts. Notice the pretty perforations on the gleaming patent leather, cleverly topped by reptile embossed calfskin. 1¾-inch covered heel. Marcelle last.

*Personality Plus!* **$3.48**

**15N2294** C-D-E width. Sizes, 2½ to 8.
**15N2295** A-B width. Sizes, 3 to 8.

**Be sure to state size and width, mentioning all numbers in a shoe that fits you.** *Shipping wt., 1½ lbs.*

Our most exquisitely styled fancy Lace Tie in brilliant black patent leather. Worthy adornment for the feet of discriminating women everywhere for every social event. The distinction portrayed by the 2-inch covered spike heel and the Parisian last is enriched by the "bow and buckle" effect cleverly produced by novelty side stitching. Winsome for all wear.

*Tomorrow's Style—Today!* **$3.98** →

**15N2296**—C-D-E width. Sizes, 2½ to 8.
**15N2297**—A-B width. Sizes, 3 to 8.

**Be sure to state size and width, mentioning all numbers in a shoe that fits you.**

*Shipping wt., 1½ lbs.*

Direct from the Avenue of Fashion and the Land of Skylines comes this most advance mode for style lovers of even the smallest hamlets, mid peaks or prairies. Everywhere the personal importance of a pleasing FOOTLINE is acknowledged—hence, this latest black patent leather One-Strap will be appreciated. It features embossed leather in snakeskin design for the strap, vamp and quarter, touched off smartly by unrivaled cutouts as firm as they are lovely. The 2-inch covered spike heel is a fitting companion to the fashionable Savoy last.

*Faultless Fashion* **$4.79**

**Brown Suede**
**15N2290**—C-D-E width. Sizes, 2½ to 8.
**15N2291**—A-B width. Sizes, 3 to 8.

**Patent Leather**
**15N2292**—C-D-E width. Sizes, 2½ to 8.
**15N2293**—A-B width. Sizes, 3 to 8.

**State size and width, mentioning all numbers in a shoe that fits you.** *Shipping wt., 1½ lbs.*

One's "footline" approaches perfection in faultless style and trim beauty in this smart One-Strap. Brown suede with "Sun Snake" pattern embossed calfskin trim, or black patent leather with embossed "Water Snake" design are both destined as social favorites. Popular Vanity last and 1¾-inch military heel convey grace.

***Your Orders Shipped Within 24 Hours!***

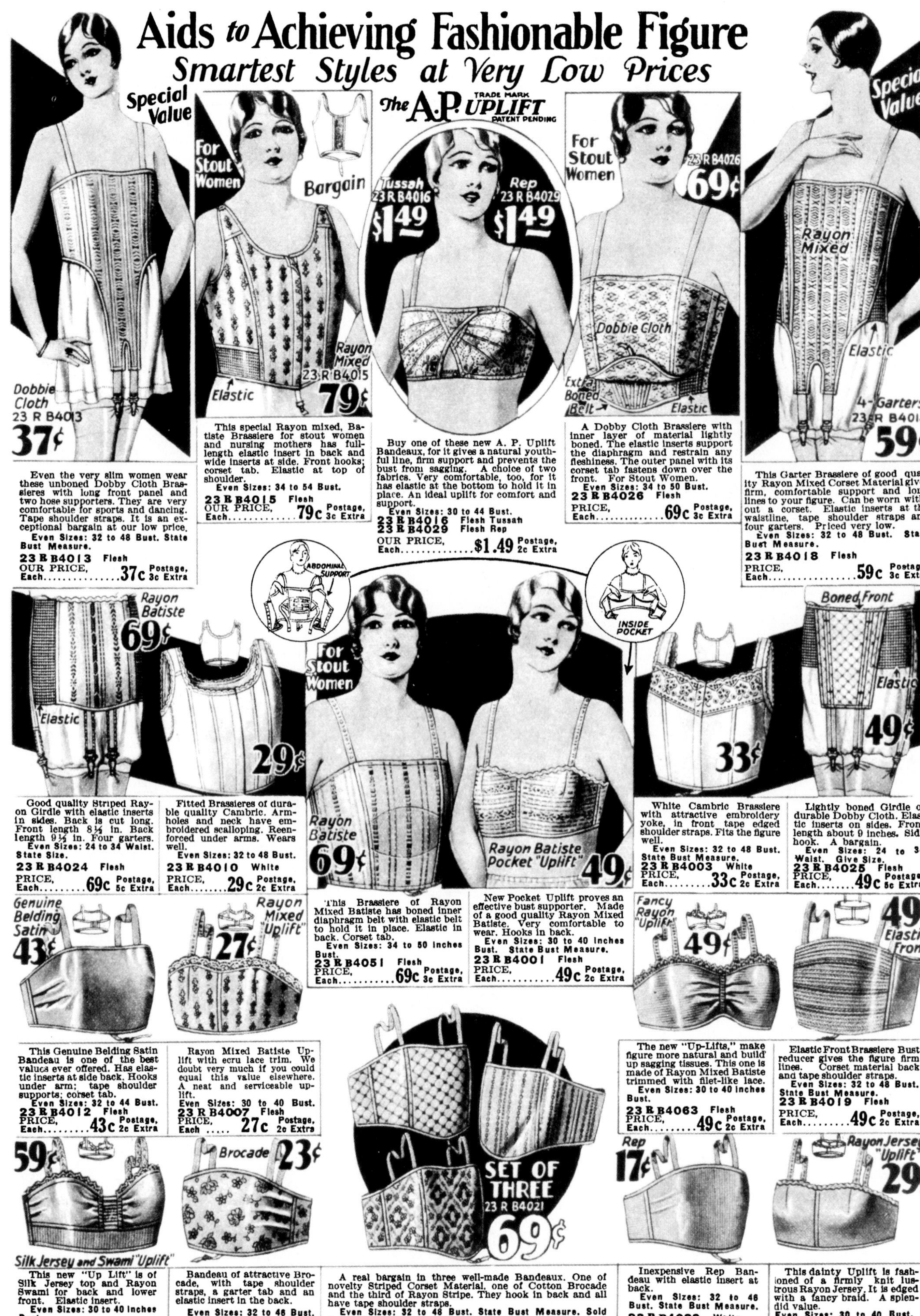
Aids to Achieving Fashionable Figure
Smartest Styles at Very Low Prices
Special Value
For Stout Women
Bargain
The A.P. UPLIFT TRADE MARK PATENT PENDING
Tussah 23 R B4016 $1.49
Rep 23 R B4029 $1.49
For Stout Women
23 R B4026 69¢
Special Value
Rayon Mixed
Rayon Mixed 23 R B4015 79¢
Elastic
Dobbie Cloth
Dobbie Cloth 23 R B4013 37¢
Extra Boned Belt
Elastic
Elastic
4-Garters 23 R B4018 59¢
This special Rayon mixed, Batiste Brassiere for stout women and nursing mothers has full-length elastic insert in back and wide inserts at side. Front hooks; corset tab. Elastic at top of shoulder.
Even Sizes: 34 to 54 Bust.
23 R B4015 Flesh
OUR PRICE, Each............79c Postage, 3c Extra
Buy one of these new A. P. Uplift Bandeaux, for it gives a natural youthful line, firm support and prevents the bust from sagging. A choice of two fabrics. Very comfortable, too, for it has elastic at the bottom to hold it in place. An ideal uplift for comfort and support.
Even Sizes: 30 to 44 Bust.
23 R B4016 Flesh Tussah
23 R B4029 Flesh Rep
OUR PRICE, Each.............$1.49 Postage, 2c Extra
A Dobby Cloth Brassiere with inner layer of material lightly boned. The elastic inserts support the diaphragm and restrain any fleshiness. The outer panel with its corset tab fastens down over the front. For Stout Women.
Even Sizes: 34 to 50 Bust.
23 R B4026 Flesh
PRICE, Each............69c Postage, 3c Extra
Even the very slim women wear these unboned Dobby Cloth Brassieres with long front panel and two hose supporters. They are very comfortable for sports and dancing. Tape shoulder straps. It is an exceptional bargain at our low price.
Even Sizes: 32 to 48 Bust. State Bust Measure.
23 R B4013 Flesh
OUR PRICE, Each...............37c Postage, 3c Extra
This Garter Brassiere of good quality Rayon Mixed Corset Material gives firm, comfortable support and long lines to your figure. Can be worn without a corset. Elastic inserts at the waistline, tape shoulder straps and four garters. Priced very low.
Even Sizes: 32 to 48 Bust. State Bust Measure.
23 R B4018 Flesh
PRICE, Each................59c Postage, 3c Extra
ABDOMINAL SUPPORT
INSIDE POCKET
Rayon Batiste 69¢
Elastic
29¢
For Stout Women
33¢
Boned Front
Elastic
49¢
Rayon Batiste 69¢
Rayon Batiste Pocket "Uplift" 49¢
Good quality Striped Rayon Girdle with elastic inserts in sides. Back is cut long. Front length 8¼ in. Back length 9½ in. Four garters.
Even Sizes: 24 to 34 Waist. State Size.
23 R B4024 Flesh
PRICE, Each........69c Postage, 5c Extra
Fitted Brassieres of durable quality Cambric. Armholes and neck have embroidered scalloping. Reenforced under arms. Wears well.
Even Sizes: 32 to 48 Bust.
23 R B4010 White
PRICE, Each.......29c Postage, 2c Extra
White Cambric Brassiere with attractive embroidery yoke, in front tape edged shoulder straps. Fits the figure well.
Even Sizes: 32 to 48 Bust. State Bust Measure.
23 R B4003 White
PRICE, Each.........33c Postage, 2c Extra
Lightly boned Girdle of durable Dobby Cloth. Elastic inserts on sides. Front length about 9 inches. Side hook. A bargain.
Even Sizes: 24 to 34 Waist. Give Size.
23 R B4025 Flesh
PRICE, Each.......49c Postage, 5c Extra
Genuine Belding Satin 43¢
Rayon Mixed "Uplift" 27¢
This Brassiere of Rayon Mixed Batiste has boned inner diaphragm belt with elastic belt to hold it in place. Elastic in back. Corset tab.
Even Sizes: 34 to 50 Inches Bust.
23 R B4051 Flesh
PRICE, Each..........69c Postage, 3c Extra
New Pocket Uplift proves an effective bust supporter. Made of a good quality Rayon Mixed Batiste. Very comfortable to wear. Hooks in back.
Even Sizes: 30 to 40 Inches Bust. State Bust Measure.
23 R B4001 Flesh
PRICE, Each..........49c Postage, 2c Extra
Fancy Rayon "Uplift" 49¢
49¢ Elastic Front
This Genuine Belding Satin Bandeau is one of the best values ever offered. Has elastic inserts at side back. Hooks under arm; tape shoulder supports; corset tab.
Even Sizes: 32 to 44 Bust.
23 R B4012 Flesh
PRICE, Each........43c Postage, 2c Extra
Rayon Mixed Batiste Uplift with ecru lace trim. We doubt very much if you could equal this value elsewhere. A neat and serviceable uplift.
Even Sizes: 30 to 40 Bust.
23 R B4007 Flesh
PRICE, Each .....27c Postage, 2c Extra
The new "Up-Lifts," make figure more natural and build up sagging tissues. This one is made of Rayon Mixed Batiste trimmed with filet-like lace.
Even Sizes: 30 to 40 Inches Bust.
23 R B4063 Flesh
PRICE, Each.........49c Postage, 2c Extra
Elastic Front Brassiere Bust reducer gives the figure firm lines. Corset material back and tape shoulder straps.
Even Sizes: 32 to 48 Bust. State Bust Measure.
23 R B4019 Flesh
PRICE, Each.........49c Postage, 2c Extra
59¢
Brocade 23¢
SET OF THREE 23 R B4021 69¢
Rep 17¢
Rayon Jersey "Uplift" 29¢
Silk Jersey and Swami "Uplift"
This new "Up Lift" is of Silk Jersey top and Rayon Swami for back and lower front. Elastic insert.
Even Sizes: 30 to 40 Inches Bust.
23 R B4058 Flesh
PRICE, Each........59c Postage, 2c Extra
Bandeau of attractive Brocade, with tape shoulder straps, a garter tab and an elastic insert in the back.
Even Sizes: 32 to 46 Bust.
23 R B4020 Flesh
PRICE, Each.........23c Postage, 2c Extra
A real bargain in three well-made Bandeaux. One of novelty Striped Corset Material, one of Cotton Brocade and the third of Rayon Stripe. They hook in back and all have tape shoulder straps.
Even Sizes: 32 to 48 Bust. State Bust Measure. Sold only in Sets of Three of One Size.
23 R B4021 Flesh
OUR PRICE, Set of...............3 for 69c Postage, 5c Extra
Inexpensive Rep Bandeau with elastic insert at back.
Even Sizes: 32 to 46 Bust. State Bust Measure.
23 R B4022 White
23 R B4023 Flesh
PRICE, Each........17c Postage, 2c Extra
This dainty Uplift is fashioned of a firmly knit lustrous Rayon Jersey. It is edged with a fancy braid. A splendid value.
Even Sizes: 30 to 40 Bust.
23 R B4017 Flesh
PRICE, Each..........29c Postage, 2c Extra
The Charles William Stores Inc. New York City
IF POSTAGE IS LESS THAN WE SPECIFY, WE WILL REFUND THE DIFFERENCE

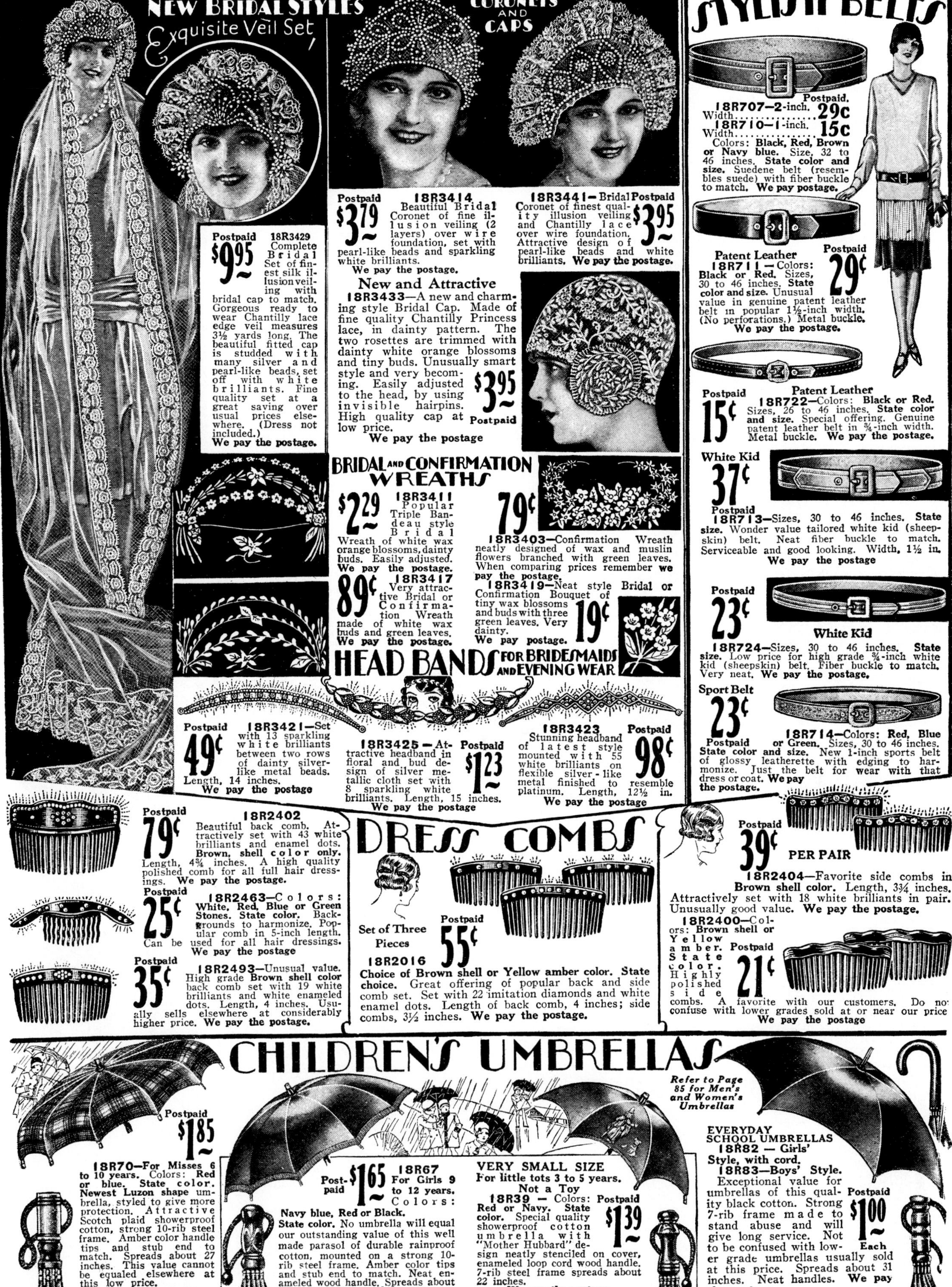
NEW BRIDAL STYLES
Exquisite Veil Set
Postpaid 18R3429 $9.95 Complete Bridal Set of finest silk illusion veiling with bridal cap to match. Gorgeous ready to wear Chantilly lace edge veil measures 3½ yards long. The beautiful fitted cap is studded with many silver and pearl-like beads, set off with white brilliants. Fine quality set at a great saving over usual prices elsewhere. (Dress not included.) We pay the postage.
CORONETS AND CAPS
Postpaid $3.79 18R3414 Beautiful Bridal Coronet of fine illusion veiling (2 layers) over wire foundation, set with pearl-like beads and sparkling white brilliants. We pay the postage.
18R3441—Bridal Coronet of finest quality illusion veiling and Chantilly lace over wire foundation. Attractive design of pearl-like beads and white brilliants. Postpaid $3.95 We pay the postage.
New and Attractive
18R3433—A new and charming style Bridal Cap. Made of fine quality Chantilly Princess lace, in dainty pattern. The two rosettes are trimmed with dainty white orange blossoms and tiny buds. Unusually smart style and very becoming. Easily adjusted to the head, by using invisible hairpins. High quality cap at low price. $3.95 Postpaid We pay the postage
BRIDAL AND CONFIRMATION WREATHS
$2.29 18R3411 Popular Triple Bandeau style Bridal Wreath of white wax orange blossoms, dainty buds. Easily adjusted. We pay the postage.
89¢ 18R3417 Very attractive Bridal or Confirmation Wreath made of white wax buds and green leaves. We pay the postage.
79¢ 18R3403—Confirmation Wreath neatly designed of wax and muslin flowers branched with green leaves. When comparing prices remember we pay the postage.
18R3419—Neat style Bridal or Confirmation Bouquet of tiny wax blossoms and buds with three green leaves. Very dainty. 19¢ We pay postage.
HEAD BANDS FOR BRIDESMAIDS AND EVENING WEAR
Postpaid 49¢ 18R3421—Set with 13 sparkling white brilliants between two rows of dainty silver-like metal beads. Length, 14 inches. We pay the postage
18R3425—Attractive headband in floral and bud design of silver metallic cloth set with 8 sparkling white brilliants. Length, 15 inches. Postpaid $1.23 We pay the postage
18R3423 Stunning headband of latest style mounted with 55 white brilliants on flexible silver-like metal finished to resemble platinum. Length, 12½ in. Postpaid 98¢ We pay the postage
STYLISH BELTS
Postpaid. 18R707—2-inch. Width 29c
18R710—1-inch. Width 15c
Colors: Black, Red, Brown or Navy blue. Size, 32 to 46 inches. State color and size. Suedene belt (resembles suede) with fiber buckle to match. We pay postage.
Patent Leather Postpaid 29¢ 18R711—Colors: Black or Red. Sizes, 30 to 46 inches. State color and size. Unusual value in genuine patent leather belt in popular 1½-inch width. (No perforations.) Metal buckle. We pay the postage.
Postpaid 15¢ Patent Leather 18R722—Colors: Black or Red. Sizes, 26 to 46 inches. State color and size. Special offering. Genuine patent leather belt in ¾-inch width. Metal buckle. We pay the postage.
White Kid 37¢ Postpaid 18R713—Sizes, 30 to 46 inches. State size. Wonder value tailored white kid (sheepskin) belt. Neat fiber buckle to match. Serviceable and good looking. Width, 1½ in. We pay the postage
Postpaid 23¢ White Kid 18R724—Sizes, 30 to 46 inches. State size. Low price for high grade ¾-inch white kid (sheepskin) belt. Fiber buckle to match. Very neat. We pay the postage.
Sport Belt 23¢ Postpaid 18R714—Colors: Red, Blue or Green. Sizes, 30 to 46 inches. State color and size. New 1-inch sports belt of glossy leatherette with edging to harmonize. Just the belt for wear with that dress or coat. We pay the postage.
DRESS COMBS
Postpaid 79¢ 18R2402 Beautiful back comb. Attractively set with 43 white brilliants and enamel dots. Brown, shell color only. Length, 4¾ inches. A high quality polished comb for all full hair dressings. We pay the postage.
Postpaid 25¢ 18R2463—Colors: White, Red, Blue or Green Stones. State color. Backgrounds to harmonize. Popular comb in 5-inch length. Can be used for all hair dressings. We pay the postage
Postpaid 35¢ 18R2493—Unusual value. High grade Brown shell color back comb set with 19 white brilliants and white enameled dots. Length, 4 inches. Usually sells elsewhere at considerably higher price. We pay the postage.
Set of Three Pieces 18R2016 Postpaid 55¢ Choice of Brown shell or Yellow amber color. State choice. Great offering of popular back and side comb set. Set with 22 imitation diamonds and white enamel dots. Length of back comb, 4 inches; side combs, 3½ inches. We pay the postage.
Postpaid 39¢ PER PAIR 18R2404—Favorite side combs in Brown shell color. Length, 3¾ inches. Attractively set with 18 white brilliants in pair. Unusually good value. We pay the postage.
18R2400—Colors: Brown shell or Yellow amber. State color. Highly polished side combs. Postpaid 21¢ A favorite with our customers. Do not confuse with lower grades sold at or near our price We pay the postage
CHILDREN'S UMBRELLAS
Refer to Page 85 for Men's and Women's Umbrellas
Postpaid $1.85 18R70—For Misses 6 to 10 years. Colors: Red or blue. State color. Newest Luzon shape umbrella, styled to give more protection. Attractive Scotch plaid showerproof cotton, strong 10-rib steel frame. Amber color handle tips and stub end to match. Spreads about 27 inches. This value cannot be equaled elsewhere at this low price. We pay the postage
Postpaid $1.65 18R67 For Girls 9 to 12 years. Colors: Navy blue, Red or Black. State color. No umbrella will equal our outstanding value of this well made parasol of durable rainproof cotton, mounted on a strong 10-rib steel frame. Amber color tips and stub end to match. Neat enameled wood handle. Spreads about 31 inches. We pay the postage.
VERY SMALL SIZE For little tots 3 to 5 years. Not a Toy
18R39 — Colors: Red or Navy. State color. Special quality showerproof cotton umbrella with "Mother Hubbard" design neatly stenciled on cover, enameled loop cord wood handle. 7-rib steel frame spreads about 22 inches. Postpaid $1.39 We pay the postage.
EVERYDAY SCHOOL UMBRELLAS
18R82 — Girls' Style, with cord.
18R83—Boys' Style.
Exceptional value for umbrellas of this quality black cotton. Strong 7-rib frame made to stand abuse and will give long service. Not to be confused with lower grade umbrellas usually sold at this price. Spreads about 31 inches. Neat handles. Postpaid $1.00 Each We pay the postage.

# POPULAR SHELL FRAME BAGS

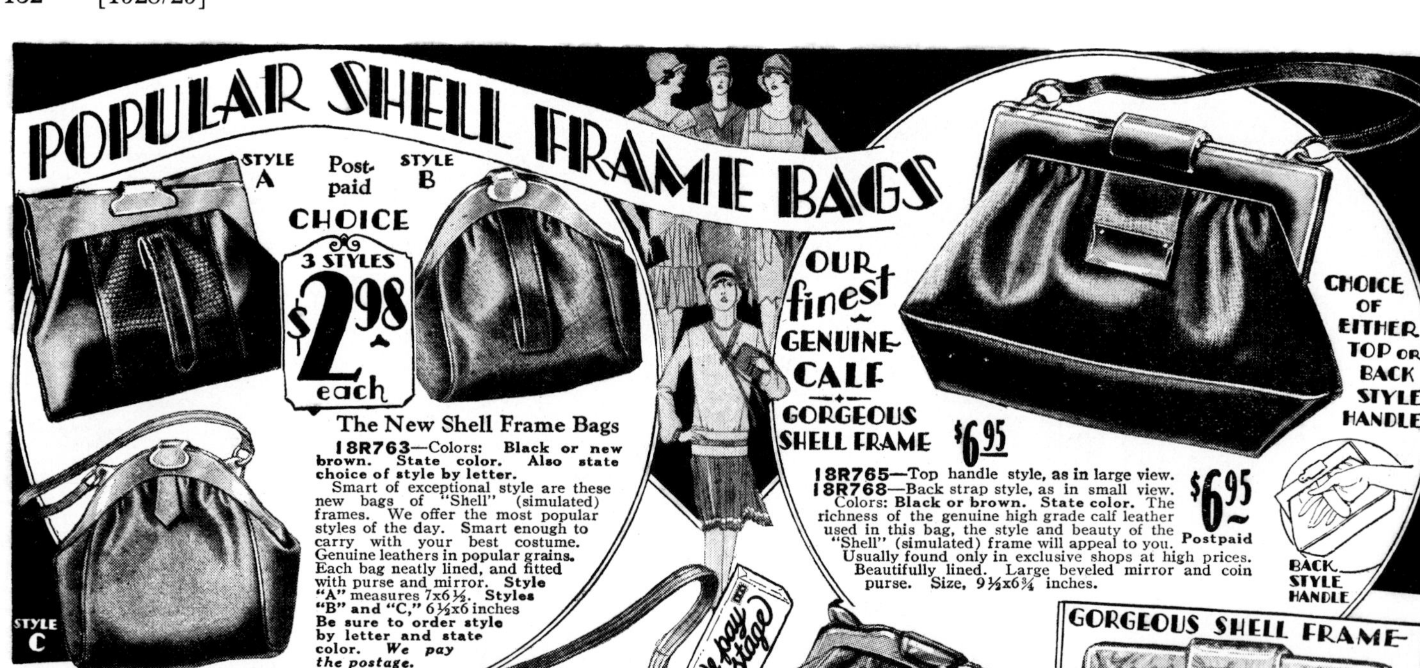


Post-paid CHOICE 3 STYLES $2.98 each

## The New Shell Frame Bags

**18R763**—Colors: **Black or new brown. State color. Also state choice of style by letter.**
Smart of exceptional style are these new bags of "Shell" (simulated) frames. We offer the most popular styles of the day. Smart enough to carry with your best costume. Genuine leathers in popular grains. Each bag neatly lined, and fitted with purse and mirror. **Style** "A" measures 7x6½. **Styles "B" and "C,"** 6½x6 inches **Be sure to order style by letter and state color.** ***We pay the postage.***

OUR finest GENUINE CALF — GORGEOUS SHELL FRAME $6.95

CHOICE OF EITHER TOP OR BACK STYLE HANDLE

**18R765**—Top handle style, as in large view.
**18R768**—Back strap style, as in small view.
Colors: **Black or brown. State color.** The richness of the genuine high grade calf leather used in this bag, the style and beauty of the "Shell" (simulated) frame will appeal to you. Usually found only in exclusive shops at high prices. Beautifully lined. Large beveled mirror and coin purse. Size, 9½x6¾ inches. **$6.95 Postpaid**

We pay postage

## WASHABLE PATENT LEATHER

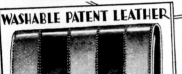

**18R770**—Colors: **Black with red; Navy with Copenhagen; sand with champagne, or all white. State color.** Smart flat frameless bag of washable glossy patent leather for spring and summer wear. Moire lined. Mirror and coin purse. Back strap, handkerchief pocket at back. Size, 7½x5¼ inches. **$2.98 Postpaid**

**18R772**—Colors: **Black or dark brown. State color.** Soft pouch style of genuine calf leather. Large size, 10x7¼ in. Triple frame. Separate compartments. Moire lined. Mirror and coin purse. **We pay the postage.** **$5.39 Postpaid**

**New Shell Frame Popular Shape**
**18R741**—Colors: **Brown or black. State color.** Rich looking back strap pouch with "Shell" (simulated) frame. Bag of high quality smooth grained genuine leather. Moire lined. Mirror and coin purse. Size, 8x6¼ inches. **We pay postage.** **$4.98 Postpaid**

## GORGEOUS SHELL FRAME

**18R790**—Colors: **Brown or black. State color.** High grade large back strap pouch of grained high quality leather. Distinctive "Shell" (simulated) frame. Silk moire lined. Mirror, coin purse. Size, 9½x7 inches. **$6.95 Postpaid**

**Smart Pouch New Grained Leather**
**18R795**—Colors: **Brown, black, navy blue, green or red. State color.** Top strap pouch. New grained genuine leather. Novel ornament. Neatly lined. Inner swinging change purse, mirror. Size, 7¾x6¼ inches. **We pay the postage.** **Postpaid $2.98**

## SILK and TAPESTRY BAGS

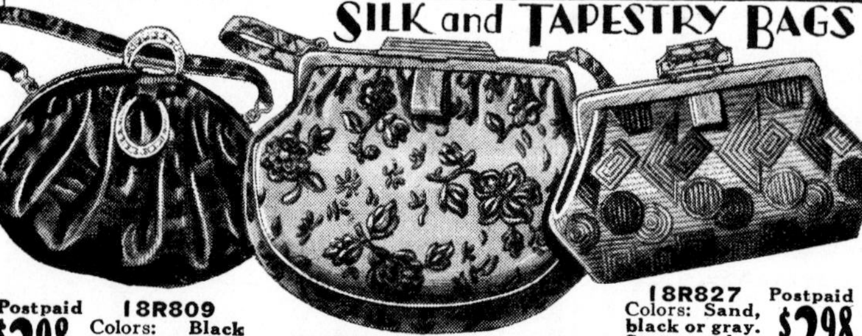

**18R809** **Postpaid $2.98**
Colors: **Black or navy blue. State color.** Medium size, silk moire pouch. Jeweled ornaments. Neatly lined. Mirror and inner swinging change purse. Size, 7¼x5¼ inches.

**18R812**—**Tapestry pouch bag.** Floral embroidered pattern over sand color background. Inner swinging change purse. Mirror. Neat lining. Size, 8⅛x6¼ inches. **Postpaid $2.98**
***Remember We Pay the Postage***

**18R827** **Postpaid $2.98**
Colors: Sand, **black or gray. State color.** Smart silk back strap bag with French Cordeaux embroidery to harmonize. Inner swinging change purse. Mirror. Moire lined. Neat clasp. Size, 8¼x4¾ inches.

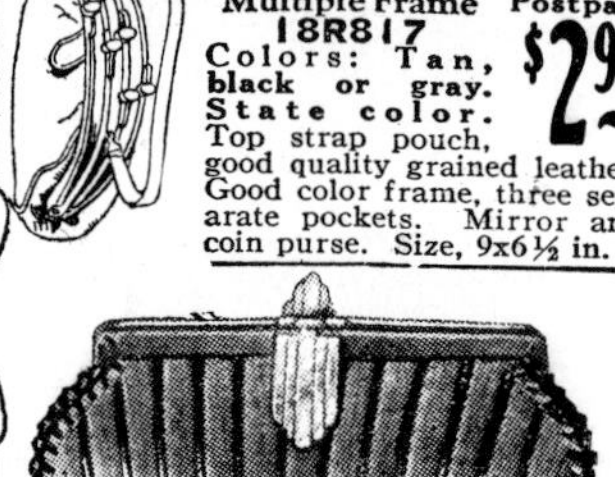

**Multiple Frame** **Postpaid $2.95**
**18R817**
Colors: **Tan, black or gray. State color.** Top strap pouch, good quality grained leather. Good color frame, three separate pockets. Mirror and coin purse. Size, 9x6½ in.

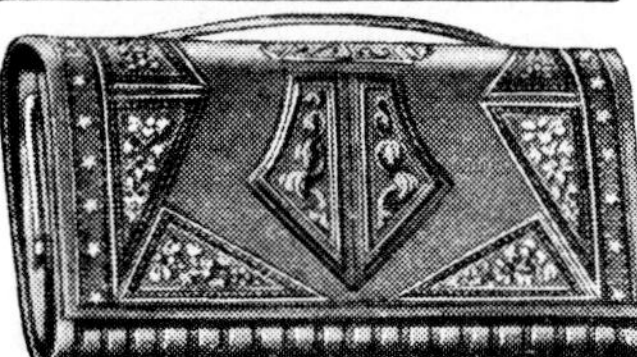

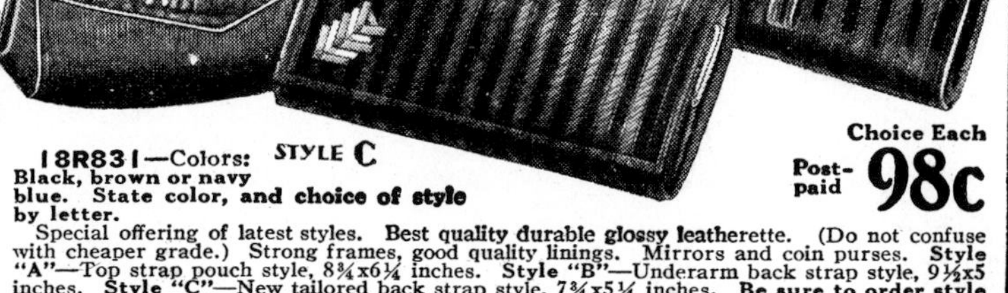

STYLE A — 98¢ Each Postpaid — STYLE B

**18R831**—Colors: **Black, brown or navy blue. State color, and choice of style by letter.** STYLE C
Special offering of latest styles. **Best quality durable glossy leatherette.** (Do not confuse with cheaper grade.) Strong frames, good quality linings. Mirrors and coin purses. **Style** "A"—Top strap pouch style, 8¾x6¼ inches. **Style "B"**—Underarm back strap style, 9½x5 inches. **Style "C"**—New tailored back strap style, 7¾x5¼ inches. **Be sure to order style by letter and state color. We pay the postage.** **Choice Each Postpaid 98c**

**18R805—Brown only.** Top ·rap of good quality leather. Em·ossed design. Three pockets. ·rong frame. Mirror. Durable ·ing. Size, 8½x4½ inches. ·e pay postage. **$1.55 Postpaid**

**Genuine Cowhide—Hand Laced**
**18R774**—Colors: **Black or brown. State color.** Tailored effect, genuine cowhide with hand lacing. Serviceable and long wearing. Back strap style, strong gold color lift lock. Size, 8¾x5½ inches. Good quality lining. Inner swinging change purse and mirror. **$3.45 Postpaid**

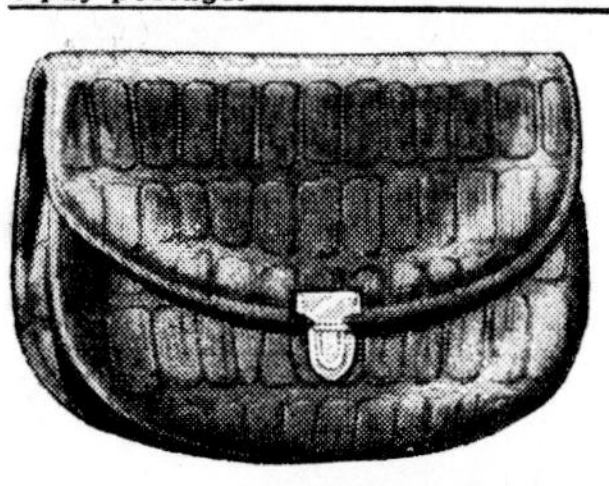

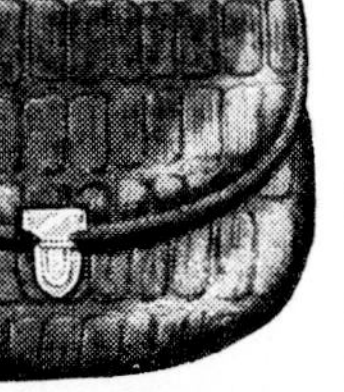

**18R807**—Colors: **Brown; green, red, navy blue or black. State color.** New Vagabond Bag. Smart frameless back strap style. New grained genuine leather. New fastener. Neatly lined. Mirror and coin purse. Size, 7¾x5⅛ in. **We pay the postage.** **$2.98 Postpaid**

**18R747**—Colors: **Brown, black or navy blue. State color.** Genuine calf, back strap bag in smart small shape. Twin clasp frame. Inner swinging change purse. Neatly lined. Mirror. Size, 7¾x4½ inches. **We pay the postage.** **$2.98 Postpaid**

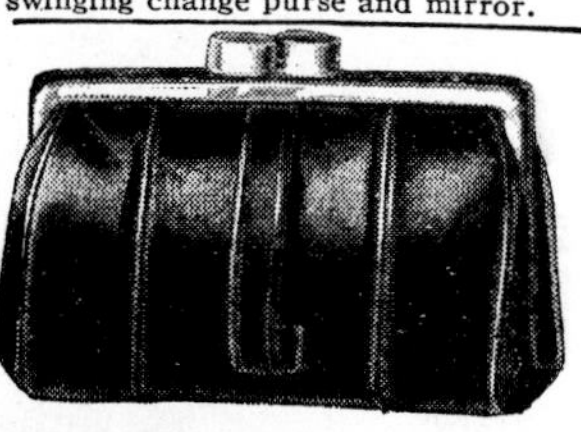

***For Brief Cases and Music Rolls See Musical Instrument Pages, or Refer to Index***

***Your Orders Shipped Within 24 Hours!***

# LAST MINUTE STYLES - EVERLASTING QUALITIES

## Broadway's Favorite—All Wool Flannel

***Choice of Brownish Tan or Blue Gray***

A sporty Suit with style, class and high quality fabric. It's so individually modeled that it's sure to win the instant admiration of your friends. A big value at the low price of $24.50.

**Coat:** Soft roll peak lapels. Half lined with silk. Novelty welt breast pocket with buckle and imitation handkerchief sewed in. Fashionable and dressy lines.

**Vest:** 2-in-1 Vest. Can be worn either side out. One side is same as suit. Other side is All Wool Fancy Vesting.

**Trousers:** Wide bottoms with black bottom cuff effect if desired or with self cloth cuffs, or plain bottoms in self material. **State which.** Two button set-on waistband; wide belt loops.

**For Sizes, See Scale at Bottom of Page.**

**4 R A751** **Brownish Tan Flannel**
**4 R A752** **Blue Gray (London Smoke) Flannel**
OUR PRICE, **The Suit**.......... **$24.50** **Postage. 20c Extra**

## New Handsome Double-Breasted Model

**All Wool Dark or Medium Gray Cassimere**

Desirable fabrics carefully selected from the products of the country's leading woolen mills, and fine custom tailoring according to our own specifications, are outstanding features of these handsome suits. Made of All Wool Cassimere in medium Gray or Dark Oxford Gray Herringbone designs. This model is a great favorite with fashionably dressed men.

**Coat:** Three-button double-breasted style with only two buttons to fasten. Half lined with wool alpaca. Broad, soft-rolling lapels.

**Vest:** Regulation style.

**Trousers:** Wide, 19-inch cuff bottoms.

**For Sizes: See Scale at bottom of Page.**

**4 R A770** **Dark Oxford Gray**
OUR PRICE.................... **$22.50**
**4 R A838** **Medium Gray**
OUR PRICE.................... **$21.75**
**Postage, each suit, 20c Extra.**

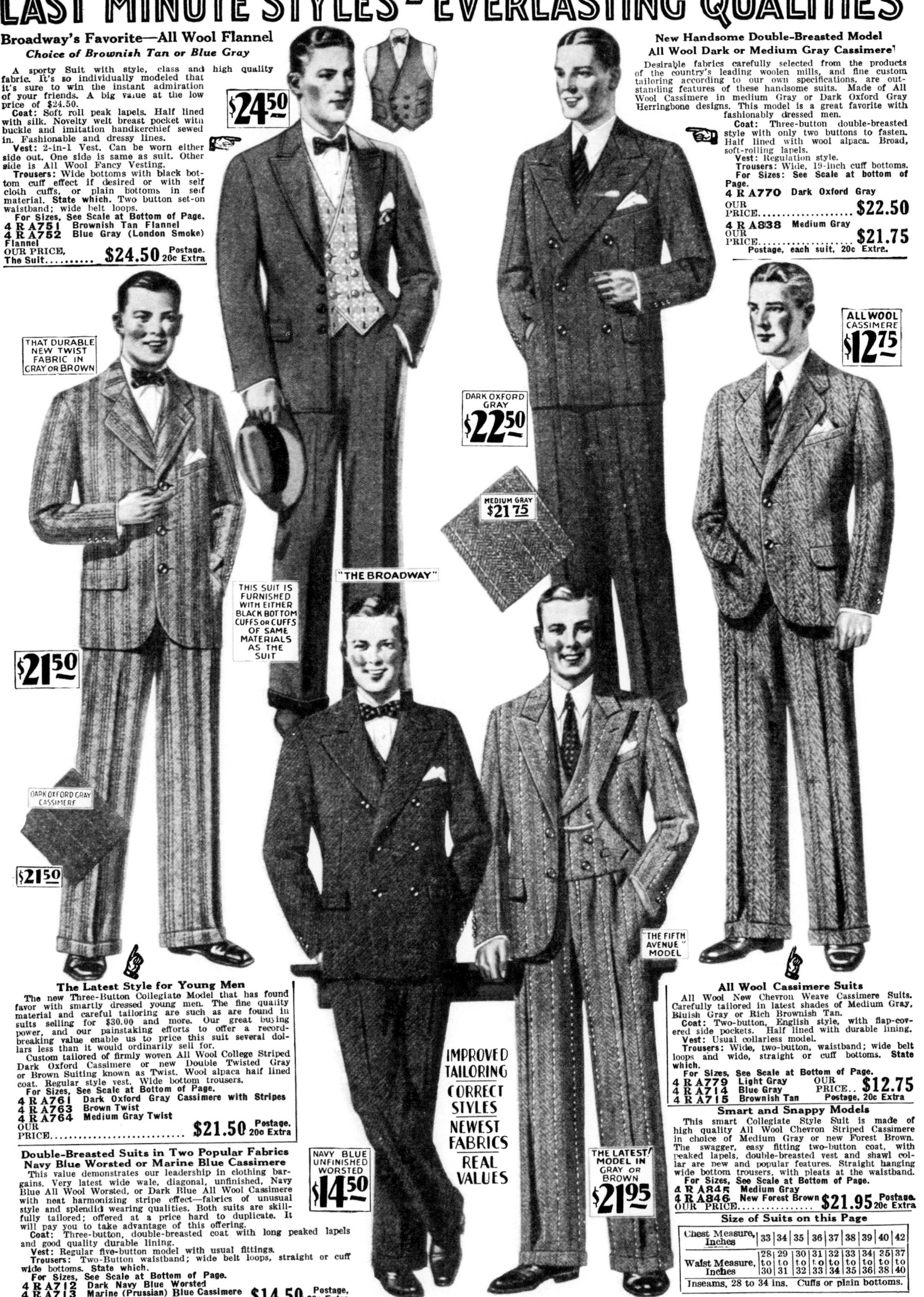


## The Latest Style for Young Men

The new Three-Button Collegiate Model that has found favor with smartly dressed young men. The fine quality material and careful tailoring are such as are found in suits selling for $30.00 and more. Our great buying power, and our painstaking efforts to offer a record-breaking value enable us to price this suit several dollars less than it would ordinarily sell for.

Custom tailored of firmly woven All Wool College Striped Dark Oxford Cassimere or new Double Twisted Gray or Brown Suiting known as Twist. Wool alpaca half lined coat. Regular style vest. Wide bottom trousers.

**For Sizes, See Scale at Bottom of Page.**

**4 R A761** **Dark Oxford Gray Cassimere with Stripes**
**4 R A763** **Brown Twist**
**4 R A764** **Medium Gray Twist**
OUR PRICE.......................... **$21.50** **Postage. 20c Extra**

## Double-Breasted Suits in Two Popular Fabrics

**Navy Blue Worsted or Marine Blue Cassimere**

This value demonstrates our leadership in clothing bargains. Very latest wide wale, diagonal, unfinished, Navy Blue All Wool Worsted, or Dark Blue All Wool Cassimere with neat harmonizing stripe effect—fabrics of unusual style and splendid wearing qualities. Both suits are skillfully tailored; offered at a price hard to duplicate. It will pay you to take advantage of this offering.

**Coat:** Three-button, double-breasted coat with long peaked lapels and good quality durable lining.

**Vest:** Regular five-button model with usual fittings.

**Trousers:** Two-Button waistband; wide belt loops, straight or cuff wide bottoms. **State which.**

**For Sizes, See Scale at Bottom of Page.**

**4 R A712** **Dark Navy Blue Worsted**
**4 R A713** **Marine (Prussian) Blue Cassimere**
OUR PRICE................................ **$14.50** **Postage, 20c Extra.**

## All Wool Cassimere Suits

All Wool New Chevron Weave Cassimere Suits. Carefully tailored in latest shades of Medium Gray, Bluish Gray or Rich Brownish Tan.

**Coat:** Two-button, English style, with flap-covered side pockets. Half lined with durable lining.

**Vest:** Usual collarless model.

**Trousers:** Wide, two-button, waistband; wide belt loops and wide, straight or cuff bottoms. **State which.**

**For Sizes, See Scale at Bottom of Page.**

**4 R A779** **Light Gray**
**4 R A714** **Blue Gray**
**4 R A715** **Brownish Tan**
OUR PRICE.. **$12.75** **Postage, 20c Extra**

## Smart and Snappy Models

This smart Collegiate Style Suit is made of high quality All Wool Chevron Striped Cassimere in choice of Medium Gray or new Forest Brown. The swagger, easy fitting two-button coat, with peaked lapels, double-breasted vest and shawl collar are new and popular features. Straight hanging wide bottom trousers, with pleats at the waistband.

**For Sizes, See Scale at Bottom of Page.**

**4 R A845** **Medium Gray**
**4 R A846** **New Forest Brown**
OUR PRICE................ **$21.95** **Postage. 20c Extra**

### Size of Suits on this Page

| Chest Measure, Inches | 33 | 34 | 35 | 36 | 37 | 38 | 39 | 40 | 42 |
|---|---|---|---|---|---|---|---|---|---|
| Waist Measure, Inches | 28 to 30 | 29 to 31 | 30 to 32 | 31 to 33 | 32 to 34 | 33 to 35 | 34 to 36 | 35 to 38 | 37 to 40 |
| Inseams, 28 to 34 ins. Cuffs or plain bottoms. | | | | | | | | | |



BE SURE TO STATE CHEST, WAIST AND INSEAM MEASURE, AS WELL AS HEIGHT AND WEIGHT

The Charles William Stores Inc. New York City

WE Pay the Postage

LIGHTFOOT OUR OWN TRADE MARK

# Canvas Footwear Cuts

## Top Favorites-Bottom Prices

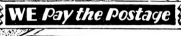

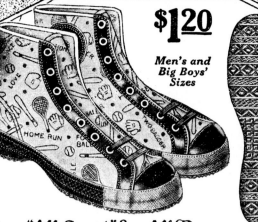

$1.20

Men's and Big Boys' Sizes

## "All Sport" for All Boys

| | |
|---|---|
| 76R9564—Men's and Big Boys'. Sizes, 6 to 10 | $1.20 |
| 76R9565—Boys'. Sizes, 1 to 5½ | 1.10 |
| 76R9566—Small Boys'. Sizes, 11 to 13½ | 1.05 |

**Wide widths only. Be sure to state size.**

*We Pay the Postage.*

Every boy will want a pair of these canvas shoes this summer. With their printed designs lettered and drawn all over the uppers, they are just his idea of what his shoes should look like. In addition to their good looks they are made of good quality materials which will stand an amazing amount of wear from hard play and all active summer sports. Come in high grade white canvas with sturdy corrugated rubber soles strongly vulcanized to uppers so they won't come loose. Made over the popular lace to toe pattern, for firm support from top to toe. The toe cap, reinforced scuffer strip and ankle patch are features which insure extra wear. The small cost and the long service will show you just how greatly canvas footwear cuts your summer shoe bill.

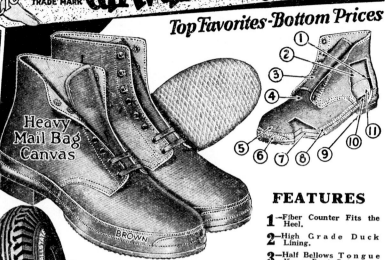

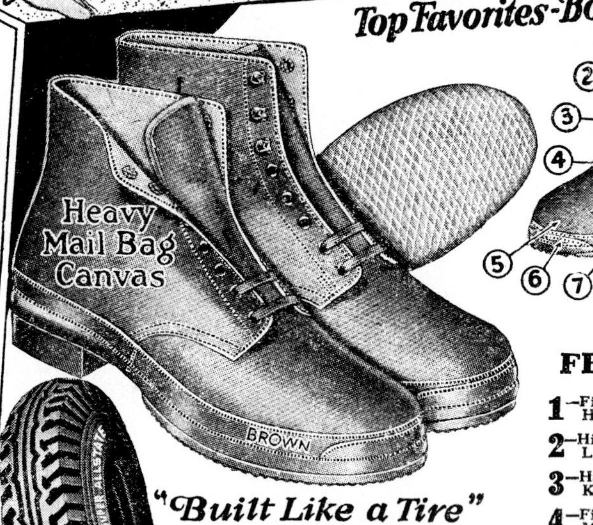


## "Built Like a Tire"

| | |
|---|---|
| 76R9632—Men's and Big Boys'. Sizes, 6 to 12 | $1.95 |
| 76R9633—Boys'. Sizes, 1 to 5½ | $1.85 |

**Wide widths only. Be sure to state size.**

*We Pay the Postage.*

Throughout the nation men and boys look for this "Old Reliable" canvas work or play shoe when selecting their summer footwear. Comfortable and unusually rugged, it is one of the finest combination work and play shoes ever sold. Not another shoe of its kind has so many features of construction and material in its favor. Look at the way it is built (see cutout view at right and explanation of each feature). That explains its increasing popularity and its sure footed dependability in every job or game. With sole and extra tap sole of **genuine tire tread rubber**, it piles up miles and miles of toughest wear. They outdistance all other canvas work shoes in their class for real value. Comparisons with the best sold anywhere prove it. Boys' sizes come in bal pattern only. Men's and boys' are blucher pattern only.

### FEATURES

1—Fiber Counter Fits the Heel.

2—High Grade Duck Lining.

3—Half Bellows Tongue Keeps Dust Out.

4—Finest Quality Heavy Mail Bag Duck Uppers.

5—Double Toe Box Keeps Its Shape.

6—Heavy Foxing Joins Sole to Upper.

7—Extra Heavy Composition Filler.

8—Sole and Tap Sole of Tire Tread Rubber.

9—Shockproof Rubber Heel.

10—High Grade Fiber Insole.

11—Leather Sock Lining.

## Women's Canvas Work Shoe

76R9634—Black.
76R9635—Brown. $1.45

Women's. **Sizes, 3 to 8. Wide widths. Be sure to state size.**

*We Pay the Postage.*

We are introducing these new Canvas Work Shoes for women to fill the need for a shoe a little stronger than the average—one durable enough to use for outdoor work as well as for inside wear. We know there is a demand for just this type of shoe for warm weather. You can now buy it here in either brown or black sturdy good grade canvas at a money-saving price. Has durable smooth and flexible rubber soles and a shockproof rubber heel.

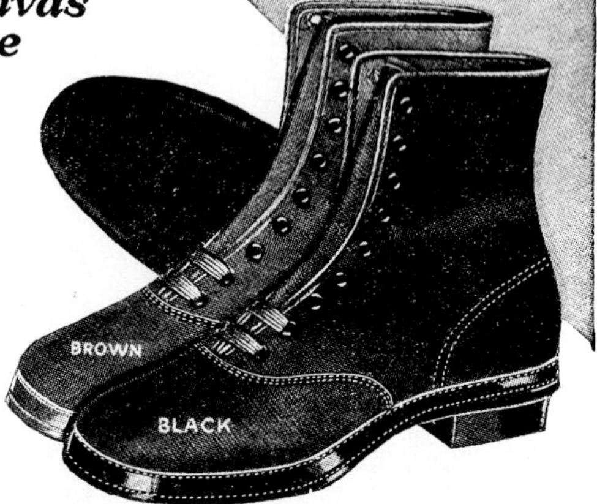


## Latest Sport Shoe

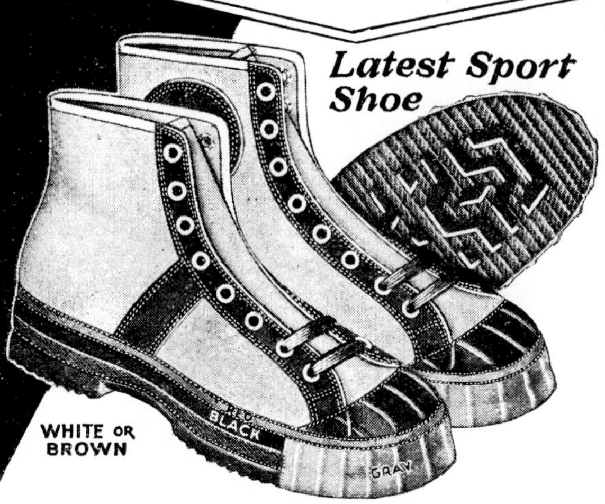


## You Can Always Depend on This New Moulded Sole

| White Canvas | | Brown Canvas | |
|---|---|---|---|
| 76R9607—Men's and Big Boys'. Sizes, 6 to 11 | $1.43 | 76R9610—Men's and Big Boys' Sizes, 6 to 11 | $1.43 |
| 76R9608—Boys'. Sizes, 1 to 5½ | 1.33 | 76R9611—Boys'. Sizes, 1 to 5½ | 1.33 |
| 76R9609—Small Boys'. Sizes, 11 to 13½ | 1.23 | 76R9612—Small Boys'. Sizes, 11 to 13½ | 1.23 |

**Wide widths only. Be sure to state size.**

*We Pay the Postage.*

Whatever sport or game you are engaged in, out of doors or in the gymnasium, on wet grass or slippery floors, you can be sure of your footwork at all times in a pair of these very latest Sport Shoes. **They are the best shoes of their kind that you can buy at any price.** Their moulded sole and heel are made doubly thick at the points where a shoe gets the most wear and their cutout pattern serves as a vacuum which clings securely to all surfaces. They are made of good grade white or brown canvas, black trimmed with a red and black double foxing which strongly fastens the soles to the uppers. Reinforced toe cap, ankle patch and ribbed bumper toe furnish added wear and protection. Lace to toe feature produces snug fit all the way up the foot, giving real support to your arches and ankles—you know how important that is in active sports.

## Popular Moulded Sole

| | |
|---|---|
| 76R9614—Men's and Big Boys'. Sizes, 6 to 11 | 93c |
| 76R9615—Boys'. Sizes, 1 to 5½ | 88c |
| 76R9616—Small Boys'. Sizes, 11 to 13½ | 83c |

**Wide widths only. Be sure to state size.**

*We Pay the Postage.*

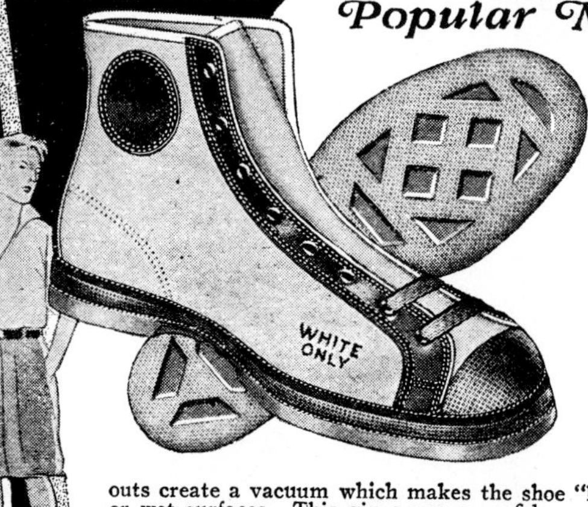


Men and boys everywhere are making Moulded Sole Sport Shoes their leading choice for summer sports and gym work. They choose it because it's a sole that can be depended upon for longer service because it is double thickness at the points where a shoe naturally gets the most wear. They also know that, because of its special construction, the cutouts create a vacuum which makes the shoe "hold its own" on the most slippery or wet surfaces. This gives you a confidence of sure footing all the time in the most energetic sports where canvas footwear is used. These shoes are made of good quality white canvas with black trimming. With lace to toe pattern they can be firmly adjusted to fit snugly from top to toe insuring proper support at ankle, at arch and at the ball of the foot. The ankle patch and extra toe cap give added reinforcement where needed. Try a pair of these shoes this summer. Get them for your boy, too. He's sure to tell others about them. You'll be more than satisfied with their long wear and the saving you make.

# ENSEMBLED *in the new modern manner*

## *Fashionable* Women assemble their costumes carefully today and this catalog has been planned to help you do it . . . . . .

WE *planned* together with definite, complete costumes for you in mind. We *bought* together. We *studied* together your preferences in *coats*, in *dresses*, in *hats*, in *shoes*, in *gloves*, in *hosiery*, in all the smart things that go into the assembling of a complete costume.

***The Result:*** every *coat*, every *frock*, every *fashion* in this entire Catalog—may be correctly combined with all of the other parts of a costume.

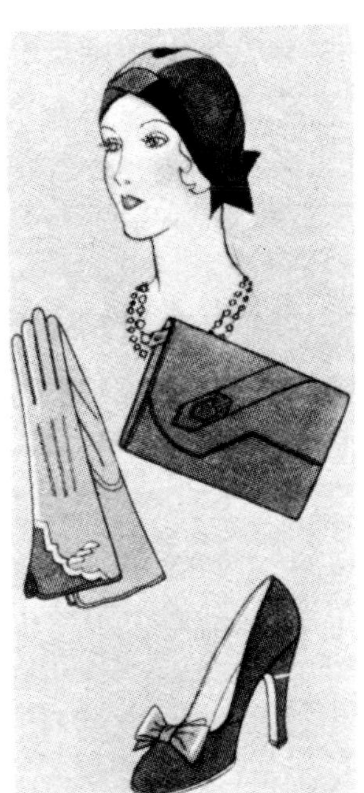

*These* SMARTLY CORRECT ACCESSORIES *can easily be found in this Catalog by referring to the* PINK INDEX *pages in center of Catalog.*

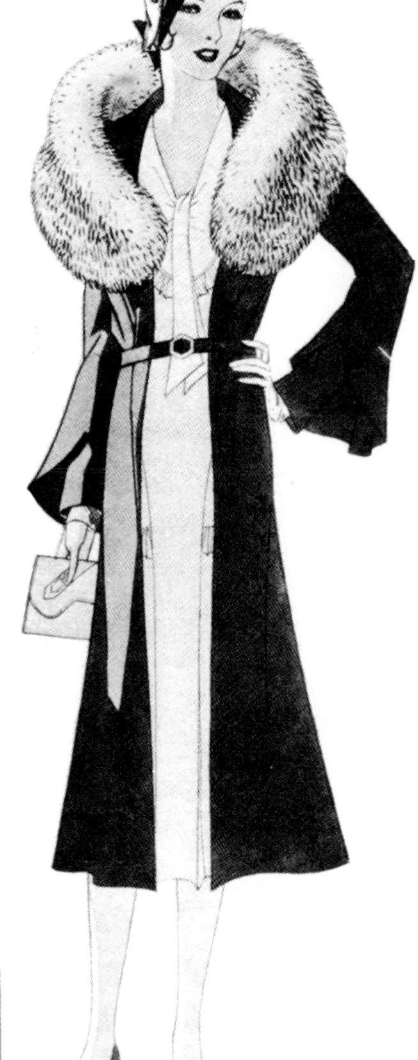

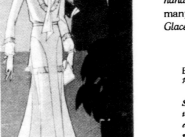

***It's so simple to assemble an outfit with***

### A BLACK COAT

. . . because any color is correct with *Black*. Choose a *Black dress* trimmed in color if possible—or select your favorite shade. Wear a *Black hat*. As for *handbag* and *shoes* both should be *Black*. *Hose* and *gloves* should harmonize with each other and the entire outfit. ALL BLACK COSTUMES WITH BLACK ACCESSORIES ARE VERY SMART.

*For complete description and price of this* ***Smart Black Coat,*** *see page*............6
***Dress*** *described on page*..................43
***Hat*** *described on page*..................82

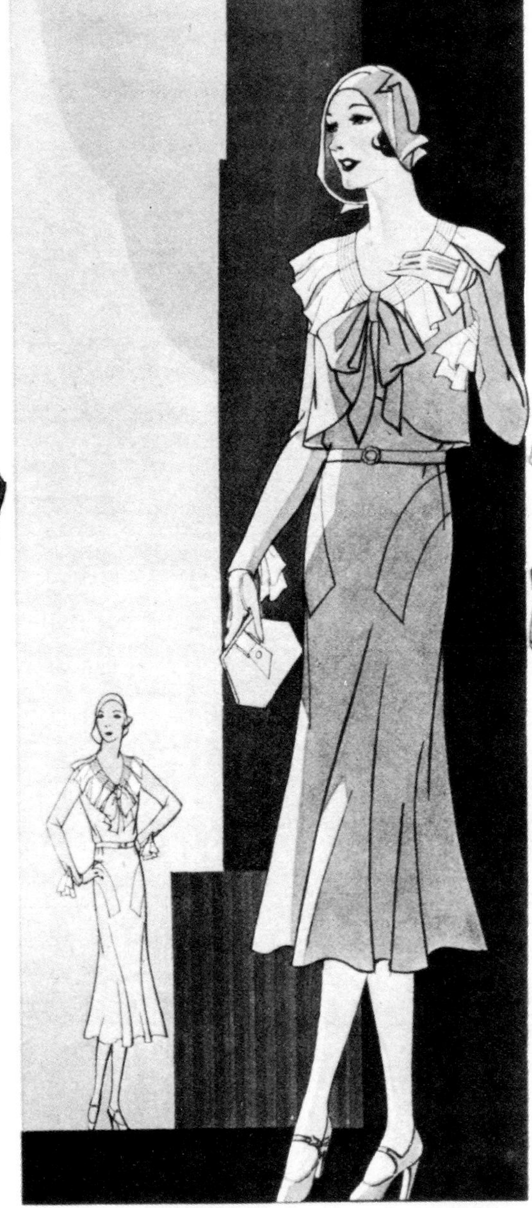

*These* CORRECT ACCESSORIES *are priced very low at Sears.*

### A MARRON GLACE COSTUME

***Seems like several with different accessories***

. . . and this is why it seems so! For instance, your *hat, shoes* and *handbag* can be a *Dark Brown* to make a dark contrast—or you can acquire a striking costume by choosing *jewelry*—a *necklace*—a *bracelet* in brilliant shades of *Green* or *Red* or *Blue* keeping *hat, shoes* and *handbag* in *Dark Brown*. So you see how many different moods your *Marron Glace costume* can have!

*For complete description and price of this* BOLERO DRESS ENSEMBLE, *see page*...............................38
***Hat*** *described on page*..........82
***Shoes, Gloves, Handbag*** *and* ***Jewelry*** *to harmonize with this dress ensemble can easily be found in their respective departments by referring to* PINK INDEX *pages.*

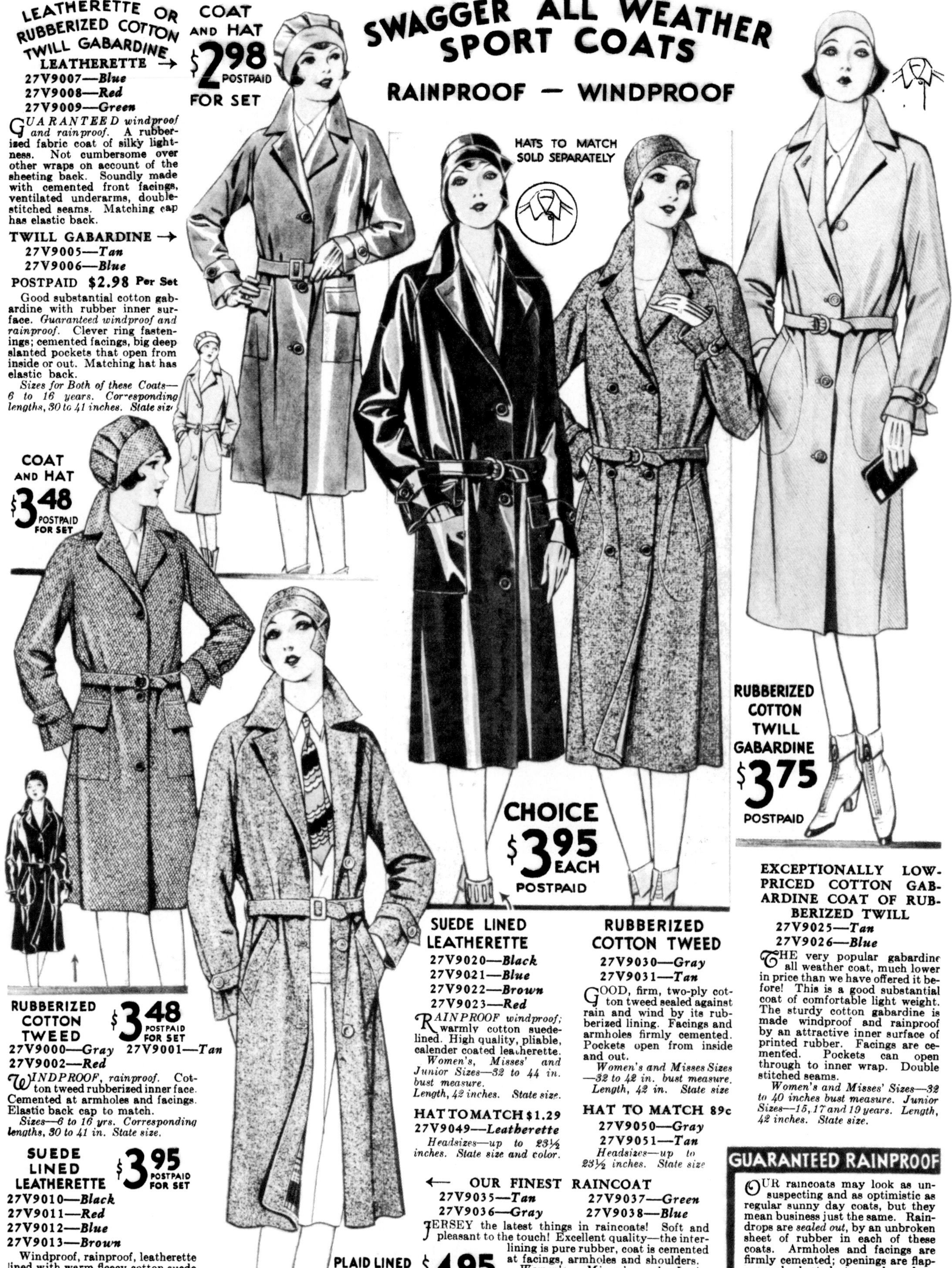


# SWAGGER ALL WEATHER SPORT COATS

## RAINPROOF — WINDPROOF

**LEATHERETTE OR RUBBERIZED COTTON TWILL GABARDINE**

**COAT AND HAT $2.98 POSTPAID FOR SET**

**LEATHERETTE →**
27V9007—*Blue*
27V9008—*Red*
27V9009—*Green*

*GUARANTEED windproof and rainproof.* A rubberized fabric coat of silky lightness. Not cumbersome over other wraps on account of the sheeting back. Soundly made with cemented front facings, ventilated underarms, double-stitched seams. Matching cap has elastic back.

**TWILL GABARDINE →**
27V9005—*Tan*
27V9006—*Blue*

**POSTPAID $2.98 Per Set**

Good substantial cotton gabardine with rubber inner surface. *Guaranteed windproof and rainproof.* Clever ring fastenings; cemented facings, big deep slanted pockets that open from inside or out. Matching hat has elastic back.
*Sizes for Both of these Coats—6 to 16 years. Corresponding lengths, 30 to 41 inches. State size.*

**COAT AND HAT $3.48 POSTPAID FOR SET**

**RUBBERIZED COTTON TWEED $3.48 POSTPAID FOR SET**
27V9000—*Gray* 27V9001—*Tan*
27V9002—*Red*

*WINDPROOF, rainproof.* Cotton tweed rubberized inner face. Cemented at armholes and facings. Elastic back cap to match.
*Sizes—6 to 16 yrs. Corresponding lengths, 30 to 41 in. State size.*

**SUEDE LINED LEATHERETTE $3.95 POSTPAID FOR SET**
27V9010—*Black*
27V9011—*Red*
27V9012—*Blue*
27V9013—*Brown*

Windproof, rainproof, leatherette lined with warm fleecy cotton suede cloth. Cemented facings and armholes. Hat to match. *Sizes—6 to 16 yrs. Corresponding lengths, 28 to 40 in. State size.*

**CHOICE $3.95 EACH POSTPAID**

**SUEDE LINED LEATHERETTE**
27V9020—*Black*
27V9021—*Blue*
27V9022—*Brown*
27V9023—*Red*

*RAINPROOF windproof;* warmly cotton suede-lined. High quality, pliable, calender coated leatherette.
*Women's, Misses' and Junior Sizes—32 to 44 in. bust measure. Length, 42 inches. State size.*

**HAT TO MATCH $1.29**
27V9049—*Leatherette*
*Headsizes—up to 23½ inches. State size and color.*

**RUBBERIZED COTTON TWEED**
27V9030—*Gray*
27V9031—*Tan*

GOOD, firm, two-ply cotton tweed sealed against rain and wind by its rubberized lining. Facings and armholes firmly cemented. Pockets open from inside and out.
*Women's and Misses Sizes—32 to 42 in. bust measure. Length, 42 in. State size*

**HAT TO MATCH 89c**
27V9050—*Gray*
27V9051—*Tan*
*Headsizes—up to 23½ inches. State size*

**RUBBERIZED COTTON TWILL GABARDINE $3.75 POSTPAID**

**EXCEPTIONALLY LOW-PRICED COTTON GABARDINE COAT OF RUBBERIZED TWILL**
27V9025—*Tan*
27V9026—*Blue*

THE very popular gabardine all weather coat, much lower in price than we have offered it before! This is a good substantial coat of comfortable light weight. The sturdy cotton gabardine is made windproof and rainproof by an attractive inner surface of printed rubber. Facings are cemented. Pockets can open through to inner wrap. Double stitched seams.
*Women's and Misses' Sizes—32 to 40 inches bust measure. Junior Sizes—15, 17 and 19 years. Length, 42 inches. State size.*

**← OUR FINEST RAINCOAT**
27V9035—*Tan* 27V9037—*Green*
27V9036—*Gray* 27V9038—*Blue*

JERSEY the latest things in raincoats! Soft and pleasant to the touch! Excellent quality—the interlining is pure rubber, coat is cemented at facings, armholes and shoulders.
*Women's, Misses' and Junior Sizes—32 to 42 inches bust measure. Length, 42 inches. State size.*

**PLAID LINED RUBBERIZED COTTON JERSEY $4.95 POSTPAID**

**GUARANTEED RAINPROOF**

OUR raincoats may look as unsuspecting and as optimistic as regular sunny day coats, but they mean business just the same. Raindrops are *sealed out,* by an unbroken sheet of rubber in each of these coats. Armholes and facings are firmly cemented; openings are flap-covered, slanted strapped, or buttoned high. There is simply *no opening* for raindrops in our coats . . . and we positively *guarantee they are windproof and rainproof*

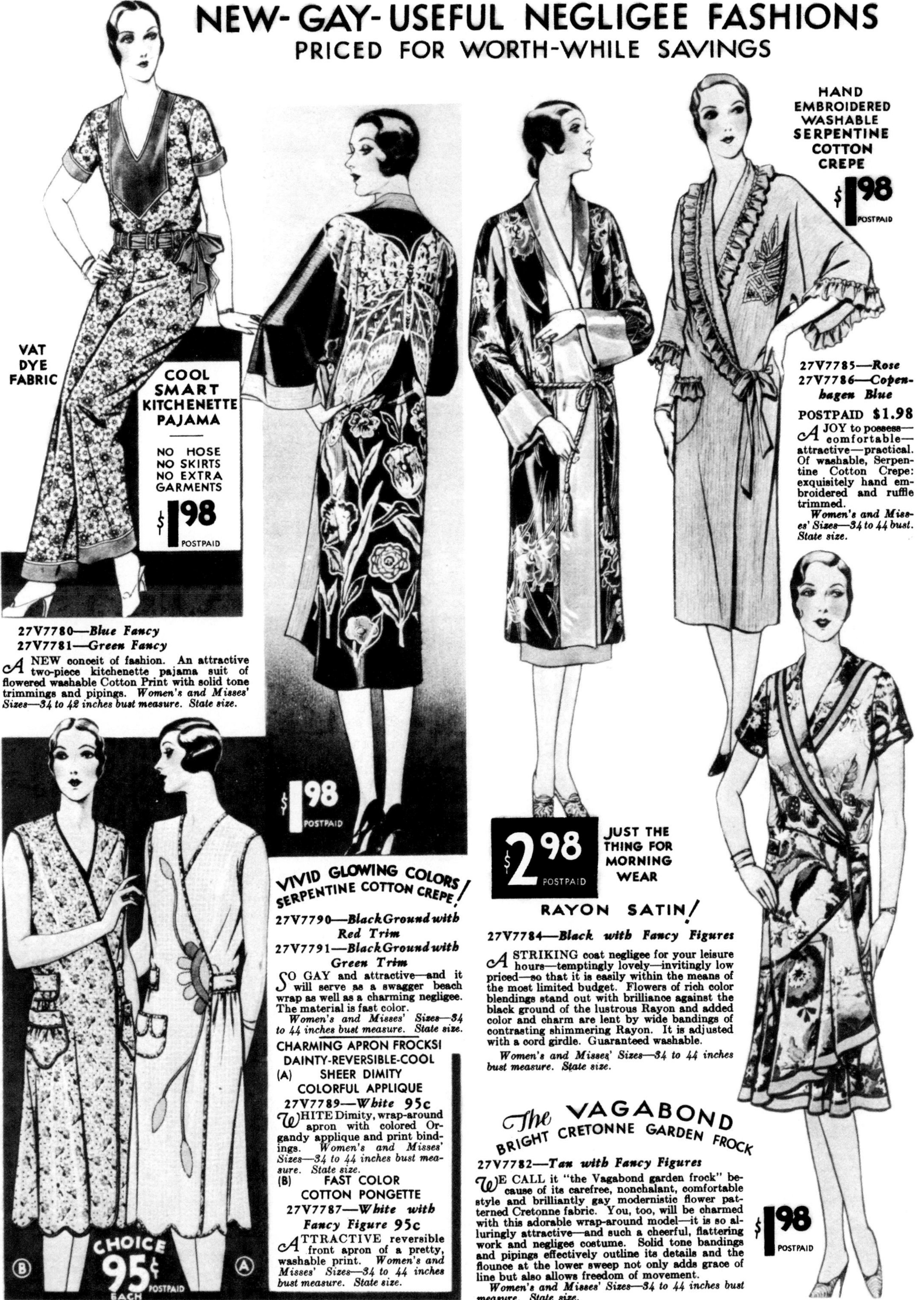
NEW-GAY-USEFUL NEGLIGEE FASHIONS
PRICED FOR WORTH-WHILE SAVINGS
VAT DYE FABRIC
COOL SMART KITCHENETTE PAJAMA
NO HOSE NO SKIRTS NO EXTRA GARMENTS
$1.98 POSTPAID
27V7780—Blue Fancy
27V7781—Green Fancy
A NEW conceit of fashion. An attractive two-piece kitchenette pajama suit of flowered washable Cotton Print with solid tone trimmings and pipings. Women's and Misses' Sizes—34 to 42 inches bust measure. State size.
$1.98 POSTPAID
VIVID GLOWING COLORS SERPENTINE COTTON CREPE!
27V7790—BlackGround with Red Trim
27V7791—BlackGround with Green Trim
SO GAY and attractive—and it will serve as a swagger beach wrap as well as a charming negligee. The material is fast color.
Women's and Misses' Sizes—34 to 44 inches bust measure. State size.
$2.98 POSTPAID
JUST THE THING FOR MORNING WEAR
RAYON SATIN!
27V7784—Black with Fancy Figures
A STRIKING coat negligee for your leisure hours—temptingly lovely—invitingly low priced—so that it is easily within the means of the most limited budget. Flowers of rich color blendings stand out with brilliance against the black ground of the lustrous Rayon and added color and charm are lent by wide bandings of contrasting shimmering Rayon. It is adjusted with a cord girdle. Guaranteed washable.
Women's and Misses' Sizes—34 to 44 inches bust measure. State size.
HAND EMBROIDERED WASHABLE SERPENTINE COTTON CREPE
$1.98 POSTPAID
27V7785—Rose
27V7786—Copenhagen Blue
POSTPAID $1.98
A JOY to possess—comfortable—attractive—practical. Of washable, Serpentine Cotton Crepe: exquisitely hand embroidered and ruffle trimmed.
Women's and Misses' Sizes—34 to 44 bust. State size.
CHARMING APRON FROCKS!
DAINTY-REVERSIBLE-COOL
(A) SHEER DIMITY
COLORFUL APPLIQUE
27V7789—White 95c
WHITE Dimity, wrap-around apron with colored Organdy applique and print bindings. Women's and Misses' Sizes—34 to 44 inches bust measure. State size.
(B) FAST COLOR
COTTON PONGETTE
27V7787—White with Fancy Figure 95c
ATTRACTIVE reversible front apron of a pretty, washable print. Women's and Misses' Sizes—34 to 44 inches bust measure. State size.
B
A
CHOICE 95¢ EACH POSTPAID
The VAGABOND
BRIGHT CRETONNE GARDEN FROCK
27V7782—Tan with Fancy Figures
WE CALL it "the Vagabond garden frock" because of its carefree, nonchalant, comfortable style and brilliantly gay modernistic flower patterned Cretonne fabric. You, too, will be charmed with this adorable wrap-around model—it is so alluringly attractive—and such a cheerful, flattering work and negligee costume. Solid tone bandings and pipings effectively outline its details and the flounce at the lower sweep not only adds grace of line but also allows freedom of movement.
Women's and Misses' Sizes—34 to 44 inches bust measure. State size.
$1.98 POSTPAID

ORDER BLANKS ARE IN BACK OF THIS CATALOG

# THE VERY LATEST FASHIONS IN CHIC GLOVES

THE LEADER

$1.00 POSTPAID

## PARISIAN SMARTNESS

### FINE QUALITY SILK

**33V3215**—Pongee color.
**33V3216**—Mode.
**33V3217**—Gray.
**33V3218**—White.

Sizes, 6 to 8½. Half sizes. **Be sure to state size.**

Fashion dictates the swagger Mousquetaire style for Gloves to correctly accompany spring and summer costumes. Made of a **good quality enduring silk,** of about four-button length, these meet approval with the style-wise woman! Undeniably smart, with their graceful scalloped cuffs bound in contrasting color, and Paris point backs. Furnished in the most seasonably smart colors! Recommended for service, too, with **double tipped fingers** for special durability. Conveniently washable. Excellent quality at this low price.

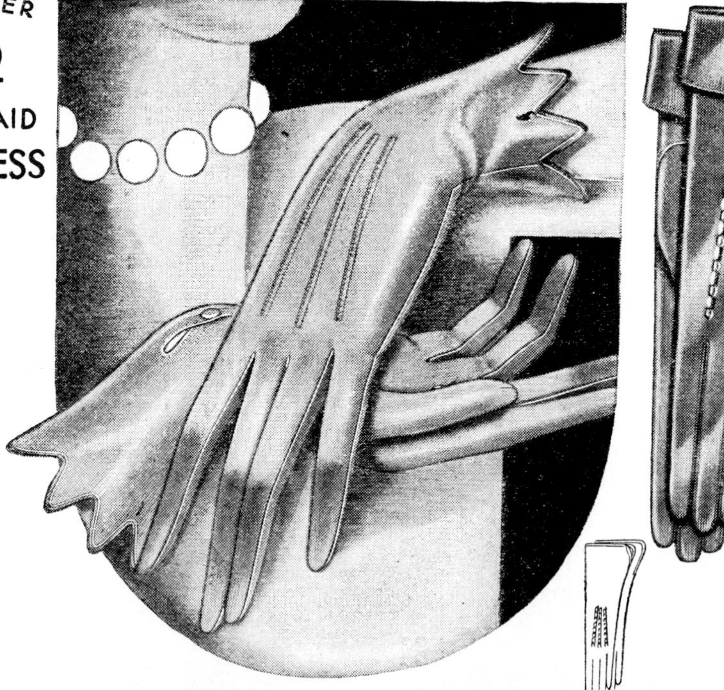

79c POSTPAID

## FOREMOST FASHIONS

### Imported Chamoisuede Fabric

**33V3305**—Sand.
**33V3306**—Gray.
**33V3307**—Mode.
**33V3308**—Nut.

Sizes, 6 to 8½. Half sizes. **Be sure to state size.**

Unusually clever styling distinguishes this new **imported** Glove creation. Gloves can be worn with cuffs turned up to show plain slip-on style (as in small illustration), or cuff turned back to show the cutout patterns, in harmonizing colors! **Faultlessly tailored of a good quality washable chamoisuede fabric.** Two-tone hairline stitching decorates the backs. Distinctive glove quality—priced so low!

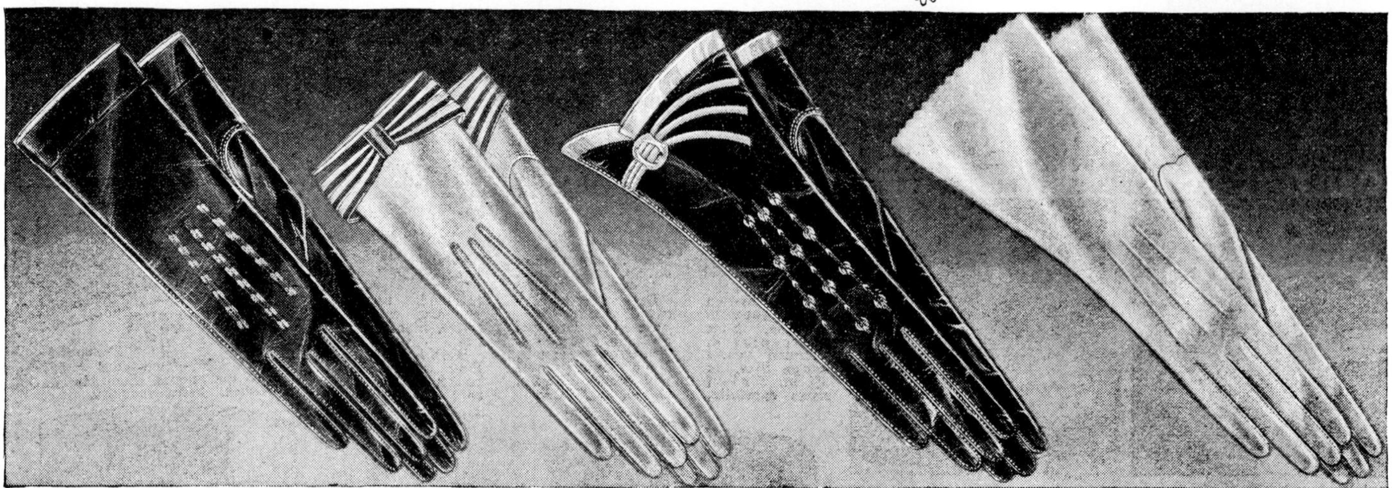

### $1.98 POSTPAID — REAL CHARM

**33V3050**—Black.
**33V3051**—Mode.
**33V3052**—Gray.
**33V3054**—Brown.

Sizes, 6 to 8. Quarter sizes. **State size.**

Simplicity marks the fashion of these clever European Glove creations. When worn in the turnover cuff style, the cuff is in beautiful contrast to the color of the glove, and matched by the two-tone embroidery on the back. Very smart looking when worn with cuff turned up. **Selected lambskin (usually called kid)** is the material used in their fine making. The seams are full pique sewed.

### $1.00 POSTPAID — STYLE AND QUALITY

**33V3360**—Sand.
**33V3361**—Gray.
**33V3362**—Mode.

Sizes, 6 to 8½. Half sizes **Be sure to state size.**

Strikingly beautiful imported Gloves of very fine quality **pre-shrunk, washable chamoisuede fabric.** Every one likes the modern touch of the two-tone horizontal striped turnover cuffs. Neat contrasting color edging in the handy single clasp wrist opening and fine stitching on the backs. **Kip-knot sewed seams Bolton thumbs** are marks of character.

### $2.98 POSTPAID — FASHIONED OF REAL KID

**33V3070**—Black.
**33V3071**—Mode.
**33V3072**—Gray.
**33V3073**—Beaver.

Sizes, 6 to 8. Quarter sizes. **Be sure to state size.**

Modern design and select quality contribute to this exceptional value! Ultra fashionable slip-on style! Made of imported, **real French washable kid,** with flaring cuffs having inverted curved tucks and hem of contrasting color. Trimmed with mother of pearl buckle and two-tone embroidered backs. Bolton thumbs and full pique sewed seams.

### $1.98 POSTPAID — FINE QUALITY DOESKIN

**33V3040**—Beige.
**33V3041**—Natural.
**33V3042**—White.

Sizes, 6 to 8. Quarter sizes. **Be sure to state size.**

Doeskin leather, soft and supple, is ingeniously fashioned into these perfect fitting accessories to every woman's ensemble. **Approved slip-on Biarritz style** of about 4-button length. Neat backs. Tailored and very fashionable; chosen for their dressy simplicity. **Remember We Pay the Postage.**

## FOR THE MISS

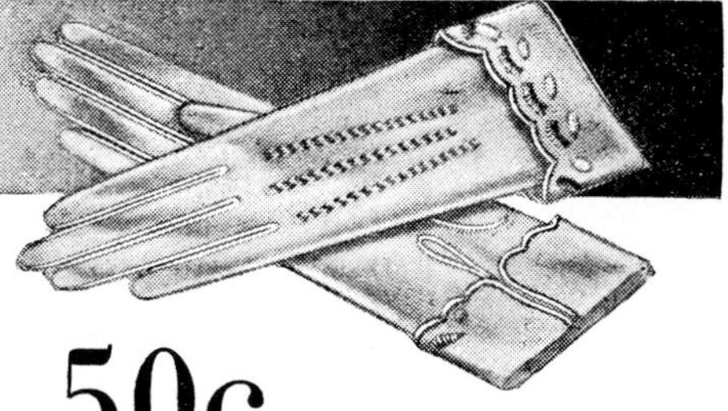

**33V3790**—Sand.
**33V3791**—Gray.
**33V3792**—Mode.

Ages, 5 to 12 years. **State age.**

Our stylists know the dash of style demanded by the modern misses. These **Imported Washable Chamoisuede Fabric** Gloves are just for them. Designed with intriguing scalloped turnover cuffs. The backs and cuffs are beautifully embroidered in the latest mode. One clasp fastener closes the wrists. Remember, they're easily washable.

50c POSTPAID

## HOW TO MEASURE YOUR HAND FOR SIZE

### Give Glove Size

HOLD HAND OUT FLAT WITH FINGERS TOUCHING, THUMB RAISED; draw ordinary tape measure close but not tight, all around hand, as shown in illustration (do not include thumb). The number of inches shown by this measurement is your correct glove size.

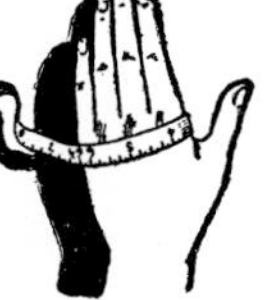

**Women's Sizes in Silk and Fabric Gloves:** 6, 6½, 7, 7½, 8 and 8½.

**Women's Sizes in Unlined Kid Gloves:** 6, 6¼, 6½, 6¾, 7, 7¼, 7½, 7¾, 8.

**For Glove Sizes for Children 5 to 12 Years of Age: GIVE AGE OF CHILD.**



*Order Blanks Are in Back of This Catalog*

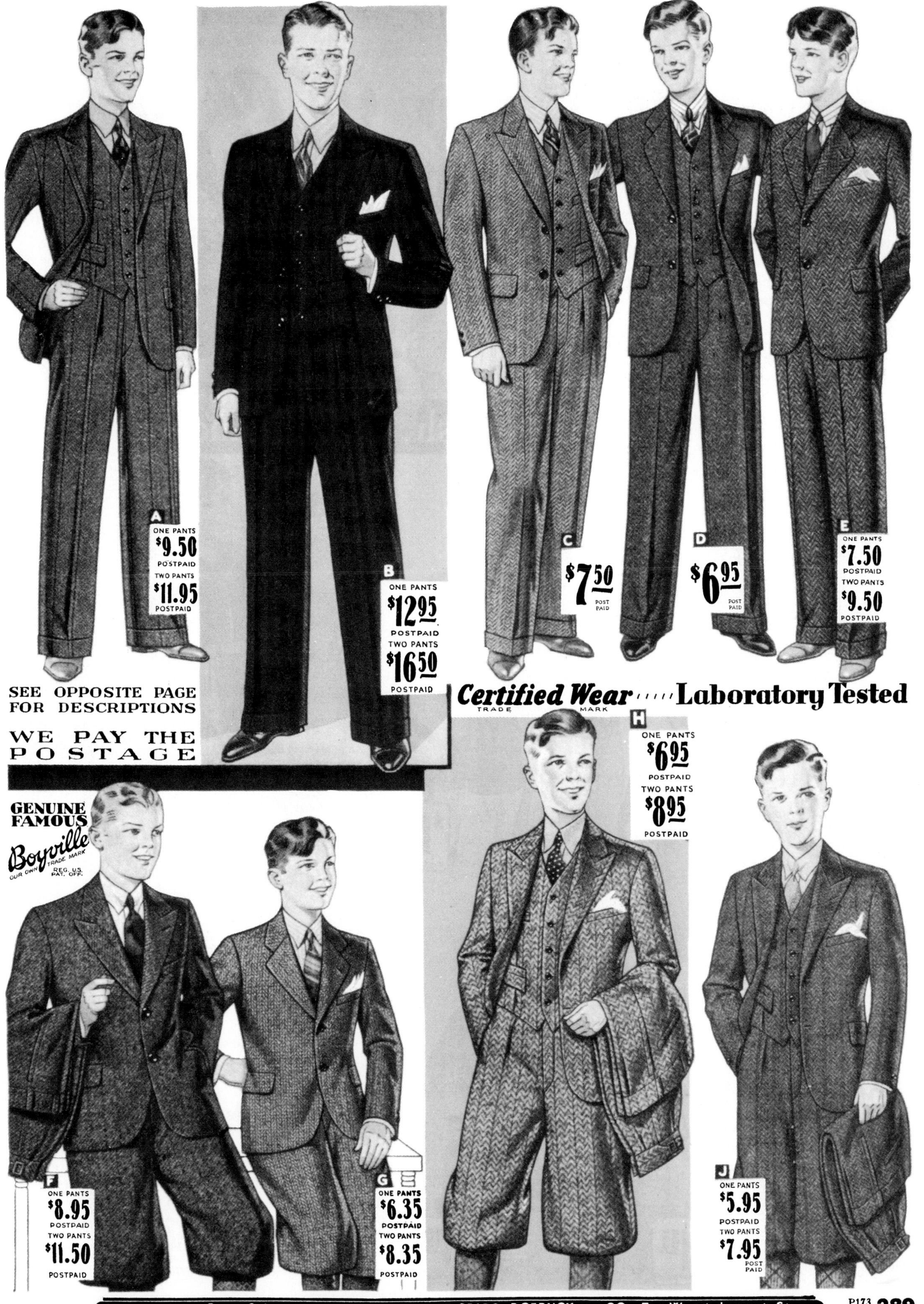
A
ONE PANTS
$9.50
POSTPAID
TWO PANTS
$11.95
POSTPAID
B
ONE PANTS
$12.95
POSTPAID
TWO PANTS
$16.50
POSTPAID
C
$7.50
POST PAID
D
$6.95
POST PAID
E
ONE PANTS
$7.50
POSTPAID
TWO PANTS
$9.50
POSTPAID
SEE OPPOSITE PAGE FOR DESCRIPTIONS
WE PAY THE POSTAGE
Certified Wear TRADE MARK ..... Laboratory Tested
H
ONE PANTS
$6.95
POSTPAID
TWO PANTS
$8.95
POSTPAID
GENUINE FAMOUS
Boyville OUR OWN TRADE MARK REG. U.S. PAT. OFF.
F
ONE PANTS
$8.95
POSTPAID
TWO PANTS
$11.50
POSTPAID
G
ONE PANTS
$6.35
POSTPAID
TWO PANTS
$8.35
POSTPAID
J
ONE PANTS
$5.95
POSTPAID
TWO PANTS
$7.95
POST PAID

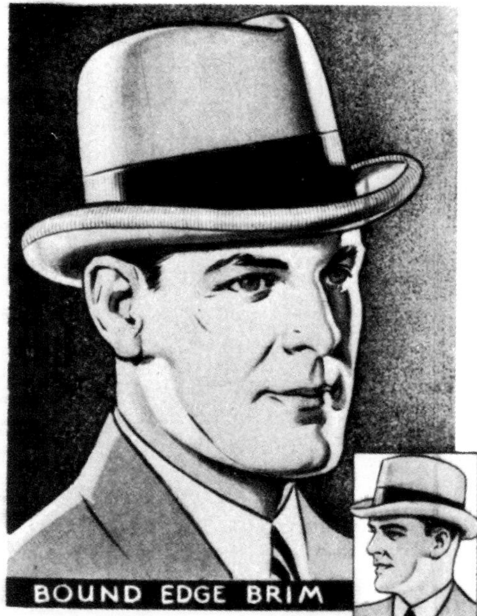


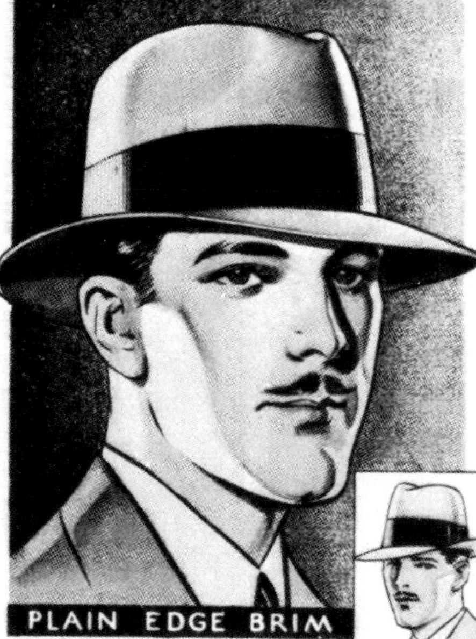


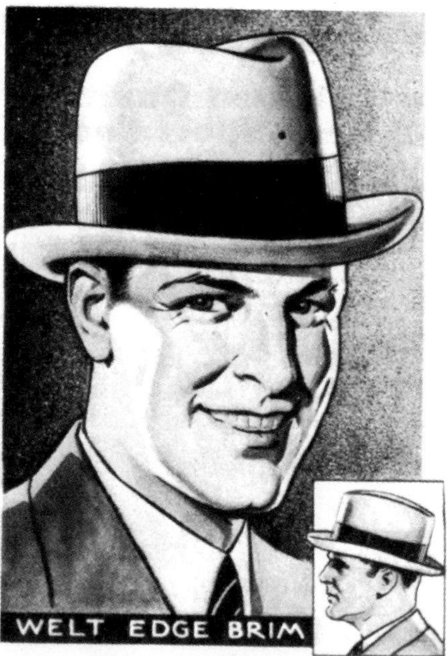


## Newest Styling

**$3.98 POSTPAID**

**93V6235—Medium gray with black band.**
**93V6236—Black.**
**93V6237—Sand tan with brown band.**
**93V6238—Dark gray with gray band.**

Sizes, 6¾ to 7½. **State size.**

Men's style dictates feature the hats with bound edge curled brims that are narrow in front and slightly wider on the sides. These hats were designed by a foremost hatter with the curled brim about 2⅜ inches in front and about 2⅝ inches on the sides. The trim tapered crown is about 5⅝ inches high. This stylish hat is made of our **Seeroe de Luxe** quality fur felt and fitted with leather sweatband and neat **silk faced lining.** Truly a surpassing value. High quality and new style at a Sears-Roebuck saving price.

## Neat Tapered Crown

**$5.00 POSTPAID**

**93V6340—Medium gray with black band.**
**93V6342—Sand tan with contrast band.**
**93V6343—Black.**
**93V6345—Dark gray with black band.**

Sizes, 6¾ to 7½. **State size.**

Men who desire the snap brim style hat with a narrower brim will choose this one of carefully styling and beautiful finish. The well matted fur felt is our **Crest de Luxe** Quality. The crown is about 5½ inches high and the plain edge snap brim is about 2⅜ inches wide. Higher quality is readily seen in the embossed and pleated **silk faced lining** and the grosgrain ribbon band. Leather sweatband. This is typical of the great values that can be found at Sears-Roebuck.

## Brisk Spring Model

**$3.98 POSTPAID**

**93V6330—Med. gray, black band.**
**93V6332—Med. tan, brown band.**
**93V6333—Dk. gray, black band.**
**93V6334—Med. brown, brown band.**

Sizes, 6¾ to 7½. **State size.**

The combination of our **Seeroe de Luxe** quality fur felt and the season's most fashionable style makes this high grade men's hat an outstanding value. The welt edge brim is about 2½ inches wide and the correctly tapered crown is only 5⅝ inches high. For fine finishing this hat has a good quality **silk faced lining** and leather sweatband. It is neatly trimmed with a grosgrain ribbon band of contrasting shade. A stylish hat for you.

## Silk Faced Lining

**$2.19 POSTPAID**

**93V6120** Med. gray, black band.
**93V6121** Dk. gray, black band.
**93V6122—Medium tan, brown band.**

Sizes, 6¾ to 7½. **State size.**

Style has been a first consideration in designing this inexpensive but very good quality Wool Felt Men's Hat. You'll like its shape. The trim tapered crown is about 5½ inches high and the smooth curved welt edge brim is about 2½ inches wide. It is complete with a **silk faced lining** and leather sweatband. This hat will be a favorite because of the reasonable price and the long satisfactory service you'll get.

## Here's Quality

**$6.98 POSTPAID**

**93V6375** Med. gray, black band.
**93V6376** Dk. gray, black band.
**93V6377—Nutria tan, brown band.**
**93V6378—Medium brown, brown band.**

Sizes, 6¾ to 7½. **State size.**

This, our finest quality snap brim hat, is designed by one of America's best hatters. At our price you will be more than pleased with the great value. A duplicate of this hat should sell for a much higher price in leading hat stores. Fashioned of perfect finish fur felt. Crown, about 5½ in. high. Plain edge brim, about 2⅜ in. wide. Heavy silk faced satin lining, leather sweatband and ribbon band.

## Here's Swagger

**$3.00 POSTPAID**

**93V6150** Med. gray, black band.
**93V6151** Dk. gray, black band.
**93V6153—Medium brown, brown band.**
**93V6154—Black.**

Sizes, 6¾ to 7½. **State size.**

Correct style in the leading spring colors. We have reproduced one of our new higher priced snap brim hats in our **Seeroe Felt** for those who want the newest style at a lower price. Fashioned with a plain edge snap brim about 2½ inches wide and a trim tapered crown about 5⅝ inches high. Has a leather sweatband and finished with a grosgrain ribbon band.

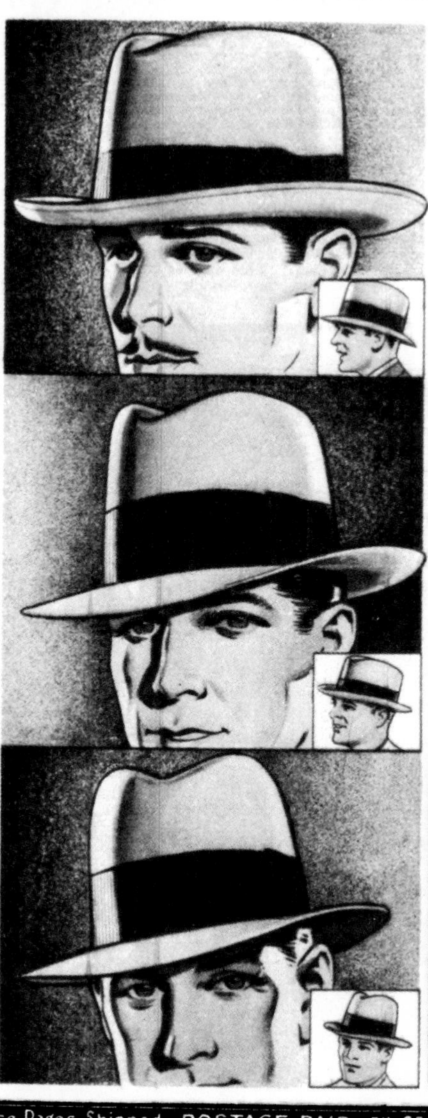

WE PAY POSTAGE

EXTRA LIGHT WEIGHT

## New Lightweight Felt!

**$3.79 POSTPAID**

**93V6214—Light pearl with black band.**
**93V6215—Medium gray with black band.**
**93V6218—Light tan with brown band.**

Sizes, 6¾ to 7½. **Be sure to state size.**

A new lightweight Hat of our **Seeroe Felt** quality for the man who wants a soft hat, comfort combined with the newest style at a popular price. Smooth finish fur felt in the beautiful light shades, generally reproduced in higher priced hats. Well shaped crown, about 5⅝ inches high, and plain edge brim is about 2⅜ inches wide. Finished with a medium width ribbon band and leather sweatband.

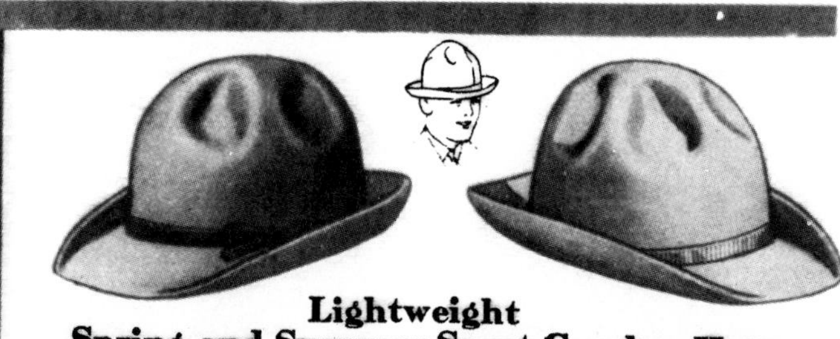

## Lightweight Spring and Summer Sport Crusher Hats

**$2.49 POSTPAID**

**93V6176—Black.**
**93V6177—Gray.**
**93V6178—Brown.**
**93V6179—Med. tan.**

Sizes, 6¾ to 7¾. **State size.**

Crushers are the style for spring and summer wear. Buy one! Excellent for motoring, golfing or other sports wear. Can be worn in any shape. Fine quality fur felt. Crown, about 5½ in. high; plain edge brim, about 2⅜ inches wide.

**98¢ POSTPAID**

**93V6184—Black.**
**93V6185—Gray.**
**93V6186—Med. tan**

Sizes, 6¾ to 7¾. **Be sure to state size.**

The ideal knockabout Wool Felt, Crusher Style Hat. Crown is about 5½ inches high, plain edge brim, about 2½ inches wide. A fine summer outing, sports or work hat at a most reasonable price. Remember, you can roll it up.

***See Measuring Chart on Opposite Page***